HEALTHCARE TECHNOLOGIES SERIES 14

Soft Robots for Healthcare Applications

Other volumes in this series:

Soft Robots for Healthcare Applications

Design, modelling, and control

S. Xie, M. Zhang and W. Meng

The Institution of Engineering and Technology

Published by The Institution of Engineering and Technology, London, United Kingdom

The Institution of Engineering and Technology is registered as a Charity in England & Wales (no. 211014) and Scotland (no. SC038698).

First published 2017

The Institution of Engineering and Technology
Michael Faraday House
Six Hills Way, Stevenage
Herts SG1 2AY, United Kingdom

www.theiet.org

British Library Cataloguing in Publication Data
A catalogue record for this product is available from the British Library

ISBN 978-1-78561-311-1 (hardback)
ISBN 978-1-78561-312-8 (PDF)

Typeset in India by MPS Limited

Contents

Preface

Robots are not new to healthcare applications. The most typical example is the Da Vinci Surgical System. This system has conducted more than 20,000 surgeries since the year of 2000 and has paved the way for robotic advancements in healthcare. Other robotic systems have also been developed to provide care to patients and help perform various surgeries and physical therapies. For instance, Magnetic Microbots are a group of tiny robots used in a variety of operations, such as removing plaque from a patient's arteries or helping with ocular conditions and disease screenings. Robots have also been used to improve the day-to-day lives of patients, such as the Bestic device to assist eating and the ReWalk Personal System 6.0 to help patients regain his/her walking ability.

Most conventional robots are constructed from stiff materials such as steel, aluminium and ABS plastics. They are usually powered directly by electric motors or by pumps forcing hydraulic fluids through rigid tubes. Such devices are capable of large forces and high speeds with great precision, which makes them very productive in factory assembly lines. However, very few of them can operate in natural environment or in close proximity to humans with interaction. In addition to safety concerns, these robots are simply not very good at adapting their behaviour when interacting with different environments. They are not well matched to the requirements due to the stiff materials used. To overcome some of these obstacles, there is an increasing interest in developing robots from soft materials.

Soft robotics is an emerging discipline that employs soft flexible materials, such as fluids, gels and elastomers, in order to enhance the use of robotics in healthcare applications. Compared to their rigid counterparts, soft robotic systems have flexible and rheological properties that are closely related to biological systems, thus allowing the development of adaptive and flexible interactions with complex dynamic environments. With new technologies arising in bio-engineering, the integration of living cells into soft robotic systems offers the possibility of accomplishing multiple complex functions such as sensing and actuating upon external stimuli. These emerging bio-hybrid systems are showing promising outcomes and opening up new avenues in the field of soft robotics for applications in healthcare and other fields.

One goal of soft robotics is to make machines that are adaptable and safe in their capabilities when interacting with human users. We take it for granted that humans can walk up and down stairs, navigate through a cluttered room or move delicate objects, but these tasks are extraordinarily difficult even for the most advanced robotic systems. The potential reason can be that stiff robots are controlled with great precision, they continuously monitor their body posture or output torque and plan out their movements with very stringent constraints. This is necessary because stiff robots can damage themselves or the world around them if in an unstable state. This issue is compounded when the robot moves into more natural or human-based environments that are filled with variety and continuously changing conditions. The robot cannot accurately predict or measure parameters that affect its performance such as surface friction, uneven floors, hard and soft obstacles, real-time interaction with environments, or moving objects, which make it simply cannot work out all required kinematic and dynamic issues to maintain precision. However, the major challenge in producing useful soft robots is to develop control systems that are suitable for highly deformable structures. Most of our existing methods cannot control high degree of freedom movements, particularly in unpredictable environments.

Complete soft robots typically resemble the animals that inspired their creation and they are constrained by the same structural considerations; soft materials do not lend themselves to building giraffe-like robots. Most soft robots are therefore terrestrial worm-like devices, although some have been built to operate underwater or to act as manipulator arms similar to those of the octopus. There are two major groups of soft devices distinguished by their mode of actuation.

The first group employed traditional motors and pumps to transfer power to the soft bodied robot using cables or pressurised air and fluid. There are designs used air-powered bladders wrapped in a braid to force the expanding bladder to shorten longitudinally. These McKibben actuators are often called pneumatic artificial muscles (PAMs). They are commercially available and have also been used to power robots with stiff skeletons. One of typical applications is to use inflatable rubber compartments carefully designed to expand in pre-arranged directions. By linking these compartments together and controlling the inflation timing these devices can be made to crawl with a variety of gaits or to generate complex movements for grasping and manipulating objects. The other group uses active materials such as electroactive polymers and shape memory alloys. These machines do not need separate motors and are potentially capable of completely soft autonomous locomotion. However, they are currently limited by poor actuator efficiency or force production and by the need to carry relatively stiff power supplies such as batteries. Designs vary from very small structures composed entirely of active gels, to aquatic jellyfish designs with embedded shape memory alloy ribs, and terrestrial caterpillar and worm-like crawling machines. Clearly these soft robots are still at an early stage of development but new devices are being designed and built remarkably quickly. A new generation of caterpillar like robots is currently being fabricated using a multimaterial three-dimensional printer that is capable of assembling completely new designs on a daily basis. Future robots are expected to combine many of these technologies, for example, the octopus arm manipulator uses both cables and shape memory alloy actuators to increase their versatility and usefulness.

This book focuses on the development of soft robotics for rehabilitation purposes. For better actuation precision and clinical outcomes, the prototypes to be reported in this book adopted soft and compliant actuators with stiff skeletons. Over the last two decades, there has been an increasing amount of research into the use of robots in physical therapy. The goal of rehabilitation is to recuperate a patient from impairment or disability and improve mobility, functional ability and quality of life. The use of soft and compliant actuators can ensure the safety of training when interacting with human users, and can also enable the implementation of wearable robotic exoskeleton.

This book systematically reviews the recent research and development of the innovative technologies for advanced robotics in healthcare applications. Through a systematic overview of the existing robotic systems and recent approaches of rehabilitation robots, interaction control, and soft and compliant healthcare robots, the problems that emerged from recent approaches have been identified. To overcome these problems and to develop a series of advanced healthcare robotics, research and development of soft robotics for human impaired limbs have been carried out. These include the review on current rehabilitation robotic systems and soft healthcare robots, the design and modelling of a novel soft actuator, the development of a soft and compliant wrist rehabilitation robot, the development of a soft and compliant ankle rehabilitation robot, and the development of a soft gait rehabilitation exoskeleton. These research topics and findings constitute the main contents of this book.

The aim of this book is to present our recent research outcomes and implementation studies in the field of advanced rehabilitation robotics by the use of soft and compliant actuators. The first chapter gives an overview of healthcare requirements, soft robots for healthcare applications, critical issues in developing soft healthcare robots, and the book outline.

The second chapter firstly presents the historical background of advanced robotics for rehabilitation purposes, including upper-limb rehabilitation exoskeletons, gait rehabilitation exoskeletons and robot-assisted ankle rehabilitation techniques. Followed is the overview of soft robotics for a variety of applications, including its definition and typical examples for healthcare applications.

Before introducing specific soft robotics for healthcare applications, Chapter 3 proposes the use of the Peano muscle, a fluid powered actuator invented by Mettam, specifically for rehabilitation devices such as robotic exoskeletons. The slim form and soft materials of this unique actuator are similar to the textiles used in clothing, lending it to use in unobtrusive and comfortable rehabilitation robots. The novel properties of the Peano muscle require new models to predict and control its behaviour. The MECHanical Approximation Lumped Parameter (MECHALP) model of the Peano muscle's static force generation was presented and validated. It models four physical effects not found in previous physics-based Peano muscle models, increasing its accuracy for control and design over these existing modelling approaches.

Following Chapter 3, Chapter 4 presents the design of the reactive Peano muscle. Inspired by biological muscles' embedded sensors, the reactive Peano muscle measures its strain, pressure and force with novel dielectric elastomer (DE) sensors. We describe how to fabricate these sensors and embed them into a Peano muscle. We then characterise the resulting Peano muscle's actuation and sensing performance and demonstrate that embedded DE sensors do not compromise its form or function. Thus, the reactive Peano muscle concept has the potential to replace passive clothing with clothing that not only actuates, but also provides feedback on the physical ability and state of its wearer.

Chapter 5 introduces the development of a soft robotic orthosis for the assessment and rehabilitation of the wrist joint. A mechanical prototype, incorporating an antagonistic setup of PAMs, will be presented. One of the main tasks of this research is the investigation of a suitable control system for the proposed prototype. Two different strategies have been implemented and compared. A feedback-based closed-loop angle and force controller was finally chosen to suit the desired system best. Experiments have been conducted on the presented system, showing that the desired measurement functionalities have been achieved.

Chapter 6 presents a soft ankle assessment and rehabilitation robot. This new design has the features of multiple degrees of freedom (DOFs), compliant actuation, appropriate workspace and actuation torque, aligned rotation centre between the robot and the ankle joint and the integration of real-time ankle assessment. This chapter mainly introduces the robot kinematics and dynamics, as well as its construction.

Chapter 7 develops control strategies on the soft-ankle rehabilitation robot (SARR). The first half of this chapter is dedicated to the development of a cascade position controller with a position loop and a force loop, which aims to implement smooth and safe robotic passive training on the SARR. The second half of this chapter proposes the active training strategies of generating an adaptive pre-defined trajectory according to the movement intention of a patient. The proposed adaptive interaction training can be then implemented by integrating it into a virtual reality-based video game to make the robotic training process more attractive to the patients.

In Chapter 8, a new robotic GAit Rehabilitation EXoskeketon (GAREX) will be presented to facilitate task-specific gait rehabilitation with controlled intrinsic compliance. The GAREX was designed for the experiments with human subjects. Several implementations ensure the safety of the subject, which is of paramount importance. The GAREX has modular design to accommodate anthropometrics of most of the population.

Chapter 9 proposes a multi-input-multi-output (MIMO) sliding mode (SM) controller which is aimed to simultaneously control the angular trajectory and compliance of the knee joint mechanism of a GAREX. The MIMO controller is developed based on the model of the GAREX system which consists of four subsystem models. Experiments with and without healthy subjects are conducted with the GAREX to validate the developed SM controller. The experimental results indicate good multivariable tracking performance of this controller.

Chapter 10 summarises the main outcomes of this book, and highlights the contributions. This chapter also provides a discussion of future directions that can be explored to extend or advance the work presented in this book. This will be used to guide coming research, or act as a reference for institutions to design and develop new medical robotic systems.

This book also contains appendices (in Chapters 6 and 9) about the materials used for the construction of the SARR, and the mechanism dynamics calculation of the GAREX system.

We would like to take this opportunity to express our deep appreciation to those who have contributed to this book. Mingming Zhang contributed to Chapters 1, 2, 6 and 10. Allan Veale contributed to Chapters 3 and 4. Jinghui Cao contributed to Chapters 8 and 9. Wei Meng contributed to Chapter 5. Mingming Zhang and Wei Meng jointly contributed to Chapter 7. Bo Sheng helped in the preparation of Chapters 2 and 6. The authors are also grateful to Jinghui Cao, Allan Veale and Bo Sheng for their assistance in compiling the book, and Ziying Lin and Shichao Peng for their help in the editing of the figures for her help in the editing of the figures. It is our sincere hope that readers will find this book useful to their study and research.

Shane (S.Q.) Xie, Mingming Zhang, and Wei Meng
Auckland, New Zealand, March 2017

Acknowledgements

The authors would like to acknowledge funding support from the Foundation for Research, Science and Technology of New Zealand, the Auckland Medical Research Foundation, the Lottery Healthcare Research Foundation and the University of Auckland.

Author Biographies

Shane (Sheng Q.) Xie has been Director of the Mechatronics and Robotics programme and Director of the Rehabilitation Robotics Lab at the University of Leeds, UK, since December 2016. He was previously Director of the Rehabilitation and Medical Robotics Centre at the University of Auckland, New Zealand (2002–2016). He received his PhD in Mechatronics Engineering from Huazhong University of Science and Technology (HUST), China, in 1998. He has published over 400 refereed papers and 7 books in the areas of advanced robotics for rehabilitation applications, and was awarded the prestigious David Bensted Fellowship for his contributions in rehabilitation robotics. He has been the Technical Editor for *IEEE/ASME Transaction on Mechatronics* and the Editor-in-Chief for the *International Journal of Biomechatronics and Biomedical Devices*.

Chair in Robotics and Autonomous Systems
School of Electronic and Electrical Engineering
University of Leeds

Dr Mingming Zhang is Executive Deputy Director of Auckland Tongji Medical & Rehabilitation Equipment Research Centre at Tongji Zhejiang College, China. He finished his PhD study at the University of Auckland in 2015, and continued to work as a research fellow until the end of 2016. He has multiple years of experience in developing novel robot-assisted rehabilitation techniques. His research interest also includes brain data mining and signal processing with different algorithms to extract meaningful neural features from large-scale brain data sets. His scientific results have been published in peer-reviewed papers in the field of mechatronics and neural engineering, and he has seven Chinese patents.

Executive Deputy Director of Auckland Tongji Medical &
Rehabilitation Research Centre, Tongji Zhejiang College Visiting Scholar,
Department of Mechanical Engineering, The University of Auckland

Dr Wei Meng is Lecturer with the School of Information Engineering, Wuhan University of Technology, Wuhan, China. From 2014 to 2016, he was a Doctoral Scholar in Mechatronics Engineering at The University of Auckland, New Zealand. His research interests include robot-assisted rehabilitation, human–robot interaction and adaptive impedance control. He is the author of two books, over twenty academic journal and conference papers, as well as three Chinese patents.

Lecturer, School of Information Engineering
Wuhan University of Technology

Chapter 1
Introduction

Much research has been conducted in the past few decades on robotics for various applications, such as industrial automation, manufacturing and healthcare. Traditional robots are mostly made of rigid materials that limit their ability to elastically deform and adapt their shape to external environments. Although they have the potential to be powerful and multifunctional with high precision of motion control, these rigid robots are more suitable for industrial applications.

In contrast to conventional machines, soft robots are primarily composed of fluids, gels, soft polymers and other easily deformable materials. These materials have the elastic property as the soft biological matter has, which makes soft robots commonly used for healthcare applications due to enhanced safety when interacting with human users. However, soft robots for healthcare applications represent an exciting new paradigm in engineering that challenges us to re-examine the materials and mechanisms to make healthcare tools more comfortable, lifelike and compatible for human interaction. This chapter introduces background information on healthcare requirements and existing soft healthcare robots, and also identifies the critical issues in developing such robots. The outline of this book is presented in this chapter.

1.1 Healthcare requirements

Healthcare is the maintenance and improvement of health via the diagnosis, treatment and prevention of disease, illness, injury and other physical and mental impairments in human beings. The ageing and disabled population is placing increasing strain on healthcare services. Physical therapy, also known as physiotherapy, is a physical rehabilitation programme that requires the use of mechanical force and movements to re-mediate impairments and promotes mobility, function and thus the quality of life. The impairments can be the results of a variety of health issues, including musculoskeletal injuries and neurological diseases. Stroke is a common cause of death and major cause of disability worldwide [1], and it can be caused by an interruption of blood flow to the brain resulting in damage to brain cells. In New Zealand, there is an estimated 8,800 people suffering from a stroke each year [2]. This figure in the United States is about 610,000 [3]. With a survival rate at 80%, it is estimated that there are 60,000 stroke survivors in New Zealand and about 7,000,000 in the United States. Many of stroke survivors are disabled and need significant daily support. According to World Health Organisation, 15 million people suffer from stroke every year globally, among whom around one-third are left permanently disabled [4].

Stroke survivors commonly experience hemiplegia, paralysis or loss of physical strength on one side of the body [1]. The impairment of the upper limb can cause difficulties in patients' daily lives such as eating, dressing and personal hygiene. The majority of stroke survivors suffer from gait disorder and around a half of these people cannot walk independently without assistance. Duncan [5] reported that the inability to walk is one of the most common problems in the population who suffered from acute stroke. Kelly-Hayes *et al.* also stated that 30% of stroke survivors are unable to walk without assistance [6]. This urges researchers to investigate enabling technologies to promote physical gait rehabilitation.

Physical therapy is the main treatment to help patients with disabilities to regain independence. Current rehabilitation services utilise manual hands-on treatment provided by physiotherapists. However, taking the treatment of ankle injuries as an example, evidence suggested that manual physiotherapy cannot provide sufficient rehabilitations [7,8], and approximately 38% of people will have recurrent activity limitations affecting their functions [9]. Furthermore, in a manual physiotherapy programme, cooperative and intensive efforts are usually required from both therapists and patients, especially over prolonged sessions [10]. Robotics technology provides a transformation for these rehabilitation clinics from labour-intensive operations to technology-assisted operations, as well as offers a rich stream of data [11]. Moreover, this kind of robot has the potential for a greater impact on rehabilitation field due to its easy deployment, high measurement reliability, applicability across a wide range of motor impairments, and capacity to deliver high dosage and high intensity training protocols [12,13]. Robot-assisted rehabilitation programmes can also be conducted without the presence of the therapists, which enables more frequent treatments and potentially reduces costs in a long term of training. The integration of virtual-reality-based games within the robot can provide a more entertaining therapy experience, thereby encouraging active engagement from patients to enhance rehabilitation efficacy [14]. The comparison of manual physiotherapy and robot-assisted rehabilitation techniques is summarised in Table 1.1.

While robot-assisted rehabilitation techniques can provide many benefits compared with manual physiotherapy, as shown in Table 1.1, a major concern is the issue of the robotic training safety when interacting with human users. In addition, the development of rehabilitation robots requires the usage of a variety of actuators and sensors, and this can be very challenging and costly with current technologies. The goal of developing assistive and rehabilitation robots is to address these key issues that are limiting manual physiotherapy.

A variety of assistive and rehabilitation robots have been developed for healthcare applications since the 1960s [15]. Robot-assisted rehabilitation techniques usually involve the development of powered feeders, wheelchair robots, mobile robots, robotic workstations, robotic orthoses and robotic rooms [16]. Typical rehabilitation robots include upper-limb exoskeletons, gait exoskeletons, and ankle rehabilitation robots. Specifically, Lo and Xie [17] presented the recent progress of

Table 1.1 Comparison of manual physiotherapy and robot-assisted physiotherapy

Evaluation index	Manual physiotherapy	Robot-assisted physiotherapy
Travelling difficulty	Travelling to rehabilitation clinics is inconvenient and time consuming, especially for patients with physical disabilities.	Rehabilitation robots allow patients to receive treatments at home or in office.
Physiotherapist availability	Manual physiotherapy is boring for patients and physiotherapists. Frequent treatment with a long-time training session is difficult due to limited availability of therapists.	Rehabilitation robots are not affected by fatigue or duration of physical exercises.
Assessment subjectivity	Qualitative assessment results from physiotherapists can be inaccurate and thus affect the treatment efficacy. Inconsistent evaluation results among different physiotherapists are also a concern.	Robot-assisted rehabilitation techniques can provide accurate quantitative assessment results based on built-in sensors.
Engagement motivation	The manual physiotherapy usually involves tedious and repetitive movements. This can lead to a reduction in the amount of voluntary effort by the patient, and thus can affect rehabilitation efficacy.	Rehabilitation robots can be used in conjunction with virtual games to encourage patients' active engagement for enhanced rehabilitation efficacy.
Treatment complexity	Physiotherapists provide basic treatments with currently available tools. It is difficult to provide a suitable amount of assistance only when required and accurately manipulate multiple joints simultaneously.	Rehabilitation robots can provide assistance only as needed through advanced control strategies. They can also be designed with multiple degrees of freedom (DOFs).

upper-limb exoskeleton robots for rehabilitation treatment of patients with neuromuscular disorders. Cao *et al.* [18] reviewed a variety of gait rehabilitation exoskeleton robots and the corresponding control strategies. Zhang *et al.* [19] compared a variety of existing ankle rehabilitation robots developed for the treatment of musculoskeletal and neurological injuries. The clinical effectiveness of these devices has been preliminarily validated on patients with disabilities.

Since rehabilitation robots need to be operated on human users, this requires the robotic design to be user friendly for training comfort and safety. Trajectory tracking controllers are generally used for passive training, such as muscle stretching exercises. Human-robot interaction forces should also be considered in controlling the robot for interactive and adaptive training. Therefore, a rehabilitation robot needs to not only be capable of moving the user's limb, but also be capable of responding to real-time human–robot interaction. Adaptive parameter adjustment of interactive controllers should be developed with the consideration of real-time disability level of the patient. These requirements introduce a number of challenges into the design and control of assistive and rehabilitation robots, as well as the selection of new actuator technologies. Some key issues or requirements in developing assistive and rehabilitation robots for healthcare applications are summarised in Table 1.2. A rehabilitation robot should conform

Table 1.2 Key issues to be considered in the development of rehabilitation robots for healthcare

Key issues/ requirements	**Specific implementation instructions**
Kinematic compatibility	A rehabilitation robot should conform to the anatomy of the human limb to maintain kinematic compatibility during training exercises. This can enhance the training safety and rehabilitation efficacy.
Training safety	Training safety should be the prime concern in the development of rehabilitation robots. While there are no rehabilitation robots with absolute training safety, some measures can be taken to minimise potential risks: • Compatible robot structure to ensure training comfort and safety; • Mechanical stops should be set up to make robots operate within safe workspace; • Emergency buttons should be available for both the physiotherapist and the patient in case any unexpected accidents; • Using soft materials to fabricate rehabilitation robots with intrinsic compliance; • Adaptive control strategies to allow adaptive training by considering real-time disability level.
Interfaces	A user interface is the space where interactions between humans and machines occur. The goal of the interaction is to allow effective operation and control of the machine from the human end, whilst the machine simultaneously feeds back information that aids the operators' decision-making process. A user-friendly interface is typically characterised by the following attributes: straightforward and well-organised, intuitive to use and reliable. Rehabilitation robots are designed to be operated by physiotherapists or patients, and thus a user-friendly interface is highly desirable for the acceptance of rehabilitation robots.
Actuators	The desired actuator attributes for a rehabilitation robot are high power–to-weight ratio, high bandwidth and low noise. The actuator is better to have intrinsic compliance to enhance the training safety.
Mechanisms	The appropriate selection of mechanisms for rehabilitation robots depends on specific applications, including serial mechanism, parallel mechanism and hybrid mechanism.
Design optimisation	Optimisation techniques should be involved to achieve appropriate robot workspace, actuation capacity, compact and efficient robotic design.
Adaptive control	The rehabilitation robot needs to be capable of interacting and responding to movements generated by human users. Adaptive adjustments of the training difficulty or amount of assistance provided by the robot are required to accommodate users with different levels of disability.

to the anatomy of the human limb to maintain kinematic compatibility during training exercises. Various precautions need to be taken to ensure the safety of training, including mechanical and control designs. A user-friendly interface is crucial to promote the acceptance of rehabilitation robots. The actuators with intrinsic compliance and high control performance have greater potential on rehabilitation robots out of the consideration of training comfort and safety. Appropriate selection of mechanisms, including serial mechanism, parallel mechanism and hybrid mechanism, depends on specific applications. Optimisation process and comparative analysis can be conducted to meet a variety of design requirements. Last but most importantly, a rehabilitation robot needs to be capable of interacting and responding to human users' movements. Robot-assisted adaptive adjustments of the training difficulty or amount of assistance are required to accommodate users with different levels of disability. These key issues should be considered and well addressed to advance robot-assisted healthcare techniques.

1.2 Soft robots for healthcare applications

From molecular machines to large-scale systems, from outer space to deep-sea exploration, robots have become ubiquitous, and their impact on our lives and society is growing at an accelerating pace [20]. Applications of robots involve the fields of medical, industrial, land, sea, air, universe and service across all scales, including the underlying principles of robotic systems covering actuation, sensor, modelling, mechanism, learning and control.

Robots can be classified as hard or soft on the basis of the compliance of their underlying materials [21]. Traditionally, engineers have employed rigid materials to fabricate a variety of robotic systems. These robots are typically used in well-defined environments in which they repetitively perform prescribed movements with high precision. This capability has been successful exploited in many applications, primarily in manufacturing. These robots are designed to be stiff so that vibration and deformation of the structure do not affect the accuracy of movement. In general, hard robots have multiple flexible joints connected by stiff links. Each joint is flexible in one rotary or translational direction for a DOF of robot motion. However, traditional robots have rigid underlying structures that limit their ability of human–robot interaction. For example, rigid robots can only manipulate objects using their specially designed end effector, which makes them often encounter difficulties when operating in unstructured environments.

In fact, natural systems often match or exceed the performance of robotic systems with deformable bodies. For example, cephalopods can achieve amazing feats of manipulation and locomotion without a skeleton. Vertebrates such as humans achieve dynamic gaits by storing elastic energy in their compliant bones and soft tissues. In recent years, researchers have been inspired by biology to design and build soft robots for various applications. With a soft structure and redundant DOFs, these robots can be used for delicate tasks in cluttered and/or unstructured environments [21]. For healthcare applications, soft robots show great potential due to their intrinsic compliance.

1.2.1 Definition of soft robots

Soft robotics is a sub-field of robotics that deals with non-rigid robots constructed with soft and deformable materials like silicone, plastic, fabric, rubber, or compliant mechanical parts like springs. A soft robot is inherently compliant and exhibits large strains in normal operation. It can interact with the environment with large deformations relying on its inherent compliance and softness. Table 1.3 compares the characteristics and capabilities of soft and hard robots.

Soft robots have a few advantages over rigid robots. First, deformable structures allow robots to deal with highly dynamic tasks and environments, for example, locomotion in rough and unknown terrain or grasping of unknown objects. Second, the usage of soft materials in the fabrication of robots allows for safe physical contact with people, which provides an opportunity to bridge the gap between robots and human users. Third, deformable materials and structures such as springs are potentially able to store and release energy, which is beneficial for energy efficient locomotion. The fourth advantage of soft robots is that soft materials are cheaper than metal parts with satisfactory actuation capacity. Lastly, soft robots have bodies made out of intrinsically soft and/or extensible materials that can absorb much of the energy arising from a collision. These features of soft robots all contribute to the improvement of robot-assisted training comfort and safety.

Table 1.3 Characteristics and capabilities of hard and soft robots [21]

	Rigid robot	**Soft robot**
Properties		
DOFs	Few	Infinite
Actuators	Few, discrete	Continuous
Materials strain	None	Large
Materials	Metal, plastics	Rubber, electroactive polymer
Capabilities		
Accuracy	Very high	Low
Load capacity	High	Lowest
Safety	Dangerous	Safe
Dexterity	Low	High
Working environment	Structured only	Structured and unstructured
Manipulable objects	Fixed size	Variable size
Conformability to obstacles	None	Highest
Design		
Controllability	Easy	Difficult
Path planning	Easy	Difficult
Position sensing	Easy	Difficult
Inspiration	Mammalian limbs	Muscular hydrostats

Soft materials are the key enablers for creating soft robot bodies. While Young's modulus is defined for homogeneous and prismatic bars that are subject to axial loading and small deformations, it is a useful measure of the rigidity of materials used in the fabrication of soft robotic systems [22,23], as in Figure 1.1. Conventionally used materials in robotics are metals or hard plastics that have moduli in the order of 10^9–10^{12} Pa, whereas natural organisms, such as skin and muscle tissue, are often composed of materials with moduli in the order of 10^4–10^9 Pa. Rus and Tolley [23] defined soft robots as systems that are capable of autonomous behaviours, and that are primarily composed of materials with moduli in the range of that of soft biological materials.

Soft robots are capable of continuum deformations, but not all continuum robots are soft. An example is the robotic elephant trunk manipulator that is a hyper-redundant continuum robot made of rigid materials [24]. The body of a soft robot may consist of multiple materials with different stiffness properties [23]. A soft robot encases in a soft body all the subsystems of a rigid robot, and these subsystems include actuation system, sensing system, computation system and driving electronic system. In this book, while some devices adopt both soft and

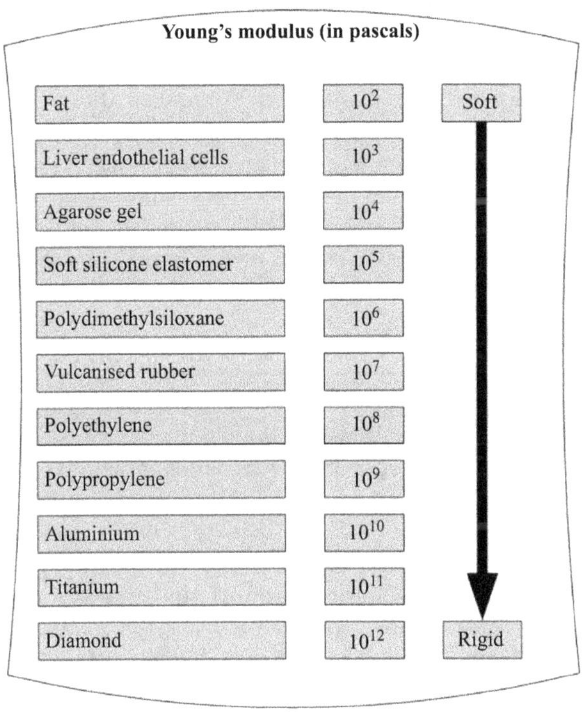

Figure 1.1 Young's modulus (in Pa) for some engineering and biological materials [22]

rigid materials (soft actuation and rigid structure), they are considered as soft robots due to the intrinsic compliance introduced by soft actuators.

The Soft Robotics Toolkit is a collection of shared resources to support the design, fabrication, modelling, characterisation and control of soft robotic devices [25]. The toolkit was developed as part of educational research being undertaken in the Harvard Biodesign Laboratory. The ultimate aim of the toolkit is to advance the field of soft robotics by allowing designers and researchers to build upon each other's work. The toolkit includes an open source fluidic control board, detailed design documentation describing a wide range of soft robotic components (including actuators and sensors), and related files that can be downloaded and used in the design, manufacture and operation of soft robots. In combination with low material costs and increasingly accessible rapid prototyping technologies, the toolkit enables soft robotic components to be produced easily and affordably. This is a valuable toolkit for the development of soft healthcare robots.

1.2.2 Examples of soft robots for healthcare

An obvious advantage of soft robots over rigid devices is that they generate little resistance to compressive forces, and therefore can conform to obstacles. These robots can be able to carry soft and fragile payloads without causing damage, which makes them suitable for healthcare applications that mostly requires dynamic human–robot interaction [21]. Rigid medical devices or orthoses run the risk of causing damage or discomfort to human bodies or tissues. It can also be difficult to replicate the motion of natural human joints with rigid structures. A potential solution can be to introduce some compliance into assistive and rehabilitation devices.

A variety of soft robots have been recently developed for healthcare applications. In this chapter, four typical examples of soft healthcare robots are presented with detailed description in design, modelling and control, as well as their applications.

Example 1 A biologically inspired soft robot to perform biomimetic swallowing [26].

In order to understand fluid transport throughout oesophageal swallowing in man, a biologically inspired soft-robotic peristaltic actuator has been designed and manufactured by Dirven *et al.* [26] to perform biomimetic swallowing. The capability of the device was examined to achieve sinusoidal transport waves with variations of clinically significant parameters. It was found that the device is capable of achieving propagation of similar wave shapes with less than 5% full-scale mean error, which improves for increasing wave-front length and reducing amplitude. The device is aimed to overcome limitations of current investigation techniques by transporting boluses in a repeatable, reliable and biologically faithful manner whilst performing objective evaluation of the bolus.

Example 2 A soft robotic glove developed by Polygerinos *et al.* [27].

The soft robotic glove was developed by Polygerinos *et al.* [27] using inexpensive hydraulic soft actuators for combined assistance and at-home rehabilitation, as in Figure 1.2. These actuators were made from elastomeric materials with fibre reinforcements to control the fingers. Integrated fluidic pressure sensors measure the internal pressure of soft actuators and allow control of finger flexion/extension.

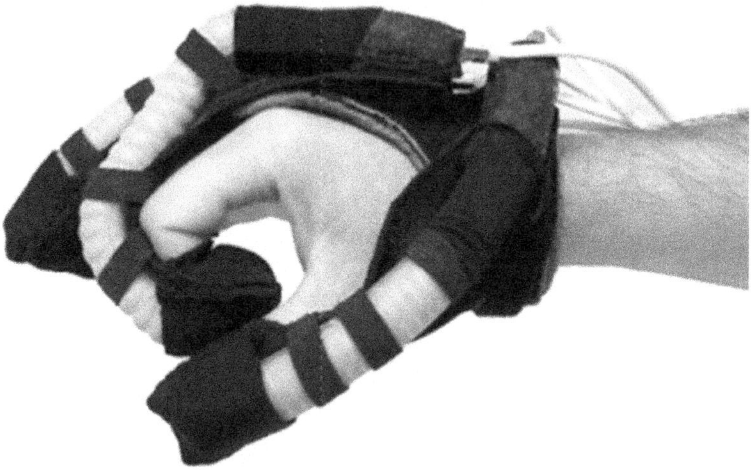

Figure 1.2 A soft robotic glove. © 2015 Elsevier. Reprinted with permission from [27]

Example 3 An improved powered ankle-foot orthosis developed by Ferris *et al.* [28].

This is an improved pneumatically powered ankle-foot orthosis (Figure 1.3) based on a previous prototype [29]. The orthosis is intended as a tool for studying gait biomechanics and rehabilitation for neurologically injured patients. The previous design had univalve shank and foot sections made from carbon fibre and connected by a plastic hinge joint. It had two pneumatic artificial muscles (PAMs) to provide dorsiflexion and plantarflexion torques about the ankle. While the previous prototype was effective in providing high actuation torque for the ankle joint, some limitations exist. First, it is difficult to don and doff due to the univalve designs for shank and foot sections. Second, changing PAMs and force sensors was time consuming because of attachment mechanisms. Third, the proportional myoelectric control was functional but produced a high degree of co-activation when the two antagonistic PAMs were on the orthosis at the same time.

The improved pneumatically powered ankle-foot orthosis overcomes limitations in the previous design and utilises a new myoelectric control strategy

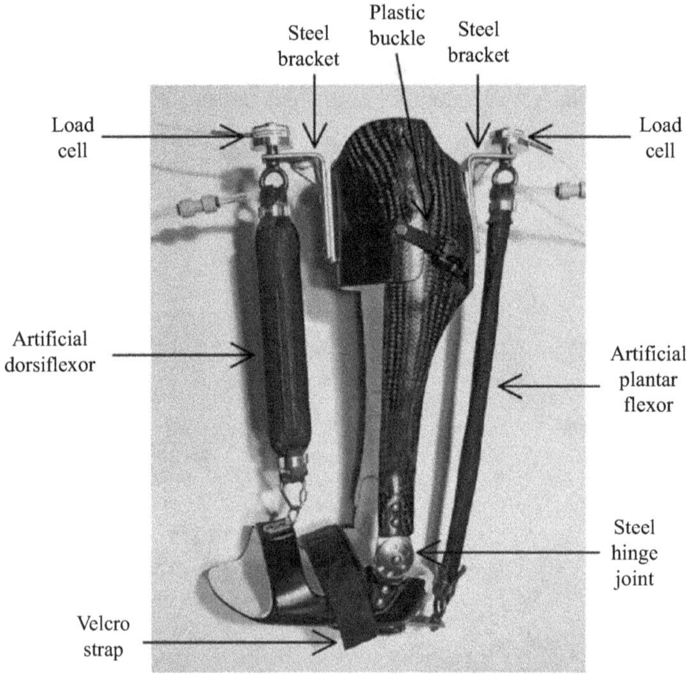

Figure 1.3 The improved pneumatically powered ankle-foot orthosis. © 2006 Elsevier. Reprinted with permission from [28]

facilitating walking [28]. The kinematic, kinetic and electromyographic data were collected for a naive healthy subject walking with the orthosis, which can be helpful in studying human walking biomechanics and assisting patients during gait rehabilitation. This new controller also allowed naive wearers to quickly adapt to the orthosis without artificial muscle co-contraction.

Example 4 A compliant ankle assessment and rehabilitation robot developed by Zhang [30].

An intrinsically compliant ankle assessment and rehabilitation robot were developed by Zhang [30] based on two critical reviews [19,31]. This ankle robot is characterised by compliant actuation, compatible robot structure that has aligned rotation centre between the robot and the ankle joint, three rotational DOFs for three-dimensional exercises, real-time biomechanical assessment and adaptive interaction training schemes, as in Figure 1.4. The function of real-time ankle assessment can be conducted using three magnetic rotary sensors measuring the position of the end effector and a six-axis load cell measuring patient–robot interaction. Its preliminary training efficacy was also validated on subjects.

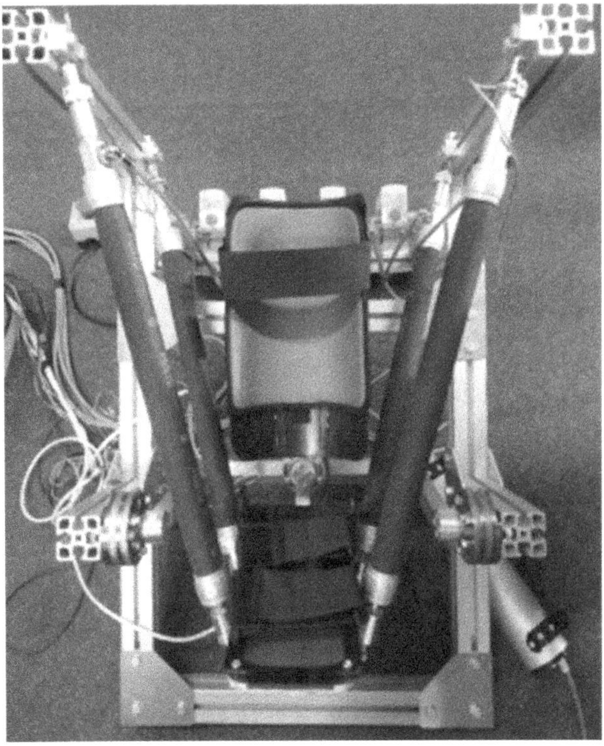

Figure 1.4 A compliant ankle assessment and rehabilitation robot by Zhang [30]

1.2.3 Motivation of soft robots for healthcare

One of the main motivations behind the adoption of robots for rehabilitation applications is the potential improvement in productivity [32,33]. Physical therapy normally requires manual manipulation of the patient's affected limb, and these manipulations can be rather repetitive and labour-intensive [34,35]. As a result, such exercises for physiotherapy can lead to the fatigue of the therapist, thus limiting the duration and intensity of the rehabilitation training. From this point of view, robot-assisted rehabilitation techniques are quite suitable for repetitive tasks if designed to have appropriate workspace and actuation capacity. Thus this can reduce the physical workload of therapists, and can potentially allow them to oversee the treatment of multiple patients simultaneously [32,35].

The use of robots in physiotherapy also has other advantages due to their high repeatability and ability for quantitative assessment of patients' health condition from built-in sensors. Physiotherapists conduct assessment mainly based on their own experiences, which may make the evaluation subjective and even inaccurate.

In contrast, the usage of robotic devices allows for objective evaluation based on quantitative data from sensors [35,36].

Active engagement in physiotherapy from patients contributes to enhanced rehabilitation efficacy [11,37,38]. Robot-assisted rehabilitation techniques can be designed with an attractive graphical user interface to capture the attention of the patient. Many rehabilitation robots have been developed for various training strategies with the integration of virtual games [17–19,39]. This has made rehabilitation exercises more engaging for long duration and intensity, thus leading to better rehabilitation efficacy.

Soft technologies are clearly going to change many aspects of our lives. Recent developments in soft robots have opened up unprecedented opportunities to transform healthcare sector in a number of areas including, but not limited to remote physical examination, rehabilitation and prosthetics. One of the driving forces behind soft robots is the necessity for machines that can work closely with humans rather than in competition with them. By incorporating soft materials into robots, they will be more compliant, adaptable, robust, safe and compatible with human activities, which makes soft robots suitable for healthcare industry. Soft robots can be personal assistants for able-bodied people, as well as the elderly and disabled. They can also support medical diagnosis and surgery, and the technology lends itself to making more functional prosthetics, synthetic organs and rehabilitation robots.

1.3 Critical issues in developing soft robots for healthcare

1.3.1 Acceptance of healthcare robots

Robotic techniques have been proposed to assist people to stay healthy and safe, and support their daily lives. Human–robot interaction and user acceptance become critical when service robots start to provide a variety of assistance to users on a personal level. However, despite the need for such assistive devices and the success of some healthcare robots, there is still a lot of work to get healthcare robots well accepted by doctors and patients.

Many studies have been conducted to investigate potential factors that may affect the acceptance of healthcare robots. A systematic literature review by Flandorfer [40] investigated how evaluations of the acceptance of socially assistive robots by older people take into account socio-demographic factors. The results indicated that while some factors (such as age, gender and education) have impacts, the relations are complex and the experience with technology mitigates the influence of socio-demographic factors on acceptance. Broadbent *et al.* [41] reviewed the literature about human responses to healthcare robots. To increase acceptance of healthcare robots, assessing the needs of human users properly and then matching the robot's role, appearance and behaviour to these needs should be conducted. We have to admit that robot-assisted healthcare techniques are not absolutely perfect. Thus another way to increase acceptance may be to modify the expectations of human users to better match robots' abilities. Broadbent *et al.* [42] also investigated the perceptions and emotions towards the utilisation of healthcare robots among individuals over the age of 40 years. It was found that participants' perceptions about robots are influenced by their prior exposure to robots in the literature or entertainment media. Participants saw many benefits and applications of healthcare robots, including simple medical procedures and physical assistance, but had some concerns about the reliability, safety and loss of personal care. Kuo *et al.* [43] found few differences between the two age groups (40–65 years and over 65 years) in attitudes and reactions to healthcare robots, and a significant gender effect with males having a more positive attitude towards healthcare robots than females. This study revealed that gender issues should be considered in the design of healthcare robots. More inter-activeness and a better voice from the robot will also promote the acceptance of healthcare robots.

To summarise, to increase the acceptance of healthcare robots, a variety of factors should be considered in the development of the robot. Specific factors include age, gender and education information of the potential human users. More importantly, assessing the needs of human users properly and then matching the robot's role, appearance and behaviour to these needs can promote the acceptance of healthcare robots. It is also possible to modify the expectations of human users to better match robots' abilities.

1.3.2 Soft actuators

Soft robots face challenges in a number of aspects, such as the range of forces they can exert on an object, precision of position and force control, hysteresis, repeatability and difficulty to develop analytical models. The availability of appropriate soft actuators is critical to the development of soft robots for healthcare applications. Soft actuation is now an emerging research area which has a wide range of applications, especially to robotics. It is not like conventional actuators such as electric motors that are always rigid and heavy, and limited in DOFs and force capacity. The soft actuator is normally made of soft materials, and can generate complex motions with intrinsic compliance. In addition to the feature of softness for safe human–robot interaction, soft actuators have multiple DOFs, both active and passive, which enables them to do something that rigid actuators cannot do, such as the mimic biomotion. Actuators are key enabling components for motion generation and control with properties that greatly impact the overall performance of mechanical systems. The lack of suitable actuators has hindered the development of high performance robotic devices with capabilities comparable to humans.

Traditional robots have linkages controlled by proportional integral derivative (PID) loops with large gains that can quickly correct for disturbances. Gear-motor-driven actuators usually move the linkages while encoders track joint positions and allow position control. Actuator dynamics significantly influence the control and overall performance of the system. They impart high mechanical impedance, which makes robots resist motion when subject to an external force. The robots also have high bandwidth and quickly move to pre-defined positions. These features make traditional robots with rigid actuators suitable for industrial automation.

However, these features are not good for robots that interact with unmapped and dynamic environments, such as healthcare applications. Traditional robots with gear-motor-driven actuators cannot store and release energy or exploit natural dynamics, and their high reflected inertia may hurt people during collisions. In contrast, soft robots are better suited for uncontrolled environments. Actuators with variable impedance have received increasing attention in recent years as many novel applications involve interactions with unknown and dynamic environments including humans [44]. A variety of soft actuators have so far been developed not only from the fundamental viewpoint of basic material science, chemistry, physics and biology, but also from the engineering viewpoint for practical applications, especially for soft robotic systems.

Soft robots can be actuated in variable length tendons or pneumatic actuation [23], as in Figure 1.5. Soft actuators are frequently arranged in a biologically inspired agonist–antagonist arrangement to allow bi-directional actuation. This arrangement can also lead to adaptable compliance due to co-contraction of muscle pairs.

Pneumatic actuators such as PAMs, with the McKibben muscle being the most well-known, contract axially and expand radially when pressurised [45]. PAMs are examples of compliant linear soft actuators composed of elastomer tubes in fibre sleeves [45]. They are among the most highly developed soft actuators and have existed for more than 50 years [46]. A PAM consists of a bladder covered in a shell of braided, strong and in-extensible fibres [45]. These actuators are length-load dependent and can only contract when inflated. During the past few decades, there has been an increase use of PAMs in the industrial and medical areas due to their advantages such as high power-to-weight ratio, high strength and light weight [47]. A special type of PAM (Festo fluidic muscle) is presented in Figure 1.6, and multiple actuators acting in series or parallel are usually required for complex movements, as in Figure 1.7.

Two examples of soft actuators with intrinsic compliance are fluidic elastomer actuators (FEAs) and series elastic actuators (SEAs). The FEA is a new type of highly extensible and adaptable, low-power soft actuator [23,48]. FEAs comprise synthetic elastomer films operated by the expansion of embedded channels under pressure, and can be operated pneumatically or hydraulically. The SEA is a traditional motor-powered actuator fitted with a spring that attaches to the load [49]. The intrinsic compliance of the SEAs makes it popularly used for healthcare robots [50]. It should be noted here that the actuator stiffness is fixed and determined by the spring selection, thus the physical stiffness cannot be changed during operation.

The biomimetic linear actuator named antagonistically driven linear actuator (ANTLA) is another example of soft actuators [51], and can be directly employed in macro-scale and micro-scale of robotic applications. The ANTLA provides cost effectiveness and simple fabrication process due to its plain construction. In addition to producing basic bi-directional rectilinear motions, the ANTLA is able to modulate its compliance for biomimetic applications.

Veale and Xie [52] presented the requirements for orthosis actuators, the electric, hydraulic and pneumatic actuators currently used in orthoses and their advantages and limitations, and new actuator technologies. It was suggested that

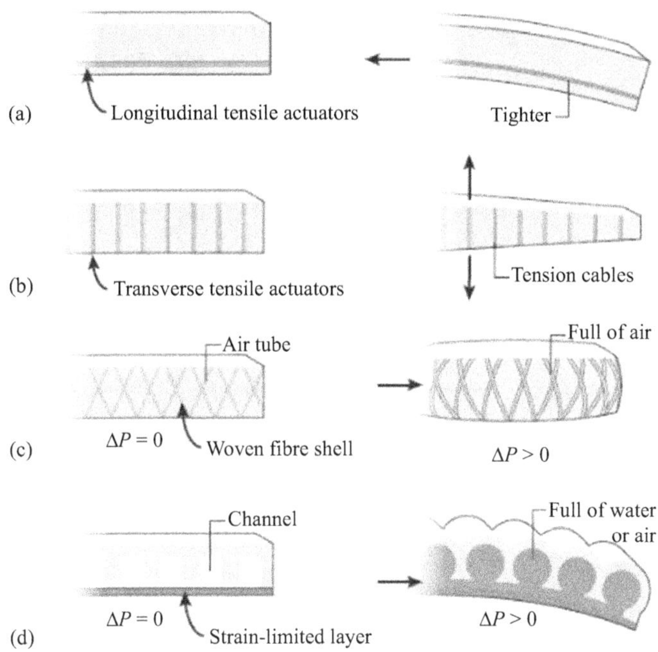

Figure 1.5 Cross-section of common approaches to actuation of soft-robot bodies in resting (left) and actuated (right) states [23]. (a) Longitudinal tensile actuators along a soft-robot arm cause bending when activated (e.g., tension cables or shape-memory alloy actuators, which contract when heated); (b) transverse tensile actuators cause a soft-robot arm to extend when contracted; (c) pneumatic artificial muscles (PAMs) are composed of an elastomeric tube in a woven fibre shell. A pressure applied internally causes the tube and shell to expand radially, causing longitudinal contraction; (d) fluidic elastic actuator or Pneu-Net design consisting of a pneumatic network of channels in an elastomer that expand when filled with a pressurised fluid, causing the soft body to bend towards a strain-limited layer. © 2015 Nature Publishing Group. Reprinted with permission from [23]

researchers should further investigate the possibilities of synergistically hybridising traditional and new actuator technologies for orthosis actuation. Pursuing these research avenues would provide valuable contributions to orthosis and robotic actuation in general and bring us closer to realising the enormous potential of robotic orthoses to change the lives of people with physical disabilities. Following the review, Veale *et al.* [53] explored the basic static and dynamic behaviour of a hydraulically actuated Peano muscle, and how its geometry affected key static and dynamic performance metrics. The Peano muscle is essentially a fluid powered

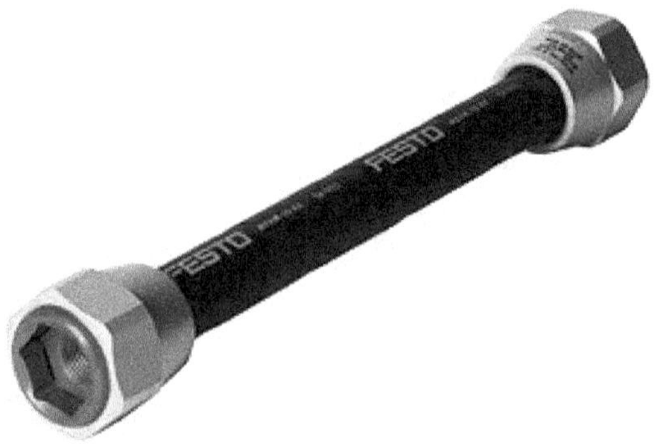

Figure 1.6 *Festo fluidic muscle. © 2017. Reprinted with permission from Festo Corporation*

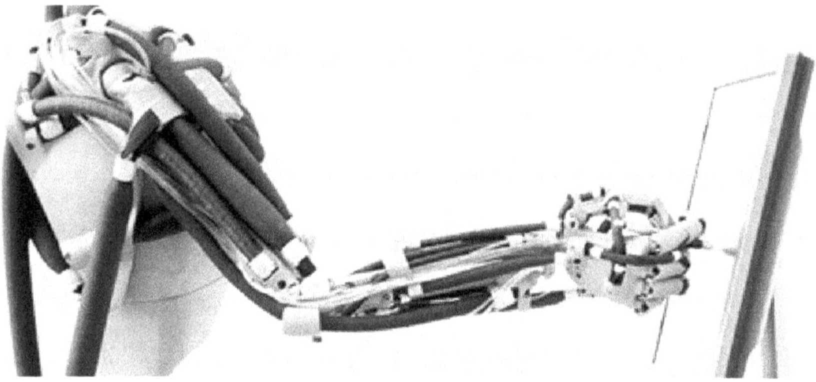

Figure 1.7 *Multiple Festo fluidic muscles for complex movements. © 2017. Reprinted with permission from Festo Corporation*

artificial muscle. Similar to McKibben PAMs, it has the ability to generate the high forces of biological muscles with the low-threshold pressure of pleated PAMs, but in a slim, easily distributed form. It was found that Peano muscles had similar characteristics to other PAMs, but produced lower-free strains.

In general, there has been an increasing interest in the development of robot-assisted healthcare techniques, arising from increasing demands in the areas of fitness and healthcare. While still at an early stage, enabling technology on soft actuation has enormous potential, especially for healthcare applications where safe control for human–robot interaction is required. Yeo *et al.* [54] anticipated further significant breakthroughs and potential uses of wearable micro-fluidics in active drug delivery patches, soft robotics sensing and control, and even implantable artificial organs in the near future.

1.3.3 Modelling and control of soft actuators

A disadvantage of soft robotics is that their soft structures are difficult to model and, therefore, hard to control. Since the field is quite young, most of soft robots are in the prototype stage and still have to be demonstrated useful under real-world conditions for various applications. However, soft robots are starting to overcome the challenges of low controllability (low bandwidth), complexity and cost.

Unlike the control of rigid bodies, the movements of which can be described by six DOFs (three rotations and three translations), the movements of soft bodies cannot be confined to planar motions. Soft materials are elastic and can bend, twist, stretch, compress, buckle and wrinkle, which makes the control very challenging. These robots usually contain some passive DOFs and their motions can be thus viewed as offering an infinite number of DOFs. The final shape of the soft robot can be described by a continuous function, and modelling this behaviour requires continuous mathematics [23]. A variety of models (static, dynamic or kinematic) have been developed to capture the ability of soft actuators for bending and flexing [55]. However, robots made from soft elastomer and powered by fluids do not yet have well-understood models or control algorithms, primarily because their intrinsic deformation is continuous, complex and highly non-linear. Controlling soft robots requires new approaches for modelling, control, dynamics and high-level planning.

Further, characterising and predicting the behaviour of soft actuators is challenging due to the non-linear nature of both the hyper-elastic material and the large bending motions they produce. A variety of modelling methods, including analytical, numerical and experimental approaches, have been proposed to describe the principle of operation of these actuators. These methods characterise the actuators' outputs (motion and force) as a function of input pressure as well as geometrical and material parameters. Currently, researchers often use piece-wise constant curvature models to estimate kinematics and dynamics of soft robots. An important aspect of these algorithms is the usage of compliance when the robot interacts with its environment. Compliance allows the robot to adapt its shape and function to objects of unknown or uncertain geometry. For example, soft robots can execute pick and place operations without precise positioning or accurate geometric models of the object to be grasped [56].

The PAMs have a high power-to-weight ratio and can be directly coupled to the joint without gearing, but each joint needs two actuators and the resultant characteristics can be highly nonlinear. The drawbacks of a joint actuated by two PAMs are the non-linear characteristics, the slow dynamics and the presence of hysteresis. While air compressibility makes them inherently compliant and spring-like, braid friction can cause hysteresis problems and dead bands making their control difficult.

1.4 Book outline

The aim of this book is to present our recent research outcomes and implementation studies in the field of advanced rehabilitation robotics by the use of soft and compliant actuators. The first chapter gives an overview of healthcare requirements, soft robots for healthcare applications, and the critical issues in developing such robots. Chapter 2 firstly presents the historical background of advanced robotics for rehabilitation purposes. Followed is the overview of soft robotics for a variety of applications, including its definition and typical examples for healthcare applications. Chapters 3 and 4 present the design analysis and development of the Peano muscle, a fluid-powered actuator, for rehabilitation devices such as robotic exoskeletons. Chapter 5 introduces a soft wrist rehabilitation robot. Chapters 6 and 7 present the design and control of a soft ankle rehabilitation robot, respectively. Chapters 8 and 9 present the development and control of a new robotic GAit Rehabilitation EXoskeketon (GAREX). Chapter 10 summarises the main outcomes and contributions of this book, and also identifies future research directions in the field of soft robotics for healthcare.

1.5 Summary

This chapter describes the main motivations and objectives of this book through an overview of healthcare requirements and soft healthcare robots. The main incentives for the usage of soft robotic devices for healthcare applications can be summarised as: their ability to reduce physical workload of physiotherapists, intrinsic compliance for safe patient–robot interaction, light weight, objective assessment and rehabilitation from built-in sensors, and great potential in making wearable devices. Some typical examples of existing soft robots used in the field of healthcare applications are presented to give readers an intuitive understanding. The key challenges in the design and control of soft healthcare robots are also discussed in the chapter.

References

[1] Donnan GA, Fisher M, Macleod M, Davis SM. Stroke. Lancet. 2008; 371(9624):1612–23.

[2] Stroke Foundation of New Zealand. Facts about stroke in New Zealand, http://www.stroke.org.nz/stroke-facts-and-fallacies; 2014 [accessed 27.04.2017].

[3] Roger VL, Go AS, Lloyd-Jones DM, *et al.* Heart disease and stroke statistics – 2012 update a report from the American Heart Association. Circulation. 2012;125(1):e2–e220.

[4] Organization WH. The atlas of heart disease and stroke, http://www.who.int/cardiovascular_diseases/resources/atlas/en. 2013 [accessed 27.04.2017].

[5] Duncan PW. Stroke disability. Phys Ther. 1994;74(5):399–407.

[6] Kelly-Hayes M, Beiser A, Kase CS, Scaramucci A, D'Agostino RB, Wolf PA. The influence of gender and age on disability following ischemic stroke: the Framingham study. J Stroke Cerebrovasc Dis. 2003;12(3):119–26.

[7] Dettori J, Basmania C. Early ankle mobilization, part II: a one-year follow-up of acute, lateral ankle sprains (a randomized clinical trial). Mil Med. 1994;159 (1):15–20.

[8] Trevino S, Davis P, Hecht P. Management of acute and chronic lateral ligament injuries of the ankle. Orthop Clin North Am. 1994;25(1):1–16.

[9] Braun BL. Effects of ankle sprain in a general clinic population 6 to 18 months after medical evaluation. Arch Fam Med. 1999;8(2):143–48.

[10] Jamwal PK. Design analysis and control of wearable ankle rehabilitation robot [PHD thesis]. Auckland, New Zealand: The University of Auckland; 2011.

[11] Krebs HI, Palazzolo JJ, Dipietro L, *et al.* Rehabilitation robotics: performance-based progressive robot-assisted therapy. Auton Robot. 2003;15(1):7–20.

[12] Huang VS, Krakauer JW. Robotic neurorehabilitation: a computational motor learning perspective. J Neuroeng Rehabil. 2009;6(1):5.

[13] Krebs HI, Volpe BT, Aisen ML, Hogan N. Increasing productivity and quality of care: robot-aided neuro-rehabilitation. J Rehabil Res Dev. 2000;37(6):639.

[14] Laver K, George S, Ratcliffe J, Crotty M. Virtual reality stroke rehabilitation – hype or hope? Aust Occup Ther J. 2011;58(3):215–19.

[15] Harwin WS, Rahman T, Foulds RA. A review of design issues in rehabilitation robotics with reference to North American research. IEEE Trans Rehabil Eng. 1995;3(1):3–13.

[16] Tejima N. Rehabilitation robotics: a review. Adv Robotics 2000;14:551–64.

[17] Lo HS, Xie SQ. Exoskeleton robots for upper-limb rehabilitation: state of the art and future prospects. Med Eng Phys. 2012;34(3):261–68.

[18] Cao J, Xie SQ, Das R, Zhu GL. Control strategies for effective robot assisted gait rehabilitation: the state of art and future prospects. Med Eng Phys. 2014;36(12):1555–66.

[19] Zhang M, Davies TC, Xie S. Effectiveness of robot-assisted therapy on ankle rehabilitation–a systematic review. J Neuroeng Rehabil. 2013;10:30.

[20] Yang GZ, Bellingham J, Choset H, *et al.* Science for robotics and robotics for science. Sci Robot. 2016;1(1).

[21] Trivedi D, Rahn CD, Kier WM, Walker ID. Soft robotics: biological inspiration, state of the art, and future research. Appl Bio Biomech. 2008; 5(3):99–117.

[22] Carmel M. Soft robotics: a perspective – current trends and prospects for the future. Soft Robot. 2014;1(1):5–11.

[23] Rus D, Tolley MT. Design, fabrication and control of soft robots. Nature. 2015;521(7553):467–75.

[24] Hannan MW, Walker ID. Kinematics and the implementation of an elephant's trunk manipulator and other continuum style robots. JRoS. 2003; 20(2):45–63.

[25] Toolkit SR. What is the soft robotics toolkit? http://softroboticstoolkit.com; 2017 [accessed 27.04.2017].

[26] Dirven S, Xu W, Cheng LK. Sinusoidal peristaltic waves in soft actuator for mimicry of esophageal swallowing. IEEE/ASME Transact Mechatr. 2015; 20(3):1331–37.

[27] Polygerinos P, Wang Z, Galloway KC, Wood RJ, Walsh CJ. Soft robotic glove for combined assistance and at-home rehabilitation. Robot Auton Syst. 2015;73:135–43.

[28] Ferris DP, Gordon KE, Sawicki GS, Peethambaran A. An improved powered ankle-foot orthosis using proportional myoelectric control. Gait Posture. 2006;23(4):425–28.

[29] Ferris DP, Czerniecki JM, Hannaford B, University of M, University of W, System VAPSH. An ankle-foot orthosis powered by artificial pneumatic muscles. J Appl Biomech. 2005;21(2):189–97.

[30] Zhang M. Improving effectiveness of robot-assisted ankle rehabilitation via biomechanical assessment and interaction control. Auckland, New Zealand: University of Auckland; 2016.

[31] Zhang M, Davies TC, Zhang Y, Xie S. Reviewing effectiveness of ankle assessment techniques for use in robot-assisted therapy. J Rehabil Res Dev. 2014;51(4):517–34.

[32] Krebs HI, Volpe BT, Aisen ML, Hogan N. Increasing productivity and quality of care: robot-aided neuro-rehabilitation. J Rehabil Res Dev. 2000; 37(6):639–52.

[33] Saglia JA, Tsagarakis NG, Dai JS, Caldwell DG. Control strategies for ankle rehabilitation using a high performance ankle exerciser. IEEE international conference on robotics and automation. IEEE: Anchorage, Alaska; 2010.

[34] Duschau-Wicke A, Von Zitzewitz J, Caprez A, Lunenburger L, Riener R. Path control: a method for patient-cooperative robot-aided gait rehabilitation. IEEE Transact Neural Syst Rehabil Eng. 2010;18(1):38–48.

[35] Riener R, Frey M, Bernhardt M, Nef T, Colombo G, editors. Human-centered rehabilitation robotics. London: IEEE International Conference on Rehabilitation Robotics; 2005.

[36] Roy A, Krebs HI, Patterson SL, *et al.*, editors. Measurement of human ankle stiffness using the anklebot. London: International Conference on Rehabilitation Robotics; 2007.

[37] Vallery H, Duschau-Wicke A, Riener R, editors. Generalized elasticities improve patient-cooperative control of rehabilitation robots. London: IEEE International Conference on Rehabilitation Robotics; 2009.

[38] Marchal-Crespo L, Reinkensmeyer DJ. Review of control strategies for robotic movement training after neurologic injury. J Neuroeng Rehabil. 2009;6(1):20.

[39] Zhang M, Nandakumar A, Xie S. A virtual-reality tracking game for use in robot-assisted ankle rehabilitation. 10th IEEE/ASME international conference on mechatronic and embedded systems and applications. IEEE/ASME: Senigallia, Italy; 2014.

[40] Flandorfer P. Population ageing and socially assistive robots for elderly persons: the importance of sociodemographic factors for user acceptance. Int J Population Res. 2012;2012:13.

[41] Broadbent E, Stafford R, MacDonald B. Acceptance of Healthcare robots for the older population: review and future directions. Int J Social Rob. 2009; 1(4):319.

[42] Broadbent E, Kuo IH, Lee YI, *et al.* Attitudes and reactions to a healthcare robot. Telemed J E-health. 2010;16(5):608–13.

[43] Kuo IH, Rabindran JM, Broadbent E, *et al.*, editors. Age and gender factors in user acceptance of healthcare robots. RO-MAN 2009 – the 18th IEEE International Symposium on Robot and Human Interactive Communication; September 27 to October 2, 2009.

[44] Vanderborght B, Albu-Schaeffer A, Bicchi A, *et al.* Variable impedance actuators: a review. Robot Auton Syst. 2013;61(12):1601–14.

[45] Ching-Ping C, Hannaford B. Measurement and modeling of McKibben pneumatic artificial muscles. IEEE T Robotic Autom. 1996;12(1):90–102.

[46] Schulte HF. The application of external power in prosthetics and orthotics: a report. Washington, DC: National Academy of Sciences, National Research Council; 1961.

[47] Frank D, Dirk L. Pneumatic artificial muscles: actuators for robotics and automation. Eur J Mech Envir Eng. 2002;47(1):11–21.

[48] Marchese AD, Onal CD, Rus D. Autonomous soft robotic fish capable of escape maneuvers using fluidic elastomer actuators. Soft Robot. 2014;1(1):75–87.

[49] Pratt GA, Williamson MM, editors. Series elastic actuators. Proceedings 1995 IEEE/RSJ international conference on intelligent robots and systems human robot interaction and cooperative robots; 1995.

[50] Yu H, Huang S, Chen G, Thakor N. Control design of a novel compliant actuator for rehabilitation robots. Mechatronics. 2013;23(8):1072–83.

[51] Hyouk Ryeol C, Kwangmok J, Ryew S, *et al.* Biomimetic soft actuator: design, modeling, control, and applications. IEEE/ASME Transact Mechatr. 2005;10(5):581–93.

[52] Veale AJ, Xie SQ. Towards compliant and wearable robotic orthoses: a review of current and emerging actuator technologies. Med Eng Phys. 2016;38(4):317–25.

[53] Veale AJ, Xie SQ, Anderson IA. Characterizing the Peano fluidic muscle and the effects of its geometry properties on its behavior. SmMaS. 2016; 25(6):065013.

[54] Yeo JC, Kenry, Lim CT. Emergence of microfluidic wearable technologies. Lab Chip. 2016;16(21):4082–90.

[55] Webster RJ, Jones BA. Design and kinematic modeling of constant curvature continuum robots: a review. Int J Rob Res. 2010;29(13):1661–83.

[56] Brown E, Rodenberg N, Amend J, *et al.* Universal robotic gripper based on the jamming of granular material. Proc Nati Acad Sci. 2010;107(44):18809–14.

Chapter 2
State of the art

A comprehensive literature review on rehabilitation robots and soft healthcare robots is carried out to identify the key issues. It begins with a survey of existing robot-assisted rehabilitation techniques proposed for human assistance and treatment. Three typical types of rehabilitation devices are upper-limb rehabilitation robots, gait rehabilitation exoskeletons and ankle rehabilitation robots. Following it, a variety of existing soft robots are presented, especially for healthcare applications.

2.1 Rehabilitation robots for healthcare

Rehabilitation robotics can be considered as a specific focus of biomedical engineering, and a part of human–robot interaction. In this field, clinicians, therapists and engineers collaborate to help rehabilitate patients with movement disabilities. Rehabilitation robotics is a field of research dedicated to understanding and augmenting rehabilitation through the application of robotic devices. Rehabilitation robotics mainly includes development of robotic devices tailored for assisting sensorimotor functions [1–3], development of various schemes of assisting therapeutic training [4,5], and assessment of sensorimotor performance of patients [6,7]. Rehabilitation robots can be used for the delivery of active-assisted, active-constrained, active-resistive, passive and adaptive exercises.

Robots have been developed for upper-limb rehabilitation [8], gait rehabilitation [5] and ankle therapy [9] for patients with a variety of disabilities. These techniques are well tolerated by patients and have been found to be an effective adjunct to therapy in individuals suffering from motor impairments.

2.1.1 Upper-limb rehabilitation exoskeletons

The upper-limb rehabilitation exoskeleton has a structure which resembles the human upper limb, and has robot joint axes that match the upper-limb joint axes. Exoskeletons are designed to operate side-by-side with the human upper limb, and therefore can be attached to the upper limb at multiple locations. Operating alongside the human limb, exoskeletons need to be able to produce similar movements to those of the upper limb. The human upper limb has a total of nine degrees of freedom (DOFs) excluding the finger joints [10]. The gleno-humeral joint at the shoulder complex is a ball-and-socket joint which enables the humerus to rotate about the gleno-humeral head in three DOFs. These movements are commonly referred to

Table 2.1 Degrees of freedom (DOFs) and actuation modes of typical upper-limb rehabilitation exoskeletons. © 2012 Elsevier. Reprinted with permission from [8]

Upper-limb exoskeletons	DOFs	Actuators	Other features and comments
IntelliArm [15]	8	Electric motors	To diagnose the biomechanical changes and abnormal couplings at the shoulder, elbow, wrist and finger joints of the impaired arm of stroke survivors.
SUEFUL-7 [16]	7	Electric motors	To assist the motions of shoulder, elbow, forearm and wrist of patients.
CADEN-7 [13] (Figure 2.1)	7	Electric motors	A therapeutic and diagnostic device for physiotherapy; an assistive device for human power amplifications; a haptic device in virtual reality simulation; a master device for teleoperation.
ARMin III [17]	6	Electric motors	The ARMin III robot provides three DOFs for the shoulder and one for the elbow joint.
Arm exoskeleton [18]	7	PAM actuators	The exoskeleton provides natural motions of the human arm from the shoulder to the wrist.
RUPERT IV [14] (Figure 2.2)	5	PAM actuators	To assist in repetitive therapy tasks related to activities of daily living, which has been advocated for enhanced training efficacy.

as shoulder flexion/extension, abduction/adduction and medial/lateral rotation. The sterno-clavicular joint has two DOFs, commonly known as shoulder elevation/depression and retraction/protraction, which moves the gleno-humeral head. Thus the shoulder complex has a total of five DOFs. An interesting phenomenon of the shoulder is that the abduction of the upper arm above the horizontal plane occurs simultaneously with the sterno-clavicular elevation [11]. The elbow complex is capable of two DOFs, and they are elbow flexion/extension and forearm pronation/supination. The wrist joint has two DOFs, wrist flexion/extension and radial/ulnar deviation. The axes of rotation of both DOFs of the wrist pass through the capitate carpal bone [12]. Existing upper-limb exoskeletons focus on movements of the shoulder, elbow and/or wrist complex, as summarised in Table 2.1. These devices have been reviewed by Lo and Xie [8], of them two typical examples are the CADEN-7 [13] (Figure 2.1) and the RUPERT IV [14] (Figure 2.2).

Many of existing upper-limb rehabilitation exoskeleton robots have been reviewed by Lo and Xie [8]. The advancements in upper-limb rehabilitation robots and the fundamental challenges in developing such devices were also discussed. It was found that majority of existing upper-limb exoskeletons are actuated by electric motors while a few of these devices adopt soft actuators, such as pneumatic artificial muscles (PAMs). The PAM has several advantages over electric motors with the most significant one being its high power-to-weight ratio. The soft nature of PAM actuators makes robotic exoskeletons intrinsically compliant and safe

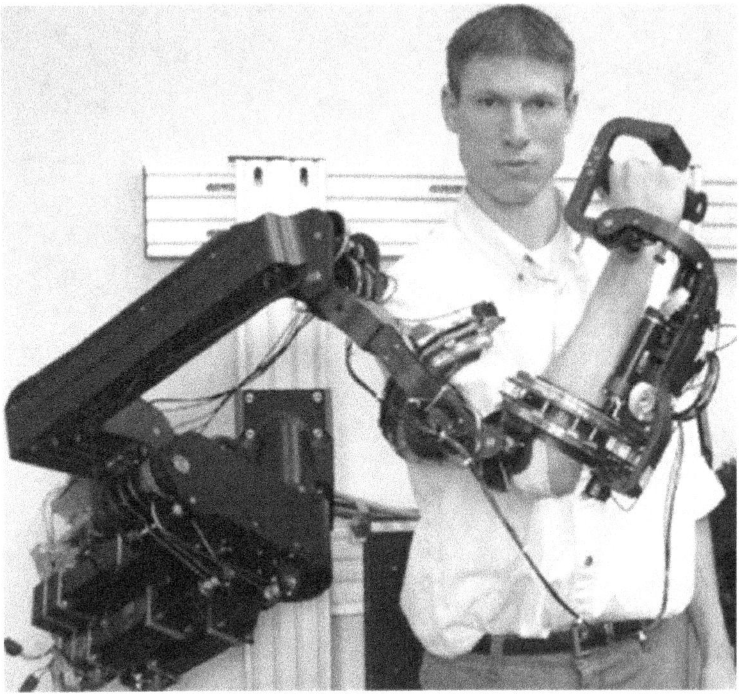

Figure 2.1 The CADEN-7 as an example of typical upper-limb exoskeletons actuated by electric motors. © 2012 Elsevier. Reprinted with permission from [8]

when interacting with human users, which makes the usage of PAMs to be increasingly popular for the development of rehabilitation robots. However, PAM actuators exhibit highly non-linear actuation characteristics making them difficult to control. Typical upper-limb exoskeletons actuated by PAMs include an arm exoskeleton [18] and the RUPERT IV [14]. The lightweight RUPERT IV exoskeleton is a portable device that uses PAM actuators to provide five-DOF training exercises of the upper limb. An example of commercial upper-limb rehabilitation robots is the Hand Mentor that uses pneumatic actuators for wrist flexion/extension movement. This can be used on patients who need rehabilitation to help restore range of motion and strengthen muscles of their wrists and hands.

2.1.2 Gait rehabilitation exoskeletons

The development of new rehabilitation techniques should consider the underlying recovery mechanism [19]. Gait rehabilitation training or locomotor recovery is a process of neurological rehabilitation. Neuro-scientists and physiotherapists have been working together to investigate the neurological theories behind the rehabilitation. Rehabilitation is essentially a process of re-learning how to move to carry

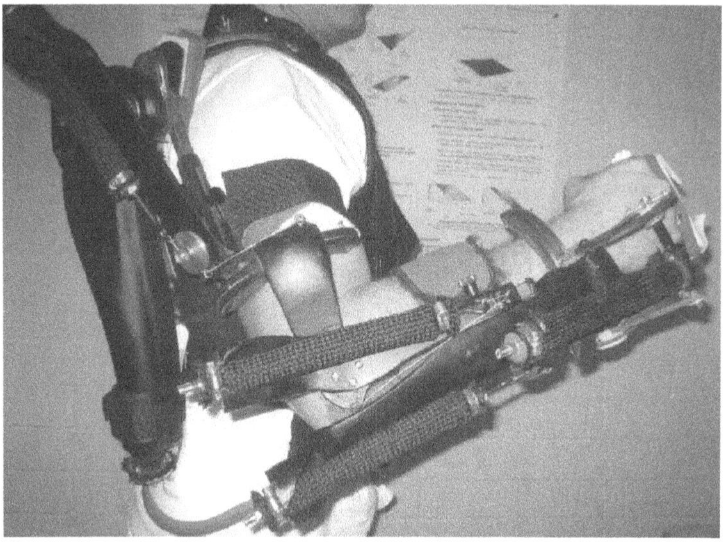

Figure 2.2 The RUPERT IV as an example of typical upper-limb exoskeletons actuated by PAMs. © 2012 Elsevier. Reprinted with permission from [8]

out their needs successfully [20]. Motor learning is thought to be a pre-requisite factor in the development of representational plasticity in the central nervous system [21]. General motor learning principles are hypothesised to be still valid for motor recovery [22]. One fundamental principle is that the degrees of performance improvement are dependent on the amount of practice [23]. Large amount of practice or repetition alone is not enough to induce ideal motor learning outcomes [24]. Animal experiments conducted by Plautz *et al.* [21] indicated that practice needs to be task-related to produce representational plasticity in motor cortex. Introducing training variability in the skill acquisition session improves the overall session performance compared to single task repetition in one session [25]. Motor learning theories have driven the development of both conventional and robotic rehabilitation strategies.

Neuro-scientists have proven that repetition plays a major role in inducing and maintaining brain changes [26]. Bayona *et al.* [27] reviewed related experiments and concluded that tasks are meaningful to animals rather than repetitions alone, which is more likely to generate functional re-organisation. For humans, daily practice of task-specific motor activities can also lead to re-organisation of the adult primary motor cortex [28,29]. Randomised controlled trials demonstrated that task-specific training programme is more effective than Bobath programme for acute patients [30,31].

Body weight support treadmill training (BWSTT), which was first proposed by Finch and Barbeau in 1986 [32], is a well-researched task-specific repetitive gait rehabilitation strategy. The BWSTT can enable patients to practice complex gait pattern repetitively. During the training, a patient walks on the treadmill with a body weight support system attached via harness. Physiotherapists guide patients' legs to follow pre-defined training trajectories with correct pelvis and trunk movements [33]. By comparing the BWSTT with conventional physiotherapy based on the Bobath concept, it was concluded that BWSTT is superior with regards to restoration of gait and improvement of over ground walking speed. These investigations also indicated that more gait cycles were achieved by the BWSTT for the sessions with same duration [34,35].

During the BWSTT, patients are trained to produce rhythmic gait cycles. On one hand, it is a tiring job for physiotherapists since they have to manually move the patients' paretic legs continuously. There could also be patients with excessive spasticity, for whom manual training is nearly impossible [36]. On the other hand, physiotherapists are required to provide optimal and identical leg swing in every gait cycle. However, assistances provided by physiotherapists largely depend on their experience, and thus optimal gait movements cannot always be achieved due to inter-/intra-physiotherapist variances. Robotic training has provided a solution to these problems with the integration of a variety of enabling technologies, for example, dynamic feedback [37], biological feedback [38] and virtual reality [39].

To date, a number of robotic gait trainers have been developed and some of them are even commercially available, as reviewed by Cao *et al.* [5] and Dzahir and Yamamoto [40]. Typical gait rehabilitation robots are mostly based on treadmill. Treadmill training robots automate the process of manual BWSTT training. They have been developed to help physiotherapists for guiding patients' leg movement and body support for gait rehabilitation. As a result, such devices usually consist of the gait driving mechanism and the trunk/pelvis manipulating mechanism. A summary of typical treadmill training robots is summarised in Table 2.2, where Arabic numbers are used to represent DOFs of the gait driving mechanism, and alphabetic characters are used for DOFs of the trunk/pelvic mechanism. The matches are as follow: 1- hip flexion/extension, 2- hip adduction/abduction, 3- knee flexion/extension, 4- ankle dorsiflexion/plantarflexion, 5- ankle joint is left free to move in all DOFs. A- vertical transition; B- forward/backward transition; C- lateral transition; D- rotation about the vertical axis; E- rotation about the axis perpendicular to the sagittal plane; F- rotation about the axis perpendicular to the frontal plane. Number or character in italic font means the specific DOF is actively actuated, while that in bond font means the DOF is left free to move. In addition, the prototypes of the active leg exoskeleton (ALEX) presented in [40] and the intrinsically compliant robotic gait orthosis [41] are presented in Figures 2.3 and 2.4, respectively.

2.1.3 Ankle rehabilitation robots

The human ankle plays a significant role in maintaining body balance during ambulation, but it is particularly susceptible to musculoskeletal and neurological injuries. Robot-assisted ankle rehabilitation solutions, as therapeutic adjuncts to

Table 2.2 Degrees of freedom (DOFs) and actuation modes of typical treadmill training robots [5]. © 2014 Elsevier. Reprinted with permission from [5]

Treadmill training robots	Gait driving mechanism		Trunk/pelvic DOFs	Other features and comments
	DOFs	Actuation system		
LokoMat DGO [36]	*1 3* **5**	Motors and gear reduction units for linear actuation with levers for active DOFs.	**A B**	DGO: driven gait orthosis, the orthosis is adjustable in size so different patients can use it. Actuators at the knee and hip joints are controlled by a position controller. With the DGO, the legs of patients with different degrees of paresis and spasticity could be trained for >30 min, and physiological gait patterns were obtained.
ALEX [42] (Figure 2.3)	*1* **2** *3* **5**	Linear motor with levers for active DOFs.	**A C D E**	ALEX: active leg exoskeleton, developed as a rehabilitation robot for assistance-as-needed gait training based on a force-field controller.
LOPES [43]	*1 2 3* **5**	Series elastic actuation (SEA) with Bowden cable transmission detached motors and gear units from moving parts.	*A* **B** *C*	LOPES: lower-extremity powered exoskeleton. Elastic elements make the actuation system more compliant. Adoption of SEA reduced weight of moving parts without reducing power, thus the force bandwidth increased. These would benefit the implementation of the zero impedance control.
ARTHuR [44]	*1 3 5*	Two moving coil forcers driven by linear motors can move along a horizontal rail to drive a two-bar linkage attached to the patient's ankle.	Not available	ARTHuR: ambulation-assisting robotic tool for human rehabilitation, it does not have proper leg orthosis. The actuation mechanism can drive the foot to reach any point in the sagittal plane by moving the forcers along their rail.
PAM and POGO [45,46]	*1* **2** *3* **5**	Actuated by pneumatic cylinders.	*A B C D* **E** *F*	PAM: pelvis assistive manipulator; POGO: pneumatically operated gait orthosis.
PAM Gait Orthosis [41] (Figure 2.4)	*1* **2** *3* **4**	A pair of PAM actuators used for one active joint.	**A C**	The actuation system was inspired by the human musculoskeletal system. For a specific joint, one PAM is for flexion and the other is for extension.

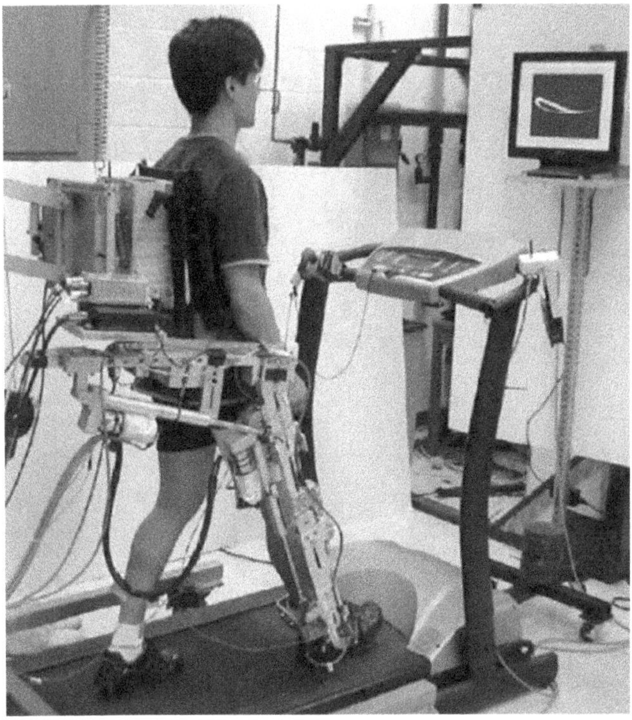

Figure 2.3 The active leg exoskeleton (ALEX) reviewed in [40]

facilitate clinical practice, have been actively researched during the past few decades. Zhang *et al.* [9] reviewed a variety of robot-assisted ankle rehabilitation techniques and demonstrated their effectiveness for clinical applications.

Existing ankle rehabilitation robots are mainly classified into two categories based on the mobility of the device during operation. They are wearable robots and platform-based ones, with some typical prototypes presented and summarised in Table 2.3. The MIT Anklebot [47], the bio-inspired soft ankle robotic device [48] and the knee-ankle exoskeleton by Yu *et al.* [49] belong to the group of wearable robots. These wearable ankle exoskeletons were normally developed to correct the user's gait pattern. The other group consists of platform-based robots that usually have a fixed platform and a moving foot plate with one or multiple DOFs [50–55]. A single-DOF device is usually actuated by a rotating motor for a specific application, for example, the device developed by Zhang *et al.* [54] for ankle stretching, while a multiple-DOF robot is mostly based on a parallel mechanism actuated by linear actuators [50–53] or motor-based linkages [55,56]. As an exception, a commercial ankle rehabilitation device is the OptiFlex Ankle CPM [57] that has two DOFs using a serial mechanism, as presented in Figure 2.5.

Robot-assisted ankle rehabilitation exercises can be delivered in a variety of ways to reduce motor impairments and enhance functional motor outcomes. While

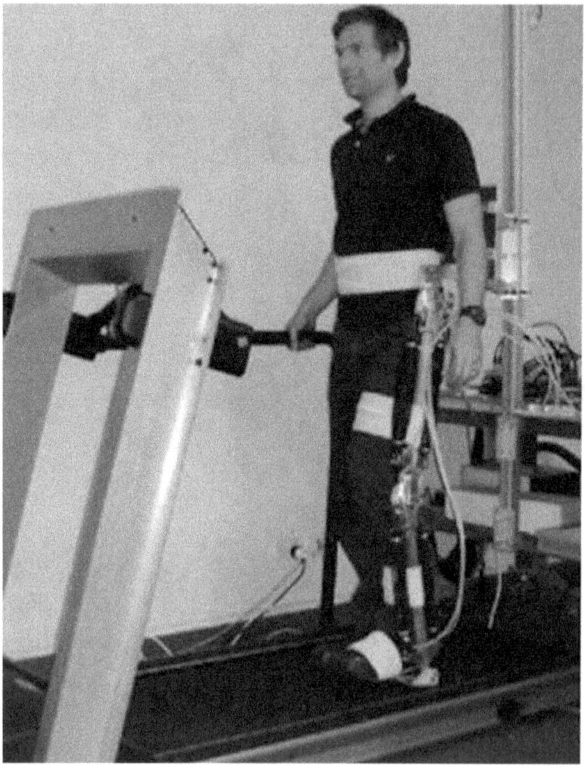

Figure 2.4 An intrinsically compliant robotic orthosis for treadmill gait training [41]. © 2012 Elsevier. Reprinted with permission from [41]

existing robot-assisted ankle rehabilitation techniques have shown great potential for treating ankle disabilities [9], few can deliver comprehensive ankle training in a three-dimensional space in passive and active modes with appropriate workspace and torque capacity. By comparing a variety of ankle rehabilitation robots, it is found that an optimal robotic design for comprehensive ankle rehabilitation should be characterised with appropriate workspace and actuation torque, aligned rotation centre between the robot and the ankle joint, and adjustable robot posture.

However, two more design issues should be considered towards optimal ankle rehabilitation robots. One is the fixation issue of the human foot and shank, and a commonly used method is using straps attaching the foot on a footplate and the shank on a fixed leg holder. Again since the anatomical ankle joint is not an ideal hinge joint [60], the rigid fixation of the foot and shank may result in un-comfort and even injury risk. A potential solution can be to design the leg holder with some flexibility to accommodate the difference between the robot structure and the human anatomy. The other issue is the setup of mechanical stops for training safety. Mechanical stops must be set on robotic systems whose workspace is larger than actual ankle motions, especially on motor-driven devices. By contrast, parallel

Table 2.3 Degrees of freedom (DOFs) and actuation modes of some typical treadmill training robots

Ankle robot by	DOFs	Type	Actuation system	Other features and comments
Yu *et al.* [49]	1 (for ankle)	Wearable	Series elastic actuators	This robot system consists of an ankle-foot module and a knee module, designed for gait training. This device is essentially a gait exoskeleton robot.
Park *et al.* [48]	2	Wearable	PAMs	This device generates an ankle ROM of 27° (14° dorsiflexion and 13° plantarflexion). This is acceptable for gait training rather than ankle stretching.
Roy *et al.* [47]	2 (3)	Wearable	Linear screw actuators	The MIT Anklebot allows normal ROM in all three DOFs of the foot during walking over-ground, on a treadmill, or while sitting. Two DOFs are actively actuated by motors.
Zhang *et al.* [54]	1	Platform	A servomotor	This device is portable and low cost, making it available to patients for frequent and long-term use at clinics or home.
OptiFlex Ankle CPM [57]	2	Platform	Electric motors	A commercial device for ROM exercises along ankle dorsiflexion/plantarflexion and inversion/eversion.
Girone *et al.* [53]	6	Platform	Pneumatic cylinders	Limited robot workspace if controlled for aligned rotation centre between the robot and the ankle joint.
Saglia *et al.* [52] Saglia *et al.* [58]	2	Platform	Customised linear actuators	This robot used customised linear actuator to meet the required forces and torques for strengthening and balance exercises.
Tsoi *et al.* [51]	3 (6)	Platform	DC motor-driven linear actuators	This robot itself has six DOFs and three rotational DOFs if considering the human ankle as a constraint. It can be only used in an upright posture.
Jamwal *et al.* [50]	3	Platform	PAMs	Limited actuation torque.
Zhang [59]	3	Platform	PAMs	Optimisation techniques should be involved to enhance the usability and functionality of this robot.
Wang *et al.* [56] Wang *et al.* [55]	2 or 3	Platform	Electric motors connected to the limbs by gearboxes	This device has the flexibility of reconfiguring into either a two-DOF rehabilitation device or a three-DOF one depending on the specific exercise mode. But it has not been clinically validated.

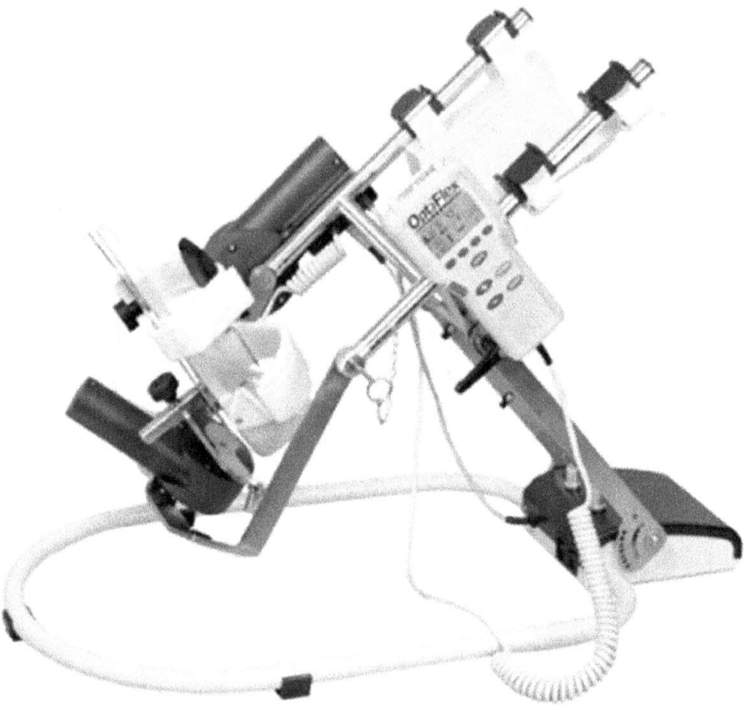

Figure 2.5 The OptiFlex Ankle CPM [57]. © 2017. Reprinted with permission from DJO Global ANZAsia

ankle rehabilitation robots do not have to set mechanical stops if they are designed with appropriate workspace.

It is believed that no 'one-size-fits-all' design exists for optimal robot-assisted ankle rehabilitation, and therapy should be essentially tailored to each patient's needs and disabilities. Therefore, a mechanical design with re-configurability can be a good solution to allow ankle rehabilitation robots used on a large population of patients.

2.2 Soft robots for healthcare

Soft robots have a number of advantages over rigid ones. For example, deformable structures play an important role on robots that have to deal with and highly dynamic tasks and environments. The usage of soft materials in the robot design allows for safe physical contact with living cells and human bodies. These features make them popularly used for healthcare applications. In addition, deformable materials and structures like springs are potentially able to store and release energy, which is beneficial for energy efficient locomotion. Another advantage of soft robots is that the used materials are cheaper than metal parts with comparable

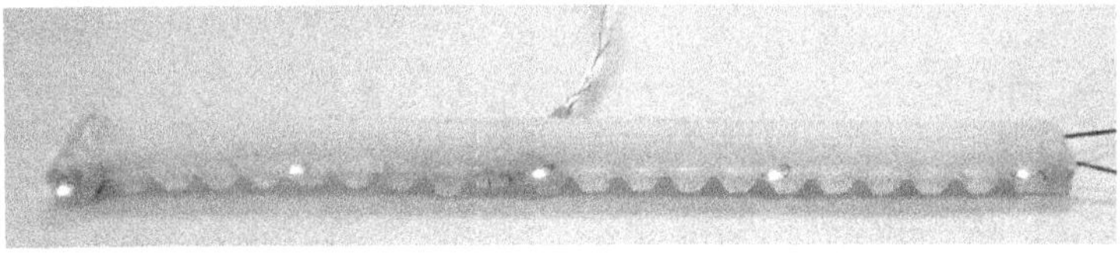

Figure 2.6 The GoQBot presented in [62]. © 2013 Elsevier. Reprinted with permission from [62]

actuation capacity. Soft robots provide an opportunity to bridge the gap between machines and people. In contrast to hard-bodied robots, soft robots have their bodies made out of intrinsically soft and/or extensible materials that can deform and absorb much of the energy arising from a collision. This section starts with some general soft robots developed for locomotion and manipulation, and followed by soft healthcare robots.

2.2.1 Soft robots for various applications

Over the last few decades, researchers have developed a variety of soft robots so far to address potential applications for locomotion, manipulation and human–machine interaction.

2.2.1.1 Locomotion

Recent work has explored the mode of locomotion possible with soft bodies. Caterpillars can curl into a wheel and generate their own rolling momentum as part of an escape repertoire. Inspired by this behaviour, Huai-Ti *et al.* [61] constructed a soft-bodied robot to explore the dynamics and control issues of ballistic rolling. This robot, called GoQBot, closely mimics caterpillar rolling, and can provide an estimate of the mechanical power for caterpillar rolling that is comparable to that of a locust jump. The prototype of the GoQBot presented in [62] is given in Figure 2.6.

Based on the antagonistic arrangement of circular and longitudinal muscle groups of Oligochaetes, Seok *et al.* [63] developed a soft robotic platform that exhibits peristaltic locomotion. The entire mechanical structure is made of flexible mesh materials and can withstand significant external impact during operation. Kwangmok *et al.* [64] developed an annelid-inspired robot driven by soft actuators based on dielectric elastomer. This device can provide a biological solution of effective locomotion adaptable to a large variety of unstructured environmental conditions. Kim *et al.* [62] reviewed the bioinspired evolution in soft robotics, of them a typical example is the worm-like robot, as presented in Figure 2.7. It mimics the mechanical actions of a lever by transforming force and displacement through Pascal's principle. The contraction of longitudinal muscles shortens the body and increases its diameter, while the contraction of circumferential muscles decreases the diameter and elongates the body.

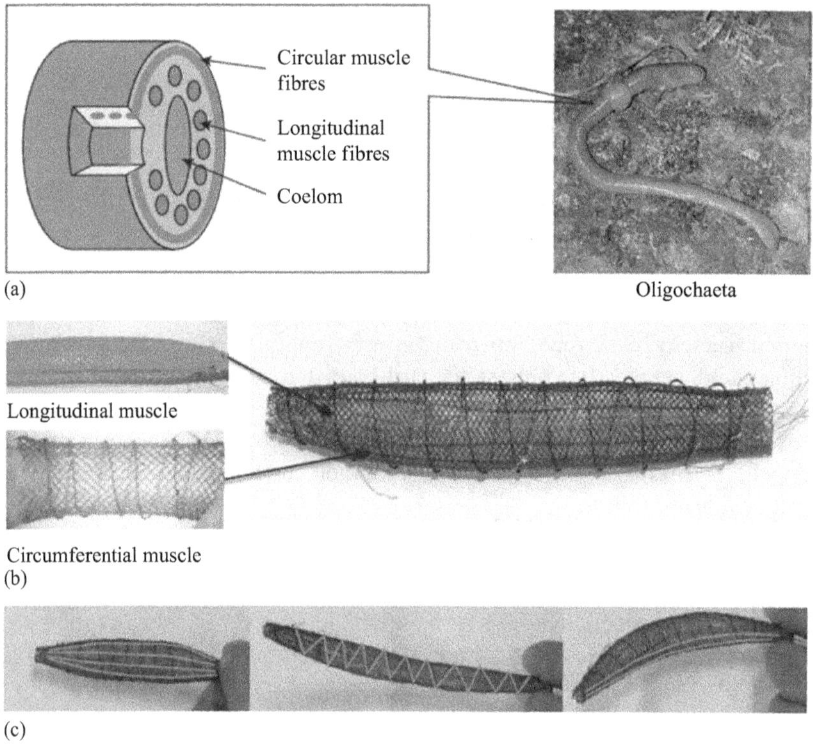

Figure 2.7 Worm-inspired robot reviewed in [62]. (a) Muscular structure of Oligochaete, which forms antagonistic pairs without skeleton or joint. (b) A mesh structure that contains longitudinal and circumferential artificial muscles, creating an antagonistic pairing similar to the pairing in Oligochaete. (c) Demonstration of various actuation modes. © 2013 Elsevier. Reprinted with permission from [62]

Cagdas and Daniela [65] developed an autonomous soft snake robot. This device consists of four bi-directional fluidic elastomer actuators in series to create a travelling curvature wave from head to tail along its body. It can undulate in a similar way to its biological counterpart using pressure for actuation power, without human intervention. Marchese *et al.* [66] constructed an autonomous robotic fish that is actuated by soft fluidic actuators and can swim forwards, turn and adjust the depth. The prototype of the soft robotic fish presented in [67] is given in Figure 2.8.

Many of the exciting applications for soft robotics require an autonomous and mobile system. However, most experimental soft robotic systems rely on power and control signals delivered through pneumatic or electrical tethers. Since typical actuation power sources (air compressors and batteries) are relatively heavy, tethers greatly simplify the system design by reducing the required carrying capacity.

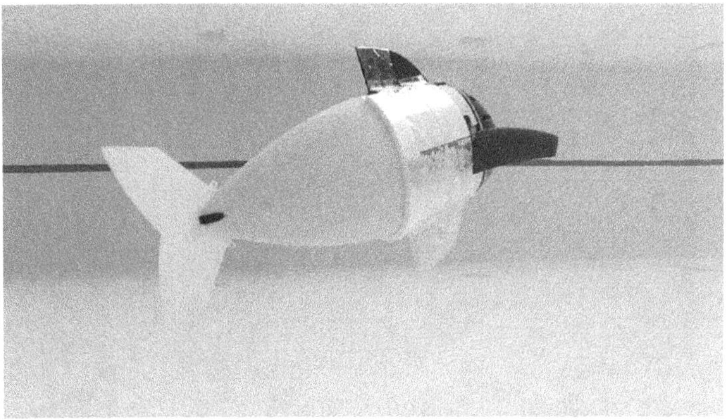

Figure 2.8 A soft robotic fish presented in [67]. © 2015 Nature Publishing Group. Reprinted with permission from [67]

2.2.1.2 Manipulation

Manipulation is one of the canonical challenges for robotics. Soft systems have a natural advantage over rigid robots in grasping and manipulating unknown objects because the compliance of soft grippers allows them to adapt to a variety of objects with simple control schemes. The OctArm has been demonstrated with the ability of the continuum robots to operate successfully both in air and water, and to maintain grasp stability under dynamic disturbances [68]. This device was constructed using air muscle extensors with three control channels per section that provide two axis bending and extension. It successfully grasped and manipulated objects over a wide range of sizes and scales, with the adaptation of their shape to that of a wide variety of payloads. An arm prototype presented in [69] is shown in Figure 2.9 with grasping a ball.

Another example is the simple gripper made based on embedded pneumatic networks (PneuNets) of channels in elastomers [70]. Figure 2.10 reproduced from [71] shows the process of the PneuNets to grip an uncooked chicken egg. While the used materials in the PneuNets are not suitable for manipulating heavy objects, the method could be extended to applications that require high loads with an appropriate choice of materials.

Abilities of soft robots such as squeezing, stretching, climbing, growing and morphing would not be possible with an approach based only on rigid links. The challenge ahead for soft robotics is to further develop the abilities to grow, evolve, self-heal, develop and biodegrade, which are the ways, that robots can adapt their morphology to the environment. However, a disadvantage of soft robots is that their soft structures are difficult to model and, therefore, hard to control. Further, since the research work in this field is still in early stage, most of soft robots are in the prototype stage and still have to be demonstrated useful under real-world conditions.

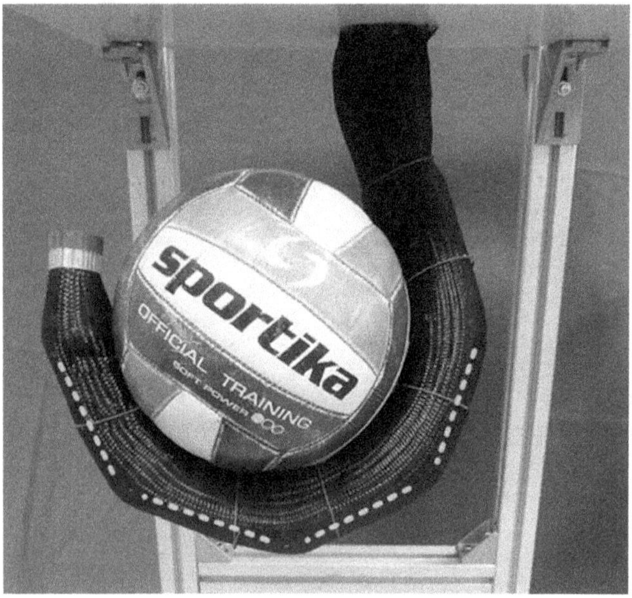

Figure 2.9 *An arm prototype is grasping a ball [69]. The activated PAMs are indicated with the dashed grey lines*

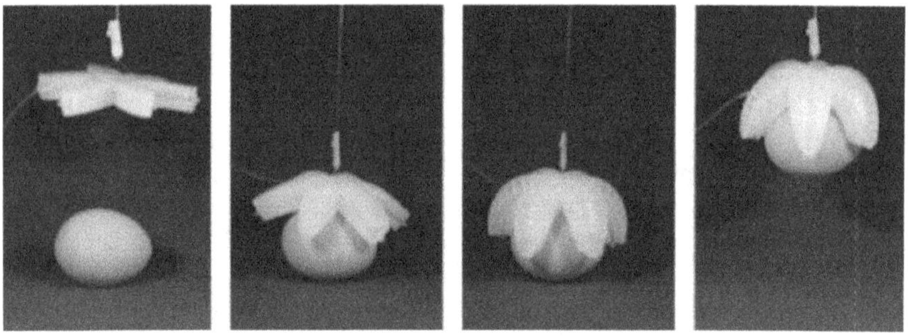

Figure 2.10 *The PneuNets to grips an uncooked chicken egg [71]*

2.2.2 Soft robots for healthcare

A variety of robots for healthcare applications have been reviewed by Bogue [72]. It was found that surgery robots are being employed in an ever-growing range of clinical procedures, and prosthetics are the topic of a major research effort and recent developments. A typical example is the da Vinci Surgical system (Figure 2.11) made by the American company Intuitive Surgical. An example of a

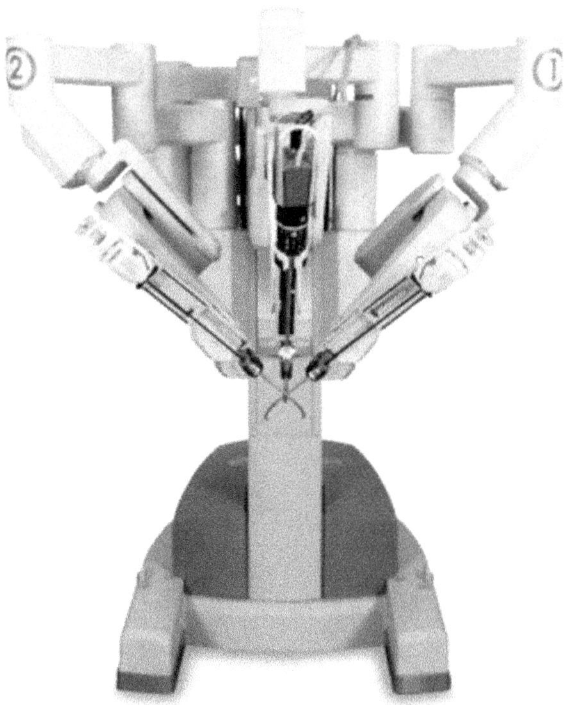

Figure 2.11 The Intuitive da Vinci Surgery robot. © 2017. Reprinted with permission from Intuitive Surgical, Inc

commercial exoskeleton is the ReWalk (Figure 2.12). This battery-powered system features a light and wearable device with motors at the hip and knee joints.

However, an obvious advantage of soft robots over rigid devices is that they generate little resistance to compressive forces and therefore can conform to obstacles. These robots carry soft and fragile payloads without causing damage, which makes them suitable for healthcare applications that interact with people [74]. Rigid medical devices or orthoses run the risk of causing damage or discomfort to human tissues. It can be also difficult to replicate the motion of natural joints with rigid actuators. One possibility is to integrate certain compliance into wearable devices, for example for orthopaedic rehabilitation.

While enabling technologies have been progressing, the soft robotics approach has been used for building integrated systems in various application scenarios. A variety of soft robots have been recently developed for healthcare applications. Kramer *et al.* [75] developed a hyper-elastic, thin and transparent pressure-sensitive keypad by embedding a silicone rubber film with conductive liquid-filled microchannels. Park *et al.* [48] presented the design and control of a wearable robotic device powered by PAM actuators for ankle-foot rehabilitation. The prototype presented in [40] is shown in Figure 2.13. This novel design was inspired by

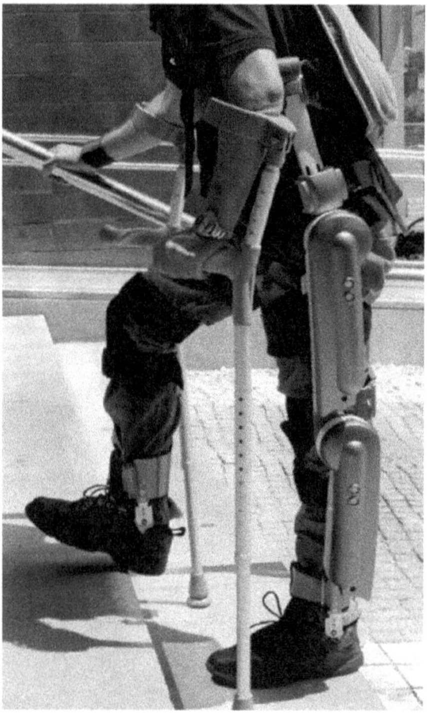

Figure 2.12 The ReWalk for all day use at home and in the community. © 2013 Nature Publishing Group. Reprinted with permission from [73]

the biological musculoskeletal system of the human leg. The soft structure of this wearable robot could provide active assistance without restricting natural ankle motions. Four PAM actuators were used to assist ankle dorsiflexion/plantarflexion and inversion/eversion. The prototype was also equipped with various embedded sensors for gait pattern analysis. Song *et al.* [76] designed a soft pneumatically actuated system for gait rehabilitation of rodents who have had their spinal cord surgically cut.

Soft actuators are also used for measurement and simulation. Mengüc *et al.* [77] developed a wearable soft sensing suit for monitoring hip, knee and ankle sagittal plane joint angles. This system consists of running tights and shoe insoles which serve as the garment base, custom electronics will collect, amplify and transmit sensor signals, and the six soft strain sensors created from liquid metal embedded in an elastomer. Roche *et al.* [78] proposed a soft system for simulation of cardiac actuation by embedding pneumatic actuators in a soft material inspired by a biological muscle fibril architecture.

Polygerinos *et al.* [79] developed a soft robotic glove for combined assistance and at-home rehabilitation using inexpensive hydraulic soft actuators. These actuators were made from elastomeric materials with fibre reinforcements to

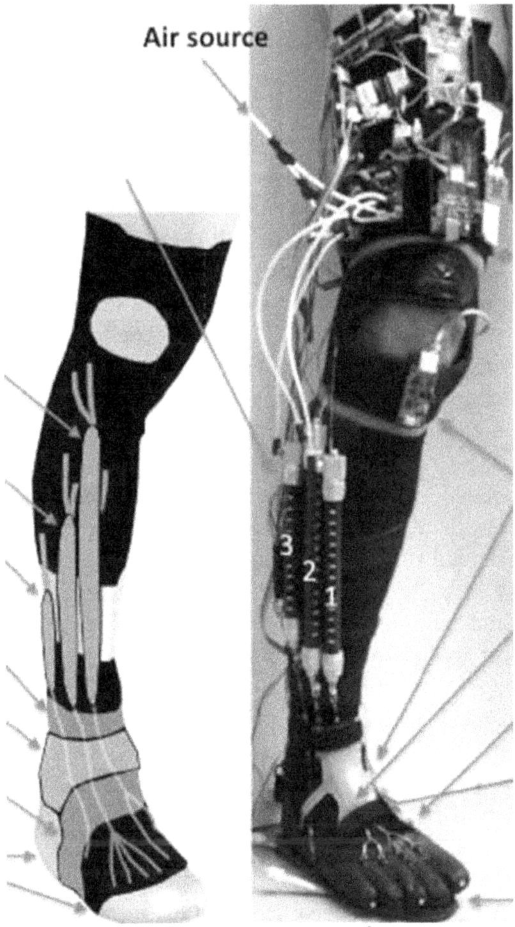

Figure 2.13 A bio-inspired wearable robotic device for ankle-foot rehabilitation presented in [40]

control the fingers (see Figure 1.2). Integrated fluidic pressure sensors measure the internal pressure of soft actuators and allow control of finger flexion/extension. Similarly, In *et al.* [80] developed a wearable hand robot called the Exo-Glove that uses a soft tendon routing system and an under-actuation adaptive mechanism. Since conventional elements of a hard exoskeleton are unsuitable for soft structure, the Exo-Glove employed a new design inspired by human finger anatomy. Due to the inherent compliance of soft actuators, no joint alignment is required between the device and the human body. In addition, Yap *et al.* [81] proposed the design of a soft wearable exoskeleton that comprises of a glove embedded with pneumatic actuators of variable stiffness for hand rehabilitation. A key feature of this exoskeleton is the variable stiffness of the actuators at different localities that not only conforms to the finger profile during actuation, but also provides customisability for different hand sizes. The actuators can achieve different bending profiles with variable stiffness implemented at different localities, which makes it be able to perform various hand therapy exercises including full fist, straight fist, hook fist and table top.

For more complex soft robotic systems for healthcare applications, Costa and Caldwell [82] developed a ten-DOF lower body exoskeleton for gait rehabilitation. The actuation is provided to the flexion and extension of the hip, knee and ankle, and abduction and adduction of the hip via PAMs. The Human Neuro-mechanics Laboratory at the University of Michigan developed a number of active orthoses, particularly focusing on ankle-foot rehabilitation [83,84]. It should be noted that this device was not designed to be fully portable with a tether to a stationary compressor. The PAM actuators were mounted to carbon fibre and poly-propylene shells, resulting in the device that is extremely lightweight and exhibiting high-power outputs. The University of Michigan has also developed a knee-ankle-foot device for gait rehabilitation [85,86], as in Figure 2.14. Both the ankle-foot and knee-ankle-foot orthoses are comfortable, lightweight and allow un-encumbered movement through a normal range of motion during walking. The orthoses were custom-built for each subject from a combination of carbon fibre and poly-propylene. Steel hinge joints allow sagittal plane movements at ankle and knee joints. It should be noted that the custom-built nature of these devices has negatives for clinical applications, since a separate device needs to be built for each patient before therapy can commence.

The MIT Bio-mechatronics Group developed a powered active ankle-foot orthosis to assist gait of patients with drop foot [87]. This device consists of a modified passive ankle-foot orthosis with the addition of a series elastic actuator to allow for the variation in the impedance of flexion/extension direction of ankle motion, and is controlled at the basis of ground force and angle position data. Clinical data demonstrated that this device could improve the gait of patients with drop foot by increasing walking speed, reducing the instances of foot slap, creating better symmetry with the unaffected leg and providing assistance during powered plantarflexion.

At Arizona State University, Bharadwaj *et al.* [88] proposed an ankle-foot-orthosis with two spring-over-muscle actuators attached to the left and right sides of the foot, forming a tripod with the heel. This orthosis is essentially a parallel robot that incorporates two pneumatically powered, double-acting, compliant and spring over muscle actuators as actuation links for ankle dorsiflexion/plantarflexion and inversion/eversion. A key feature of the tripod design is that the human anatomy is part of the robot. Hollander *et al.* [89] constructed a robotic tendon using a motor and a spring in series in which the stiffness of the spring is crucial for its successful usage in a lightweight, energy efficient and powered ankle orthosis.

The Mechatronics Laboratory of the University of Auckland also used PAMs to develop lower-limb devices for promoting robot-assisted rehabilitation techniques. Jamwal *et al.* [50] designed a novel wearable robot for the treatment of ankle sprain through physical therapy. The ankle robot has a bio-inspired design with three rotational DOFs, devised after a careful study of the improvement

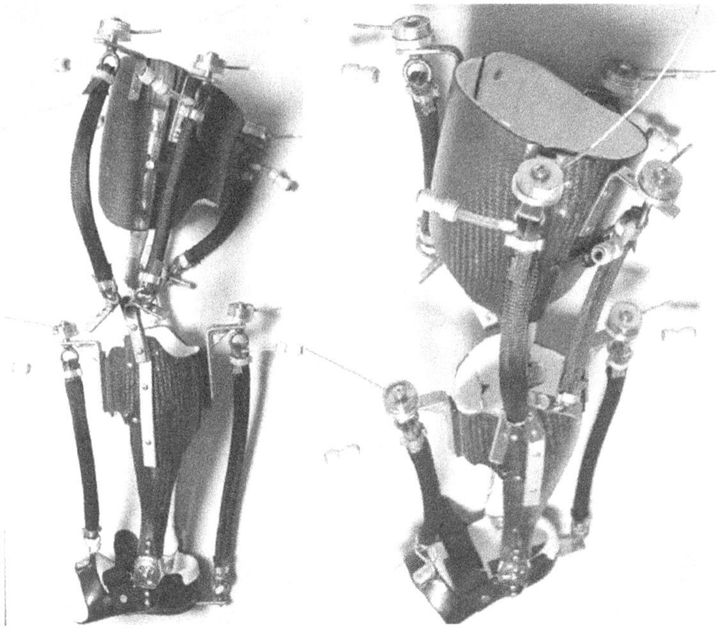

Figure 2.14 *University of Michigan Knee-Ankle-Foot Orthosis. Two pictures of the unilateral (left leg) knee-ankle-foot orthosis with artificial pneumatic muscles display the thigh and shank sections made from carbon-fibre and the foot section made from poly-propylene. The orthoses were custom moulded from a cast unique to each subject. Hinge joints at the ankle and knee allowed free motion in the sagittal plane. We used steel brackets to attach two artificial pneumatic muscles (a plantarflexor and a dorsiflexor) around the ankle and four around the knee (two extensors and two flexors). Each artificial pneumatic muscle had a compression load transducer mounted in series on the proximal steel bracket attachment and a release valve for quick connection to the pressurised air source. A special shoe was worn over the foot section during walking trials [86]*

opportunities in existing ankle robots. Four lightweight but powerful PAM actuators (Shadow Robot Company) were employed for the actuation of the ankle robot to mimic skeletal muscles. To evaluate the robot design, the disturbance observer, and the adaptive fuzzy logic controller, experiments were performed on a neurologically intact subject and showed satisfactory trajectory tracking performance in the presence of unpredicted human intervention.

An improved prototype of the ankle robot by Jamwal *et al.* [50] was also made at the University of Auckland, as in Figure 2.15. This design was a vast improvement in terms of stability and aesthetics with thicker fittings and welded

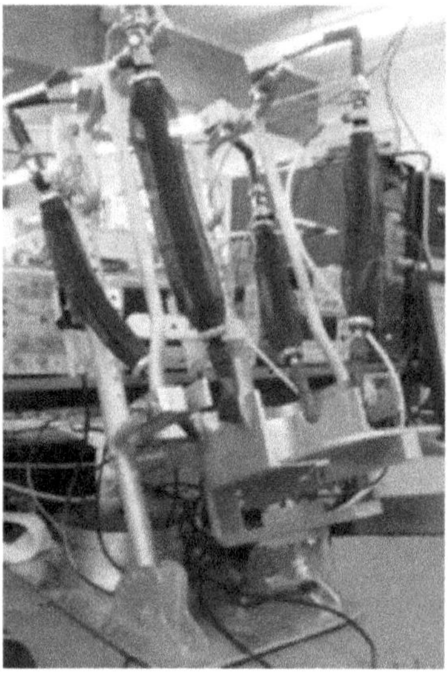

Figure 2.15 An upgraded ankle robot based on the prototype developed by Jamwal et al. [50]

joints. It incorporates more curves, giving it a friendlier and more appealing look, in particular the new footplate. This transition is vital in the continuing development of medical robots that look less intimidating to patients. This design also allows for ankle adduction and abduction due to the new layout of actuators. More recently, this prototype has been further improved by Zhang [59], as in Figure 1.4.

Hussain *et al.* [90] proposed a lightweight robotic gait training orthosis with two actuated and four passive DOFs, as in Figure 2.4. The two actuated DOFs were powered by PAM actuators (Shadow Robot Company). An assistance-as-needed gait training paradigm was developed based on adaptive impedance control for providing interactive robotic gait training. The robotic orthosis can be operated in two gait training modes, namely, inactive mode and active mode, to evaluate the performance of the proposed control scheme. Experimental results on ten healthy subjects demonstrated that an increase in voluntary participation of human subjects resulted in a decrease of the robotic assistance and vice versa for enhanced training efficacy.

Park *et al.* [91] presented a soft wearable robotic device composed of elastomeric artificial muscle actuators and soft fabric sleeves for active assistance of knee motions. A key feature of the device is the two-dimensional design of the elastomer muscles that not only allows the compactness of the device, but also significantly simplifies the manufacturing process. Four elastomer actuators were employed for assisted knee extension and flexion. The robotic device was tested on a printed leg model with an articulated knee joint, and the results showed maximum extension and flexion angles of 95° and 37°, respectively.

2.3 Summary

This chapter firstly presents the historical background of advanced robotics for rehabilitation purposes. Followed is the overview of soft robotics for a variety of applications, including its definition and typical examples for healthcare applications. Comparison analysis demonstrates that conventional rehabilitation robots suffer from a few limitations. Most of them used rigid actuators to achieve precise position and force. While soft robots have shown great potential in the field of robot-assisted healthcare applications, there is a long way for them to be well used in real-word conditions.

Soft robots can be divided into two categories. The first group uses active materials such as electroactive polymers and shape memory alloys. These machines do not need separate motors and are potentially capable of completely soft autonomous locomotion. However, they are currently limited by poor actuation efficiency or force production, and by the need to carry relatively stiff power supplies such as batteries. The research in this field is still in an early stage. The other group employs traditional motors and pumps to transfer power to the soft bodied robot using cables or pressurised air/fluid. One of typical applications is to use inflatable rubber compartments designed to expand in pre-arranged directions. By linking these compartments together and controlling the inflation timing, these devices can be made to crawl with a variety of gaits or to generate complex movements for grasping and manipulating objects. This book focuses on the use of soft robotics for rehabilitation purposes. For better actuation precision and clinical applications, the prototypes to be reported in this book adopt soft and compliant actuators with stiff skeleton.

References

[1] Brewer BR, McDowell SK, Worthen-Chaudhari LC. Poststroke upper extremity rehabilitation: a review of robotic systems and clinical results. Top Stroke Rehabil. 2007;14(6):22–44.

[2] Michmizos KP, Rossi S, Castelli E, Cappa P, Krebs HI. Robot-aided neurorehabilitation: a pediatric robot for ankle rehabilitation. IEEE Trans Neural Syst Rehabil. 2015;23(6):1056–67.

[3] Balasubramanian S, Klein J, Burdet E. Robot-assisted rehabilitation of hand function. Curr Opin Neurol. 2010;23(6):661–70.

[4] Marchal-Crespo L, Reinkensmeyer DJ. Review of control strategies for robotic movement training after neurologic injury. J Neuroeng Rehabil. 2009;6(1):20.

[5] Cao J, Xie SQ, Das R, Zhu GL. Control strategies for effective robot assisted gait rehabilitation: the state of art and future prospects. Med Eng Phys. 2014;36(12):1555–66.

[6] Balasubramanian S, Colombo R, Sterpi I, Sanguineti V, Burdet E. Robotic assessment of upper limb motor function after stroke. Am J Phys Med Rehabil. 2012;91(11):S255–69.

[7] Zhang M, Davies TC, Zhang Y, Xie S. Reviewing effectiveness of ankle assessment techniques for use in robot-assisted therapy. J Rehabil Res Dev. 2014;51(4):517–34.
[8] Lo HS, Xie SQ. Exoskeleton robots for upper-limb rehabilitation: tate of the art and future prospects. Med Eng Phys. 2012;34(3):261–8.
[9] Zhang M, Davies TC, Xie S. Effectiveness of robot-assisted therapy on ankle rehabilitation - a systematic review. J Neuroeng Rehabil. 2013;10:30.
[10] Tondu B. Estimating shoulder-complex mobility. Appl Bionics Biomech. 2007;4(1):19–29.
[11] Ludewig PM, Phadke V, Braman JP, Hassett DR, Cieminski CJ, Laprade RF. Motion of the shoulder complex during multiplanar humeral elevation. J Bone Joint Surg Ser A. 2009;91(2):378–89.
[12] Neu CP, Crisco JJ, Wolfe SW. In vivo kinematic behavior of the radio-capitate joint during wrist flexion-extension and radio-ulnar deviation. J Biomech. 2001;34(11):1429–38.
[13] Perry JC, Rosen J, Burns S. Upper-limb powered exoskeleton design. IEEE/ASME Transact Mechatronics. 2007;12(4):408–17.
[14] Balasubramanian S, Ruihua W, Perez M, Shepard B, Koeneman E, Koeneman J, *et al.*, editors. RUPERT: an exoskeleton robot for assisting rehabilitation of arm functions. 2008 Virtual Rehabilitation; 25–27 August 2008.
[15] Ren Y, Park HS, Zhang LQ. Developing a whole-arm exoskeleton robot with hand opening and closing mechanism for upper limb stroke rehabilitation. 2009 IEEE international conference on rehabilitation robotics; 2009.
[16] Gopura RARC, Kiguchi K, Li Y. SUEFUL-7: a 7DOF upper-limb exoskeleton robot with muscle-model-oriented EMG-based control. 2009 IEEE/RSJ international conference on intelligent robots and systems; 2009.
[17] Nef T, Guidali M, Riener R. ARMin III – arm therapy exoskeleton with an ergonomic shoulder actuation. Appl Bionics Biomech. 2009;6(2):127–42.
[18] Caldwell DG, Tsagarakis NG, Kousidou S, Costa N, Sarakoglou I. “Soft” exoskeletons for upper and lower body rehabilitation–Design, control and testing. Int J Hum Robot. 2007;04(03):549–73.
[19] Kitago T, Krakauer JW. Motor learning principles for neurorehabilitation. In: Barnes MP, Good DC, editors. Handbook of clinical neurology. Amsterdam: Elsevier; 2013. p. 93–103.
[20] Carr JH, Shepherd RB, Gordon J, Gentile A, Held JM. Movement science: foundations for physical therapy in rehabilitation. New York, NY: Aspen Publishers; 1987.
[21] Plautz EJ, Milliken GW, Nudo RJ. Effects of repetitive motor training on movement representations in adult squirrel monkeys: role of use versus learning. Neurobiol Learn Mem. 2000;74(1):27–55.
[22] Krakauer JW. Motor learning: its relevance to stroke recovery and neuro-rehabilitation. Curr Opin Neurol. 2006;19(1):84–90.
[23] Schmidt RA, Lee TD. Motor control and learning: a behavioral emphasis. 3rd ed. New Zealand: Human Kinetics; 2011.

[24] Nudo R. Adaptive plasticity in motor cortex: implications for rehabilitation after brain injury. J Rehabil Med Suppl. 2003;(41):7–10.

[25] Shea CH, Kohl RM. Composition of practice: influence on the retention of motor skills. Res Quart Exerc Sport. 1991;62(2):187–95.

[26] Kilgard MP, Merzenich MM. Cortical map reorganization enabled by nucleus basalis activity. Science. 1998;279(5357):1714–8.

[27] Bayona NA, Bitensky J, Salter K, Teasell R. The role of task-specific training in rehabilitation therapies. Top Stroke Rehabil. 2005;12(3):58–65.

[28] Classen J, Liepert J, Wise SP, Hallett M, Cohen LG. Rapid plasticity of human cortical movement representation induced by practice. J Neurophysiol. 1998;79(2):1117–23.

[29] Ungerleider LG. Functional MRI evidence for adult motor cortex plasticity during motor skill learning. Nature. 1995;377:155–8.

[30] Langhammer B, Stanghelle JK. Bobath or motor relearning programme? A comparison of two different approaches of physiotherapy in stroke rehabilitation: a randomized controlled study. Clin Rehabil. 2000;14(4):361–9.

[31] Langhammer B, Stanghelle JK. Bobath or motor relearning programme? A follow-up one and four years post stroke. Clin Rehabil. 2003;17(7):731–4.

[32] Barbeau H, Wainberg M, Finch L. Description and application of a system for locomotor rehabilitation. Med Biol Eng Comput. 1987;25(3):341–4.

[33] Hesse S. Locomotor therapy in neurorehabilitation. NeuroRehabil. 2001; 16(3):133–9.

[34] Hesse S, Bertelt C, Jahnke M, *et al.* Treadmill training with partial body weight support compared with physiotherapy in nonambulatory hemiparetic patients. Stroke. 1995;26(6):976–81.

[35] Hesse S, Malezic M, Schaffrin A, Mauritz K. Restoration of gait by combined treadmill training and multichannel electrical stimulation in non-ambulatory hemiparetic patients. Scand J Rehabil Med. 1995;27(4):199.

[36] Colombo G, Joerg M, Schreier R, Dietz V. Treadmill training of paraplegic patients using a robotic orthosis. J Rehabil Res Dev. 2000;37(6):693–700.

[37] Lunenburger L, Colombo G, Riener R. Biofeedback for robotic gait rehabilitation. J Neuroeng Rehabil. 2007;4(1):1–11.

[38] Koenig A, Omlin X, Bergmann J, *et al.* Controlling patient participation during robot assisted gait training. J Neuroeng Rehabil. 2011;8(1):14–25.

[39] Liebermann DG, Buchman AS, Franks IM. Enhancement of motor rehabilitation through the use of information technologies. Clin Biomech. 2006; 21(1):8–20.

[40] Dzahir M, Yamamoto SI. Recent trends in lower-limb robotic rehabilitation orthosis: control scheme and strategy for pneumatic muscle actuated gait trainers. Robotics. 2014;3(2):120.

[41] Hussain S, Xie SQ, Jamwal PK, Parsons J. An intrinsically compliant robotic orthosis for treadmill training. Med Eng Phys. 2012;34(10):1448–53.

[42] Banala SK, Kim SH, Agrawal SK, Scholz JP. Robot assisted gait training with active leg exoskeleton (ALEX). IEEE Trans Neural Syst Rehabil. 2009;17(1):2–8.

[43] Veneman JF, Ekkelenkamp R, Kruidhof R, Helm FCTvd, Kooij Hvd. A series elastic- and Bowden-cable-based actuation system for use as torque actuator in exoskeleton-type robots. Int J Robot Res. 2006;25(3):261–81.
[44] Emken JL, Wynne JH, Harkema SJ, Reinkensmeyer DJ. Robotic device for manipulating human stepping. IEEE-INST Electrical Electronics Engineers Inc; 2006.
[45] Aoyagi D, Ichinose WE, Harkema SJ, Reinkensmeyer DJ, Bobrow JE. A robot and control algorithm that can synchronously assist in naturalistic motion during body-weight-supported gait training following neurologic injury. IEEE Trans Neural Syst Rehabil. 2007;15(3):387–400.
[46] Ichinose WE, Reinkensmeyer DJ, Aoyagi D, *et al.* A robotic device for measuring and controlling pelvic motion during locomotor rehabilitation. Proceedings of the 25th annual international conference of the IEEE engineering in medicine and biology society (IEEE Cat No 03CH37439); 2003.
[47] Roy A, Krebs HI, Williams DJ, *et al.* Robot-aided neurorehabilitation: a novel robot for ankle rehabilitation. IEEE Transact Robot. 2009;25(3):569–82.
[48] Park YL, Chen BR, Pérez-Arancibia NO, *et al.* Design and control of a bio-inspired soft wearable robotic device for ankle-foot rehabilitation. Bioinspir Biomim. 2014;9(1):016007.
[49] Yu H, Huang S, Chen G, Pan Y, Guo Z. Human–robot interaction control of rehabilitation robots with series elastic actuators. IEEE Trans Robot. 2015;31(5):1089–100.
[50] Jamwal PK, Xie SQ, Hussain S, Parsons JG. An adaptive wearable parallel robot for ankle injury treatments. IEEE/ASME Trans Mechatronics. 2014;19(1): 64–75.
[51] Tsoi YH, Xie SQ, Graham AE. Design, modeling and control of an ankle rehabilitation robot. Stud Comput Intell. 2009;177:377–99.
[52] Saglia JA, Tsagarakis NG, Dai JS, Caldwell DG. A high-performance redundantly actuated parallel mechanism for ankle rehabilitation. Int J Robot Res. 2009;28(9):1216–27.
[53] Girone M, Burdea G, Bouzit M, Popescu V, Deutsch JE. A stewart platform-based system for ankle telerehabilitation. Auton Robot. 2001;10(2):203–12.
[54] Zhang LQ, Chung SG, Bai Z, *et al.* Intelligent stretching of ankle joints with contracture spasticity. IEEE Trans Neural Syst Rehabil. 2002;10(3):149–57.
[55] Wang C, Fang Y, Guo S. Multi-objective optimization of a parallel ankle rehabilitation robot using modified differential evolution algorithm. Chinese J Mech Eng. 2015;28(4):702–15.
[56] Wang C, Fang Y, Guo S, Chen Y. Design and kinematical performance analysis of a 3-RUS/RRR redundantly actuated parallel mechanism for ankle rehabilitation. J Mech Robot. 2013;5(4):041003.
[57] Chattanooga. OptiFlex Ankle CPM. 2017. <http://www.djoglobal.com/products/chattanooga/optiflex-ankle-cpm>; [accessed 02.05.2017].
[58] Saglia JA, Tsagarakis NG, Dai JS, Caldwell DG. Control strategies for patient-assisted training using the ankle rehabilitation robot (ARBOT). IEEE/ASME Trans Mechatronics. 2013;18(6):1799–808.

[59] Zhang M. Improving effectiveness of robot-assisted ankle rehabilitation via biomechanical assessment and interaction control. Auckland, New Zealand: University of Auckland; 2016.
[60] Siegler S, Chen J, Schneck CD. The three-dimensional kinematics and flexibility characteristics of the human ankle and subtalar joints – Part I: Kinematics. J Biomech Eng. 1988;110(4):364–73.
[61] Huai-Ti L, Gary GL, Barry T. GoQBot: a caterpillar-inspired soft-bodied rolling robot. Bioinspir Biomim. 2011;6(2):026007.
[62] Kim S, Laschi C, Trimmer B. Soft robotics: a bioinspired evolution in robotics. Trends Biotechnol. 2013;31(5):287–94.
[63] Seok S, Onal CD, Cho KJ, Wood RJ, Rus D, Kim S. Meshworm: a peristaltic soft robot with antagonistic nickel titanium coil actuators. IEEE/ASME Trans Mechatronics. 2013;18(5):1485–97.
[64] Kwangmok J, Ja Choon K, Jae-do N, Young Kwan L, Hyouk Ryeol C. Artificial annelid robot driven by soft actuators. Bioinspir Biomim. 2007; 2(2):S42.
[65] Cagdas DO, Daniela R. Autonomous undulatory serpentine locomotion utilizing body dynamics of a fluidic soft robot. Bioinspir Biomim. 2013; 8(2):026003.
[66] Marchese AD, Onal CD, Rus D. Autonomous soft robotic fish capable of escape maneuvers using fluidic elastomer actuators. Soft Robot. 2014; 1(1):75–87.
[67] Rus D, Tolley MT.Design, fabrication and control of soft robots. Nature. 2015;521(7553):467–75.
[68] McMahan W, Chitrakaran V, Csencsits M, *et al.* Field trials and testing of the OctArm continuum manipulator. Proceedings 2006 IEEE international conference on robotics and automation; 2006.
[69] Kang R, Guglielmino E, Zullo L, Branson DT, Godage I, Caldwell DG. Embodiment design of soft continuum robots. Adv Mech Eng. 2016;8(4): 1687814016643302.
[70] Ilievski F, Mazzeo AD, Shepherd RF, Chen X, Whitesides GM. Soft robotics for chemists. Angew Chem. 2011;123(8):1930–5.
[71] Whitesides GM. Bioinspiration: something for everyone. Interface Focus. 2015;5(4).
[72] Bogue R. Robots in healthcare. Industr Robot Int J. 2011;38(3):218–23.
[73] Gwynne P. Technology: mobility machines. Nature. 2013;503(7475):S16–S7.
[74] Trivedi D, Rahn CD, Kier WM, Walker ID. Soft robotics: biological inspiration, state of the art, and future research. Appl Bionics Biomech. 2008;5(3):99–117.
[75] Kramer RK, Majidi C, Wood RJ, editors. Wearable tactile keypad with stretchable artificial skin. 2011 IEEE International Conference on Robotics and Automation; 9–13 May, 2011.
[76] Song YS, Sun Y, Brand Rvd, *et al.* Soft robot for gait rehabilitation of spinalized rodents. 2013 IEEE/RSJ international conference on intelligent robots and systems; 2013.

[77] Mengüc Y, Park YL, Pei H, *et al.* Wearable soft sensing suit for human gait measurement. Int J Robot Res. 2014;33(14):1748–64.
[78] Roche ET, Wohlfarth R, Overvelde JTB, *et al.* A bioinspired soft actuated material. Adv Mater. 2014;26(8):1200–6.
[79] Polygerinos P, Wang Z, Galloway KC, Wood RJ, Walsh CJ. Soft robotic glove for combined assistance and at-home rehabilitation. Robot Auton Syst. 2015;73:135–43.
[80] In H, Kang BB, Sin M, Cho KJ. Exo-Glove: a wearable robot for the hand with a soft tendon routing system. IEEE Robot Autom Mag. 2015;22(1): 97–105.
[81] Yap HK, Jeong Hoon L, Nasrallah F, Goh JCH, Yeow RCH, editors. A soft exoskeleton for hand assistive and rehabilitation application using pneumatic actuators with variable stiffness. 2015 IEEE international conference on robotics and automation; 2015.
[82] Costa N, Caldwell DG, editors. Control of a Biomimetic "Soft-actuated" 10DoF Lower Body Exoskeleton. The first IEEE/RAS-EMBS international conference on biomedical robotics and biomechatronics; 2006.
[83] Ferris DP, Gordon KE, Sawicki GS, Peethambaran A. An improved powered ankle-foot orthosis using proportional myoelectric control. Gait Posture. 2006;23(4):425–28.
[84] Ferris DP, Czerniecki JM, Hannaford B, University of M, University of W, System VAPSH. An ankle-foot orthosis powered by artificial pneumatic muscles. J Appl Biomech. 2005;21(2):189–97.
[85] Sawicki GS, Gordon KE, Ferris DP, editors. Powered lower limb orthoses: applications in motor adaptation and rehabilitation. IEEE 9th international conference on rehabilitation robotics. IEEE: Chicago, IL. 2005:206–11.
[86] Sawicki GS, Ferris DP. A pneumatically powered knee-ankle-foot orthosis (KAFO) with myoelectric activation and inhibition. J Neuroeng Rehabil. 2009;6(1):23.
[87] Blaya JA, Herr H. Adaptive control of a variable-impedance ankle-foot orthosis to assist drop-foot gait. IEEE Trans Neural Syst Rehabil. 2004; 12(1):24–31.
[88] Bharadwaj K, Sugar TG, Koeneman JB, Koeneman EJ. Design of a robotic gait trainer using spring over muscle actuators for ankle stroke rehabilitation. J Biomech Eng. 2005;127(6):1009–13.
[89] Hollander KW, Ilg R, Sugar TG, Herring D. An efficient robotic tendon for gait assistance. J Biomech Eng. 2006;128(5):788–91.
[90] Hussain S, Xie SQ, Jamwal PK. Adaptive impedance control of a robotic orthosis for gait rehabilitation. IEEE Trans Cybernet. 2013;43(3):1025–34.
[91] Park YL, Santos J, Galloway KG, Goldfield EC, Wood RJ. A soft wearable robotic device for active knee motions using flat pneumatic artificial muscles. 2014 IEEE international conference on robotics and automation (ICRA); 2014.

Chapter 3

Concept and modelling of a soft rehabilitation actuator: the Peano muscle

The large, heavy and rigid form of traditional electric, hydraulic and pneumatic actuators is ill-suited to actuating rehabilitation devices worn on the body. Many alternative actuators have a more promising form, but do not share the reliability and availability of their counterparts. We propose the Peano muscle as solution. It is a soft, sheet-like fluid-powered actuator invented in 1959 by Mettam [1] that potentially shares the form, fabrication and materials of everyday clothing. Hence, it can give clothing the ability to move the body, whether for assistance or rehabilitation. As a relatively unexplored actuator, the Peano muscle lacks models that account for its material and geometry properties. We present and validate the MECHanical Approximation Lumped Parameter (MECHALP) model for accurately predicting the static force generation of Peano muscles. Its accuracy and physics-based nature makes it a useful tool that is foundational for the design and control of Peano muscle actuated rehabilitation wearables.

This chapter explains the limitations of current actuators compared to the relevant requirements of rehabilitation devices; presents the concept of the Peano muscle as a promising rehabilitation actuator; and describes the MECHALP static model and its validation.

3.1 Towards soft and wearable actuation for rehabilitation systems

Until recently, robots have been primarily used in automated manufacturing and assembly. They have been designed to accurately complete repetitive and labour-intensive work in predictable environments. To do this, their actuators need to be precise and powerful. The untiring, task-based and automatic nature of robots has driven their adoption in rehabilitative technologies. Effective rehabilitation also requires task-specific, high intensity and frequent movement sequences, but has been constrained by the limited availability and high cost of skilled therapists [2–4]. The similarities between robots' capabilities and the demands of therapy have meant that rehabilitation robots have the potential to automate therapy [5]. These rehabilitation robots are often exoskeletons that are worn on their users' limbs, and apply torques in parallel with their users' muscles to help their users move their joints.

Table 3.1 Definitions of assistive device user needs relevant to exoskeleton actuation (adapted from [10])

User need	Definition [8,9]
Affordability	The initial and ongoing financial costs of the device
Durability	The operational lifetime of the device
Easy to maintain/ repair	The ease of keeping the device functioning as designed
Effectiveness	The ability of the device to improve its user's quality of life
Operability	The ease of controlling the device and its adaptability to changes in its user's size and disability level
Physical comfort/ acceptance	The fit, appearance and sound of the device does not cause its user to feel pain or be stigmatised
Portability	The ease of transporting the device between locations
Reliability	The consistency of the device's operation in normal operating conditions
Safety	The potential for the device to harm its user (or others)

Clearly, exoskeletons and their actuators have a very different working environment and hence design requirements compared to traditional assembly line robots. For example, mounting a robot on a human raises unprecedented issues of safely harmonising the close physical interaction of the robotic exoskeleton with its user. This means putting the user at the centre of the exoskeleton design process, a lesson we can learn from history. In the past, high proportions (at least 35%) of mechanical exoskeletons have been abandoned by their users [6,7]. Research has shown that this was due to a lack of consideration of user needs in exoskeleton design. Similarly, robotic exoskeletons will be abandoned unless they are designed according to requirements that capture the needs of their users. Those needs most relevant to exoskeleton actuation are defined in Table 3.1. They are a subset of the 'necessary and sufficient' needs originally proposed by Batavia and Hammer [8], and later refined by Lane *et al.* [9]. Simply put, these needs regard an exoskeleton's functionality and how it fits into its user's life [9]. What this practically means is that to maximise an exoskeleton's acceptability, exoskeleton actuator design needs to be based on the performance, physical form and safety requirements that meet the user needs in Table 3.1.

Comparing the needs of Table 3.1 with those of a traditional factory floor robot highlights three key areas of difference: physical comfort and acceptance, portability and safety. These needs are important to rehabilitation robots, but not to traditional robots, and are reflected in unique requirements for rehabilitation actuators. First, an exoskeleton's actuator should have a minimalistic form that conforms to the body, ensuring the exoskeleton is unobtrusive [11,12] and comfortable to wear [13,14]. Second, an exoskeleton's actuators should be lightweight [15] to maximise the exoskeleton's portability. Third, an exoskeleton's actuators should share the compliance, damping and limited range of motion (ROM) of biological muscles [16]. These last requirements ensure safety by

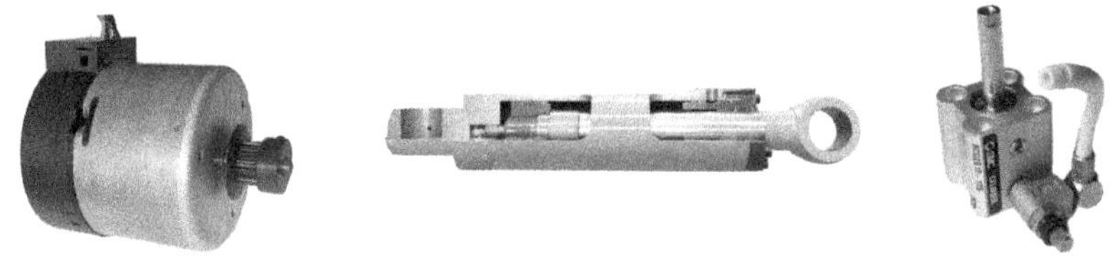

(a) (b) (c)

Figure 3.1 Traditional robots are actuated by electric servomotors (a), hydraulic cylinders (b) and pneumatic cylinders (c). Credit line: User: Hotdogcartman/Public Domain (b) [21]

inherently constraining the exchange of motion and power between the exoskeleton and its user. A more detailed investigation of these and other rehabilitation actuator requirements is in [10].

Collectively the unique requirements of exoskeleton actuators require them to have similar power and in some cases accuracy to traditional robots' actuators yet with a form that is soft with minimal size and weight. The rigid and heavy materials of the electric servomotors, and hydraulic or pneumatic cylinders used in traditional robots (Figure 3.1) make them obtrusive, uncomfortable, unportable and inherently unsafe. Recognising these limitations of traditional actuator options, researchers have sought to develop softer alternatives, or artificial muscles. Types of artificial muscles include thermally activated smart materials, ionic electroactive polymers (EAPs), electronic EAPs and electrostatic force actuators. All these artificial muscles aim to minimise the size, weight or rigidity of traditional actuators. The most promising for rehabilitation actuation are dielectric elastomers (DEs) [17], super coiled polymer [18] and PVC gel [19] actuators. However, in practice these actuators are not yet suitable for most exoskeletons. They either require complex fabrication, are unreliable or their soft materials require bulky support structures that compromise their minimalistic form. This brings us to another type of artificial muscle that is easy to make, reliable [20] and does not require a support structure: fluid powered muscles.

3.2 Fluid powered muscles for rehabilitation

Fluid powered muscles are lightweight and flexible actuators with muscle-like force, stroke and compliance [22]. They are flexible pressure vessels that contract when filled with fluid such as air or water. Although there are many variants of fluid powered muscles [23], the most commonly used in exoskeleton actuation is the McKibben pneumatic artificial muscle (PAM). It is usually made of a rubber tube sheathed in a helical braid of stiff fibres. The ends of the tube are sealed and clamped to the fibre braid by caps that also serve to connect the muscle to its load (Figure 3.2(a)). When pressurised, the tube expands radially, which causes

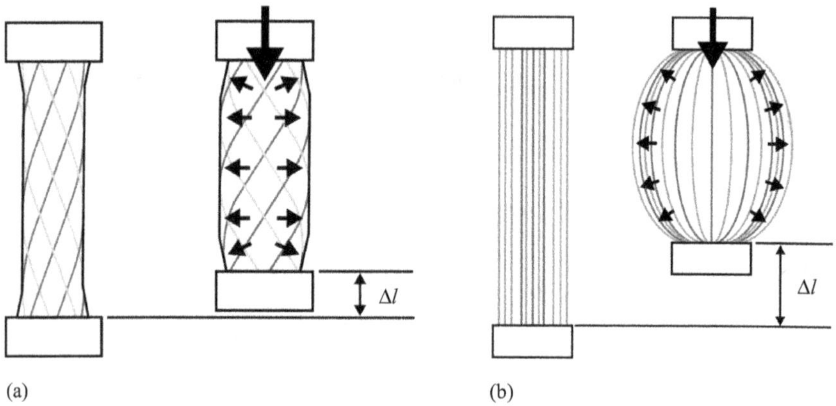

Figure 3.2 McKibben PAM (a) and PPAM (b) contract by Δl when inflated with a fluid. Fluid pressure is shown by arrows. The McKibben PAM is made of a rubber tube sheathed in a braid of stiff reinforcing fibres. The PPAM is made of an inelastic pleated membrane with reinforcing fibres running along the pleats valleys (pleat mountains are light grey and valleys with reinforcing fibres are dark grey)

the fibres in the braid to scissor, coupling the radial expansion to shortening of the tubular muscle. Another fluid powered muscle used in exoskeletons is the Daerden's pleated PAM (PPAM) [24,25]. As shown by Figure 3.2(b), it consists of a cylindrical membrane pleated about its circumference. Caps seal the membrane's ends and are connected to each other by stiff reinforcing fibres that run along the valleys of the PPAM's pleats. Inflating the PPAM causes it to form a sphere, transferring contractile forces to a load via its reinforcing fibres and end caps. The PPAM can contract more than the McKibben PAM and has lower static losses, but is bulkier and has a more complex assembly [26].

A fundamental limitation of the McKibben PAM and PPAM geometries is that the force they produce is proportional to their cross-sectional area. This means that to generate large forces they must either be too bulky for an exoskeleton or require many smaller actuators in parallel [27–29], which reduces their reliability and increases their losses and fabrication complexity. Mettam's Peano muscle [30] was proposed [31] to solve this trade-off. As shown in Figure 3.3, it is made of a series of side-by-side reinforced sealed tubes connected along their lengths. When the tubes are deflated, their initially flat cross-section tends towards a circle, shortening the width of the muscle's tubes so the muscle contracts. The advantage of this muscle geometry is that its force scales with its planform area, or the surface area of its deflated tubes. Hence, for a given Peano muscle length and thickness, its force can be increased by increasing the length of its tubes. The result is a fluid powered muscle with the biological flexibility, force, motion and compliance of McKibben PAMs and PPAMs [32] that can be made as slim and unobtrusive as materials and manufacturing techniques allow.

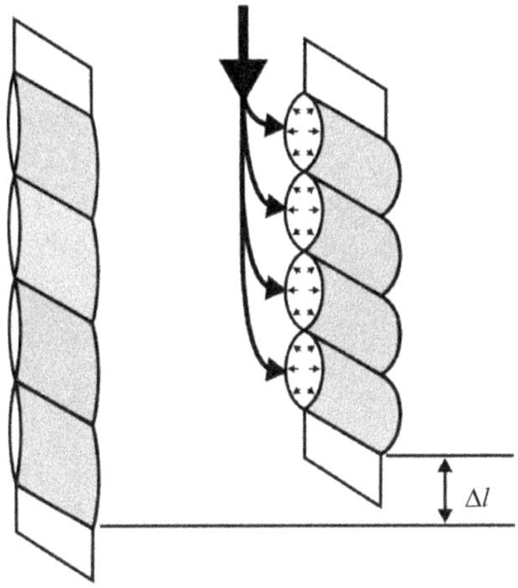

Figure 3.3 The Peano muscle contracts by Δl when inflated with a fluid. Fluid pressure is shown by arrows

3.3 Static modelling of the Peano muscle

Effective design and control of the Peano muscle requires a model that can predict its behaviour based on its physical properties. Only Mettam [1] and Niiyama *et al.* [33] have proposed a static force model for the Peano muscle. They used the virtual work method to derive a physics-based model, first Mettam for an ideal muscle, and then Niiyama *et al.* for a muscle with finite tensile stiffness. Mettam began with a Peano muscle constructed of n_t ideal tubes each generating a static force F_s when inflated to a pressure P (Figure 3.4(a)). Each muscle tube was assumed to be made of an infinitely stiff and infinitely flexible material with a deflated width w_t and length l_t. Note the terms stiff and flexible are used in the sense that such an ideal muscle tube has an infinite tensile stiffness and zero bending stiffness respectively. The normalised width of each tube is its contractile strain ε, which is measured in the units mm^{-1} or expressed as a percentage. It is related to the muscle tube's change in width Δw and deflated width by the following equation:

$$\varepsilon = \Delta w / w_t. \tag{3.1}$$

Mettam showed that an ideal muscle tube generates force according to the parametric equations (3.2) and (3.3). In these equations, the parametric variable θ is half of the included angle of the sector formed by the muscle tube's cross-section (Figure 3.4(b)).

$$F_s(P, \theta) = P w_t l_t \frac{\cos\theta}{\theta} \tag{3.2}$$

$$\varepsilon(\theta) = 1 - \frac{\sin\theta}{\theta} \tag{3.3}$$

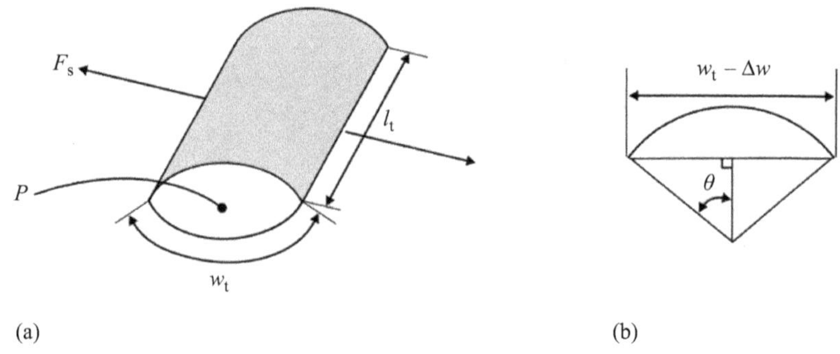

Figure 3.4 Parameters of an ideal Peano muscle tube. The tube has a deflated width w_t and length l_t (a). When inflated to a pressure P it generates a force F_s and contracts by a distance Δw. The included angle of the sector formed by half of the muscle tube is 2θ (b)

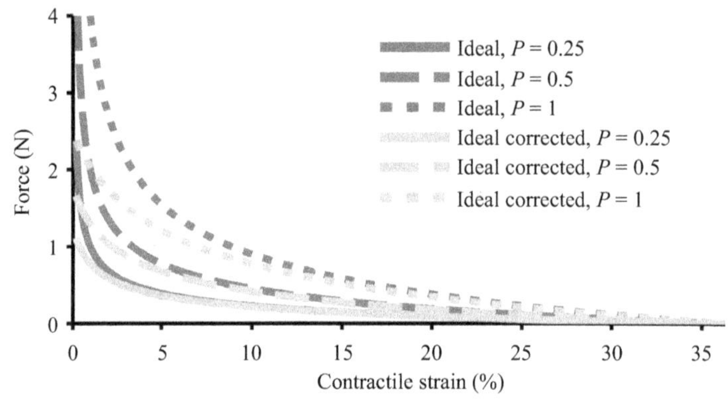

Figure 3.5 Mettam's ideal and Niiyama et al.'s ideal corrected Peano muscle models plotted for various pressures. The ideal corrected model includes the corrective coefficient $C_e = 0.025$, and in both models $w_t = 1$ and $l_t = 1$. The plot demonstrates how the corrective coefficient gives the static force model a finite blocking force

Plotting θ over the range $0 < \theta \leq \pi/2$, Figure 3.5 shows the ideal muscle tube produces a force proportional to pressure and planform area $w_t l_t$, with a free-strain of $(\pi - 2)/\pi$ or about 36%. The parametric model also predicts an infinite blocking force. Blocking force is the force produced at a given pressure when the muscle strain is zero. In contrast to the predicted behaviour of the ideal parametric model, a real muscle tube has a finite blocking force because it does not have an infinite tensile stiffness. Niiyama *et al.* dealt with this discrepancy by modifying the strain equation with a corrective coefficient C_e to get (3.4).

$$\varepsilon(P,\theta) = \left(1 - \frac{\sin\theta}{\theta}\right)\left(1 + \frac{\pi}{\pi - 2}C_eP\right) - C_eP. \tag{3.4}$$

The corrective coefficient has units of Pa^{-1} and is fitted to experimental data. Its effect on the blocking force of the parametric model is shown in Figure 3.5.

Niiyama *et al.*'s ideal corrected static model, building on the ideal model proposed by Mettam, relates the basic geometry properties of the Peano muscle to its force, strain and pressure. This makes it a useful starting point for understanding and predicting the Peano muscle's behaviour. However, it has a number of shortcomings. Although it empirically accounts for a finite blocking force, it does so through a corrective coefficient that has little physical meaning. The finite blocking force is caused by the muscle's tensile stiffness [33,34], so it is reasonable that the model should reflect this insight. Other notable characteristics of the Peano muscle are that its free-strain (maximum, unloaded contractile strain) varies with pressure, that the fluid channels interconnecting the muscle tubes reduce its force, that distortion of the muscle tube ends reduces its force, and that it acts as a spring when stretched in its deflated state [33–35]. These are the additional effects addressed by the MECHALP static model.

3.4 The MECHALP static model

The MECHALP static model is a completely new modelling tool we invented to overcome some of the limitations of Mettam and Niiyama *et al.*'s Peano muscle models. It aims to meaningfully model a Peano muscle's tensile stiffness and account for the Peano muscle tube material's non-zero bending stiffness. It also aims to model force reduction due to flow channels integrated in the muscle tubes. The MECHALP static model captures these effects through the four element approximation in Figure 3.6. Each element captures a dominant characteristic of the muscle's static force behaviour. The contractile element captures its ideal force generation. This force is reduced by the series and parallel stiffness elements that represent the Peano muscle tubes' tensile and bending stiffnesses. Finally, the extension element represents force reduction due to flow channels. Let us now examine how these work and relate to the physical properties of a Peano muscle.

The contractile element approximates the force generated by an ideal Peano muscle tube. An ideal tube that is infinitely stiff and flexible generates an infinite force in its deflated state that decreases to zero when it reaches a contractile strain of about 36%. Here this behaviour is approximated by a piston acting on a linkage with arms of length l_a. In the piston's rest position, with the linkage arms horizontal, it initially generates an infinite force against a load restraining the arms' motion. If l_a is sized correctly with respect to w_t, the linkage arms will reach their vertical zero force position when they have travelled a horizontal displacement equivalent to the muscle tube contracting by a strain of 36%. The displacement

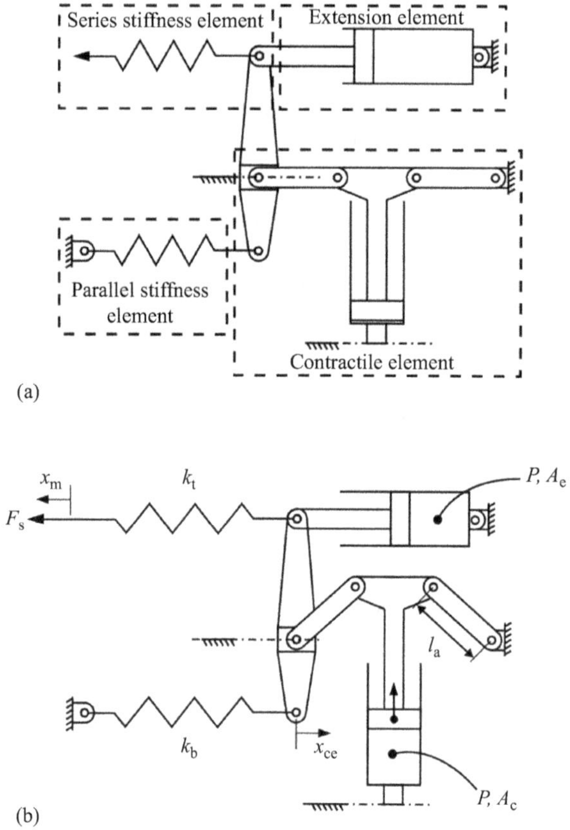

(a)

(b)

Figure 3.6 The MECHALP static model captures the behaviour of the Peano muscle as a force balance of the four mechanical lumped parameter elements in their rest (a) and partially actuated state (b). The contractile element approximates the force generation F_{ce} of an ideal Peano muscle tube. The extension element models the force reduction F_{ee} due to flow channels integrated in the muscle tubes. The series stiffness element represents the tensile stiffness of the deflated Peano muscle k_t, and the parallel stiffness, the net bending stiffness of its tubes k_b (adapted from Figure 4 in [31])

of the contractile element from its rest position is x_{ce} and the area of the piston A_c. The force generated by this element is then as in (3.5).

$$F_{ce} = PA_c \frac{l_a - (x_{ce}/2)}{\sqrt{l_a^2 - (l_a - (x_{ce}/2))^2}} \tag{3.5}$$

where the linkage arm length

$$l_a = \frac{\pi - 2}{2\pi} w_t. \tag{3.6}$$

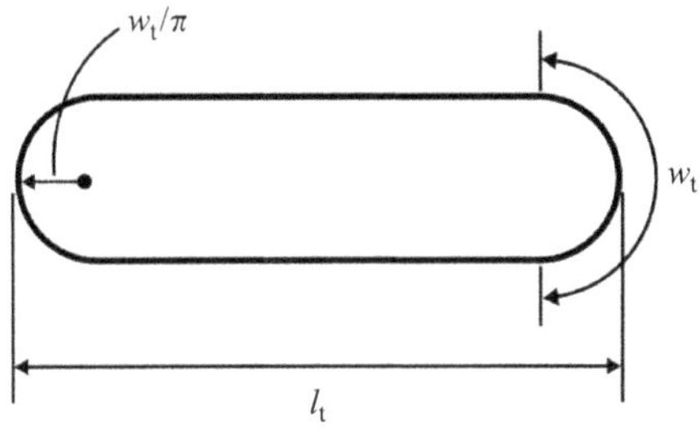

Figure 3.7 A cross-section of a fully inflated Peano muscle tube assuming hemispherical end tube distortion. With this assumption we can calculate an estimate of the tube length utilisation α. The effective length of the tube is reduced by the two tube end radii to $l_t - (2w_t/\pi)$

Noting that as in Mettam's ideal force model in (3.3) force is also proportional to area, the piston area is defined in (3.7).

$$A_c = \gamma(\alpha w_t l_t) \tag{3.7}$$

In this equation, α is the tube length utilisation, the proportion of the tube length generating force and γ is the approximation constant. In an ideal tube $\alpha = 1$, but in a real tube $\alpha \leq 1$ because of end tube distortion [34,35]. In practice, α changes as the tube inflates, but we can calculate a worst case value of α by assuming the tube ends distort to form hemispheres (see Figure 3.7), and hence

$$\alpha = 1 - \frac{2w_t}{\pi l_t}. \tag{3.8}$$

Of course, the tube length utilisation will need to be sized differently if the muscle tubes have channels running along their ends.

The approximation constant fits the force generation profile of the contractile element to approximate Mettam's ideal force equation. It does so independently of muscle pressure and geometry over the range $0.01 < \varepsilon \leq (\pi - 2)/\pi$. We ignore very low strains because the series stiffness element dominates the equation's force output in this region. Figure 3.8 shows a plot of the normalised root mean square error (NRMSE) of the contractile element over the desired strain range for different γ values. The optimal γ value to two decimal places is 0.91.

Next is the extension element, which approximates the force acting over the muscle's flow channels to extend the muscle, as in (3.9).

$$F_{ee} = PA_e. \tag{3.9}$$

For example, in Figure 3.9 the extension area is $h_c l_t$. In other muscles it may vary with inflation pressure or be zero.

The series stiffness k_t is the tensile stiffness of the muscle when it is deflated. The other material property in the MECHALP model is k_b, the parallel bending stiffness of the muscle. Although k_b does not correspond to a quantity that can be

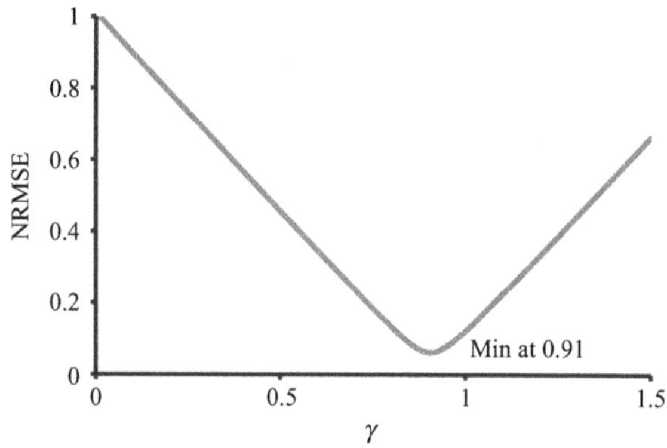

Figure 3.8 *The NRMSE of the MECHALP static model's contractile element compared to Mettam's ideal parametric model for various values of the approximation constant γ. The optimal value of γ is 0.91, when its NRMSE is at its minimum. This optimal value is independent of pressure and muscle geometry*

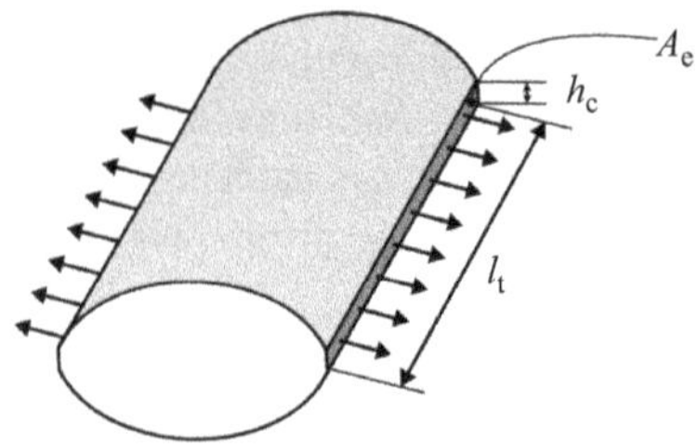

Figure 3.9 *A simple extension element area. In this case, the flow channel is along the length of the muscle tube side and has an area $A_e = h_c l_t$ acting to extend the muscle tube when it is pressurised*

directly measured from a Peano muscle, it does model the pressure dependence of the Peano muscle's free-strain. In addition, it intuitively captures the idea that the more a muscle tube inflates, the more difficult it becomes to inflate because of its increased curvature and the non-zero bending stiffness of the tube material.

Finally, we can build the complete MECHALP static model by recognising the kinematic relation between muscle tube displacement x_{m}, as measured from its deflated width, and the contractile element displacement as

$$x_{\mathrm{ce}} = F_{\mathrm{s}}/k_{\mathrm{t}} - x_{\mathrm{m}}. \tag{3.10}$$

Then we write out the complete force balance as

$$F_{\mathrm{ce}} - F_{\mathrm{ee}} - k_{\mathrm{b}}x_{\mathrm{ce}} - F_{\mathrm{s}} = 0. \tag{3.11}$$

which expands to

$$P\left(0.91aw_t l_t \frac{l_a - (F_s/k_t - x_m)/2}{\sqrt{l_a^2 - (l_a - (F_s/k_t - x_m)/2)^2}} - A_e\right)$$
$$-k_b(F_s/k_t - x_m) - F_s = 0. \tag{3.12}$$

Equation (3.12) can be rearranged to (3.13), which is suitable to be solved numerically to find F_s, noting that $x_m = -\varepsilon w_t$. In this chapter, MATLAB's (R2012b, MathWorks, MA) Levenberg–Marquardt numerical solver was used with the MECHALP static model.

$$P(0.91aw_t l_t(l_a - (F_s/k_t - x_m)/2))$$
$$-\sqrt{l_a^2 - (l_a - (F_s/k_t - x_m)/2)^2}(PA_e - k_b x_m + (1 + (k_b/k_t))F_s) = 0 \tag{3.13}$$

In summary, the MECHALP static model conceptually improves on Niiyama *et al.*'s model by modelling the channel extension force; a finite blocking force through a tensile stiffness lumped parameter and a pressure-dependent free-strain through a bending stiffness lumped parameter. It also empirically accounts for muscle tube end distortion. Given an approximate idea of a Peano muscle's design, material and hence the stiffness lumped parameters, it can be used to design the geometry or predict the force of that muscle. This sounds nice in theory, but is it supported by practice? Next, we validate the accuracy of the MECHALP static model against Niiyama *et al.*'s model.

3.4.1 Model validation method

A Peano muscle prototype with the geometry parameters in Table 3.2 was tested to obtain data for validation of the MECHALP and Niiyama *et al.*'s static models. As this was an early prototype, it featured rigid metal components as well as rubberised fabric. These metal components were used to constrain the inflated shape of the Peano muscle, maximising its contraction. However, in the next chapter a completely soft, all rubber and fabric Peano muscle design is presented. This design replaces the metal components with stitching and fabric reinforced rubber. Hence, it uses similar materials to those in everyday clothing, making it ideal for embedding into soft and wearable rehabilitation devices. The muscle tested for MECHALP's validation, shown in Figure 3.10, was placed in a tensile testing rig (described in [34]), pressurised and quasi statically unloaded to its free-strain and loaded back to its starting length. This was done at pressures of 0, 80, 200 and 500 kPa. During the experiments the muscle's force and strain was measured, yielding separate unloading and loading force–strain curves due to the muscle's hysteresis.

After the experiments, the loading and unloading curves for a given pressure experiment were averaged for fitting of the models' empirical parameters and validation of the models' accuracy. In the MECHALP model, the muscle's stiffness in the form of $k_t = ax + b$ was found from the ratio of the Peano muscle's force to

Table 3.2 Geometry and material parameters of the Peano muscle used for validation of the MECHALP static model

Geometry parameters		Material parameters
n_t	4	$k_t = 1.5 \times 10^8(x_m + x_{ce}) + 8 \times 10^4$
w_t	0.01725 m	$= \frac{1}{2}\left(8 \times 10^4 + \sqrt{6.4 \times 10^9 + 6 \times 10^8 F_s}\right)$
l_t	0.0465 m	
a	0.809	
h_c	0.002 m	$k_b = 1 \times 10^{15} x_{ce}{}^4$
A_c	$h_c l_t$ m^2	

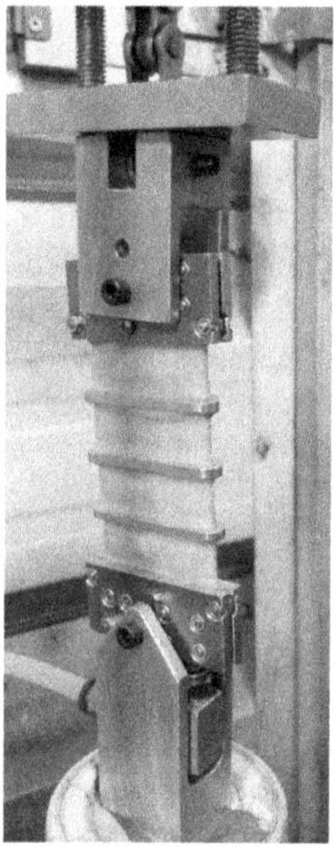

Figure 3.10 The four-tube Peano muscle used to validate the MECHALP static model

strain in the 0 kPa test. The tensile and bending stiffnesses are listed in Table 3.2. The bending stiffness was found as a function of x_{ce}, which is εw_t when the Peano muscle's force is zero. We took the free-strains from the 0, 80 and 500 kPa experiments and used (3.12) with F_s set to zero to calculate k_b at each of these pressures. From these k_b values and the corresponding x_{ce} values we fitted a curve of the form of $k_b(x_{ce}) = ax_{ce}{}^4$.

In Niiyama *et al.*'s model, we fitted C_e to the value of 1.0394×10^{-6} Pa^{-1} by minimising the NRMSE between its prediction and the 80 and 500 kPa curves. The 0 kPa curve was not used because this model predicts zero force when pressure is zero.

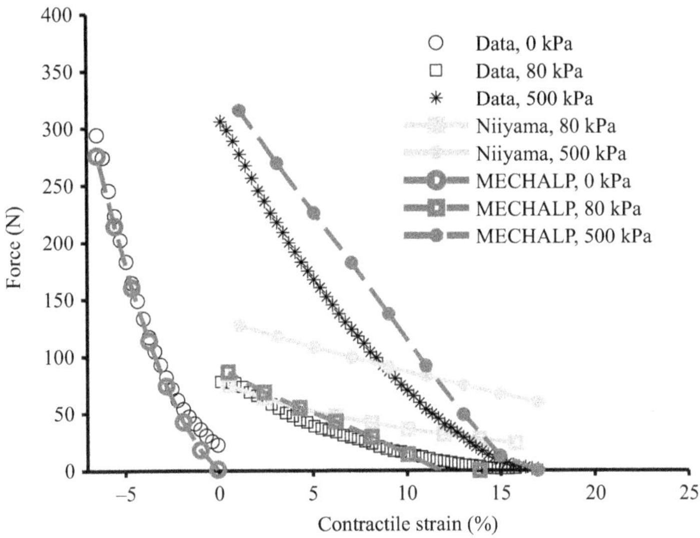

Figure 3.11 *Niiyama et al.'s ideal model (with corrective coefficient) and the MECHALP static model plotted against force–strain data from a Peano muscle. The data was the average of the loading and unloading force–strain curves of different pressure experiments. The data shown was used to fit the empirical parameters in both models: the corrective coefficient in Niiyama et al.'s model, and the series and parallel stiffness elements in the MECHALP static model*

The 200 kPa curve was not used to fit either model because it was used for their validation. Validation involved comparing the models prediction of the 200 kPa curve qualitatively and quantitatively with the NRMSE.

3.4.2 Model validation results and discussion

The fit of the MECHALP static model to the 0, 80 and 500 kPa Peano muscle data in Figure 3.11 shows the MECHALP model predicts the 0 kPa curve well, slightly overestimates blocking force and underestimates free-strain with decreasing pressure. It also overestimates force at moderate strains, and more so at higher pressures. In comparison, Niiyama *et al.*'s model cannot model the 0 kPa curve, estimates blocking force well at 80 kPa, but underestimates it severely as pressure increases to 500 kPa. Niiyama *et al.*'s model overestimates free-strain at all pressures, predicting an ideal free-strain of 36% compared to the Peano muscle's maximum free-strain of about 17%.

Qualitatively, Figure 3.12 shows the MECHALP static model and Niiyama *et al.*'s model exhibited the same prediction trends for the 200 kPa validation data as observed in the 0, 80 and 500 kPa fitting data (Figure 3.11). The MECHALP static model was more accurate, with a lower NRMSE of 9.3% compared to 19.4%

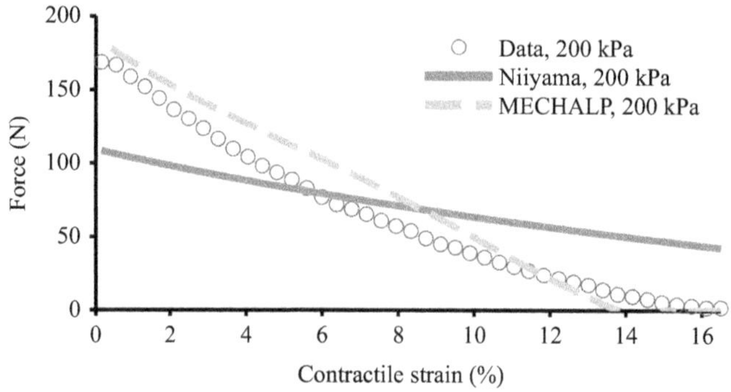

Figure 3.12 Niiyama et al.'s ideal model (with corrective coefficient) and the MECHALP static model plotted against force–strain data from a Peano muscle. The data was the average of the loading and unloading force–strain curves from a tensile test experiment. This data was not used to fit the models' parameters and was used to evaluate their accuracy

of Niiyama *et al.*'s model. As expected from the trends in the fitting data, the MECHALP model predicted blocking force well, slightly overestimated force at moderate strains and underestimated free-strain. Niiyama *et al.*'s model underestimated blocking force and overestimated free-strain.

The MECHALP static model improved on the accuracy of Niiyama *et al.*'s model by accounting for the non-ideal nature of the Peano muscle's material properties. Most notably, Niiyama *et al.*'s model assumes a Peano muscle's tubes have a zero bending stiffness. This means it predicts a free-strain of approximately 36% for all non-zero inflation pressures. In reality, the Peano muscle tested in this chapter had a maximum free-strain of 17% because of its significant bending stiffness. As Niiyama *et al.*'s model consistently underestimated free-strain over all pressures, the optimal value of its corrective coefficient did not result in a satisfactory fit of the model to the behaviour of the Peano muscle.

Although Niiyama *et al.*'s model could not accurately predict blocking force at higher pressures or free-strain, the MECHALP static model could through its inclusion of the empirically determined tensile and bending stiffnesses. Even if these stiffnesses are unknown, the ideal contractile unit of the MECHALP model (in (3.5)), is an improvement over the parametric equations of Mettam's ideal model ((3.2) and (3.3)) because (3.5) can be explicitly calculated and includes the effect of end tube distortion. Equation (3.5) can also be extended to include the extension element force F_{ee} without compromising its explicit form. The reduction in force by F_{ee} due to the Peano muscle's flow channels can be significant, and was estimated at 46.5 N at 500 kPa. Evidently, this contributed to the model's accuracy. A further advantage of the MECHALP model is its prediction of the elastic nature of the Peano muscle when it is unpressurised. It does this through the finite tensile stiffness k_t. However, care must be taken in the measurement and fitting of k_t from the muscle's 0 kPa force–strain curve because it significantly effects the force predicted by the MECHALP model at non-zero pressures. This may be why, in the experiments presented here, the MECHALP model overestimated force at moderate strains and moderate to high pressures. Care also has to be taken in estimating the bending stiffness. Here, free-strain only increased a small amount when the pressure changed from 80 to 500 kPa. The corresponding sharp change in k_b was difficult to capture with the proposed fourth-order polynomial and may be better predicted by a higher order polynomial or a linear piecewise model.

In spite of these limitations, the MECHALP static model captured the overall shape and magnitude of the Peano muscle's force generation behaviour. Hence, it could be used to design and simulate muscles of a certain geometry and material. If further precision is required, such as in particular control applications, the model should be combined with a force element that models the Peano muscle's significant hysteresis [33,34]. This could be done with the Preisach or virgin curve hysteresis models proposed by Van Damme *et al.* [36] and Vo-Minh *et al.* [37].

3.5 Summary

This chapter introduced the Peano muscle, an actuator invented by Mettam that is a soft and slim fluid powered actuator for rehabilitation devices such as exoskeletons. It also presented and validated the MECHALP static model for predicting the Peano muscle's force. The MECHALP model is a completely new physics-based lumped parameter model that improves on existing Peano muscle models by predicting a finite blocking force via the muscle's tensile stiffness; a pressure dependent free-strain through the bending stiffness parameter; and a reduction in muscle force due to flow channel area and end tube distortion. Compared to Niiyama *et al.*'s Peano muscle model's NRMSE of 19.4%, it had an NRMSE of 9.3%. This shows the additional factors in the MECHALP static model, and its reliance on material properties in particular, makes it a more accurate and realistic tool for understanding, designing and controlling Peano muscles. Also important to controlling the Peano muscle in rehabilitation applications is its ability to sense and assess its environment. The next chapter will tackle the challenge of enabling the Peano muscle with this ability, and in such a way that does not compromise its human friendly form.

References

[1] Mettam AR. Inflatable servo actuators, Ministry of Aviation, Aeronautical Research Council, England. <http://naca.central.cranfield.ac.uk/reports/arc/cp/0671.pdf>; 1964 [Accessed May 2017]

[2] Bütefisch C, Hummelsheim H, Denzler P, Mauritz K. Repetitive training of isolated movements improves the outcome of motor rehabilitation of the centrally paretic hand. J Neurol Sci. 1995;130(1):59–68.

[3] Kwakkel G, Kollen BJ, Krebs HI. Effects of robot-assisted therapy on upper limb recovery after stroke: a systematic review. Neurorehabil Neural Repair. 2008;22(2):111–21.

[4] Bayona NA, Bitensky J, Salter K, Teasell R. The role of task-specific training in rehabilitation therapies. Top Stroke Rehabil. 2005;12(3):58–65.

[5] Klamroth-Marganska V, Blanco J, Campen K, *et al.* Three-dimensional, task-specific robot therapy of the arm after stroke: a multicentre, parallel-group randomised trial. Lancet Neurol. 2014;13(2):159–66.

[6] Phillips B, Zhao H. Predictors of assistive technology abandonment. Assist Technol. 1993;5(1):36–45.

[7] Wessels R, Dijcks B, Soede M, Gelderblom GJ, De Witte L. Non-use of provided assistive technology devices, a literature overview. Technol Disabil. 2003;15(4):231–38.

[8] Batavia AI, Hammer GS. Toward the development of consumer-based criteria for the evaluation of assistive devices. J Rehabil Res Dev. 1990;27(4): 425–36.

[9] Lane JP, Usiak D, Moffat JA, Langton A. Consumer criteria for assistive devices: operationalizing generic criteria for specific ABLEDATA categories. Proceedings of the RESNA 1996 annual conference. RESNA: Salt Lake City, UT; 1996. p. 146–8.

[10] Veale AJ, Xie SQ. Towards compliant and wearable robotic orthoses: a review of current and emerging actuator technologies. Med Eng Phys. 2016;38:317–25.

[11] Kleinjan JG, Dunning AG, Herder JL. Design of a compact actuated compliant elbow joint. Int J Struct Stabil Dyn. 2014;14(8):1–16.

[12] Brown-Triolo DL, Roach MJ, Nelson K, Triolo RJ. Consumer perspectives on mobility: implications for neuroprosthesis design. J Rehabil Res Dev. 2002;39(6):659–69.

[13] Polygerinos P, Wang Z, Galloway KC, Wood RJ, Walsh CJ. Soft robotic glove for combined assistance and at-home rehabilitation. Robot Auton Sys. 2014;1:1–9.

[14] Polygerinos P, Galloway KC, Savage E, Herman M, O'Donnell K, Walsh CJ. Soft robotic glove for hand rehabilitation and task specific training. IEEE international conference on robotics and automation. IEEE: Seattle, WA. 2015. p. 2913–9.

[15] Nycz CJ, Bützer T, Lambercy O, Arata J, Fischer GS, Gassert R. Design and characterization of a lightweight and fully portable remote actuation system for use with a hand exoskeleton. IEEE Robot Autom Lett. 2016; 1(2):976–83.

[16] Sugar TG, He J, Koeneman EJ, *et al.* Design and control of RUPERT: a device for robotic upper extremity repetitive therapy. IEEE Trans Neural Sys Rehabil Eng. 2007;15(3):336–46.

[17] Kovacs G, Düring L, Michel S, Terrasi G. Stacked dielectric elastomer actuator for tensile force transmission. Sens Actuators A Phys. 2009;155(2): 299–307.

[18] Haines CS, Lima MD, Li N, *et al.* Artificial muscles from fishing line and sewing thread. Science 2014;343(6173):868–72.
[19] Li Y, Hashimoto M. Design and prototyping of a novel lightweight walking assist wear using PVC gel soft actuators. Sens Actuators A Phys. 2016; 239:26–44.
[20] Woods BKS, Gentry MF, Kothera CS, Wereley NM. Fatigue life testing of swaged pneumatic artificial muscles as actuators for aerospace applications. J Intel Mat Sys Struct. 2012;23(3):327–43.
[21] User:Hotdogcartman Cutaway Welded Hyco Cylinder, <https://en.wikipedia.org/wiki/File:Cutawayweldedcylinder544x123.jpg>; 2017 [Accessed May 2017].
[22] Chou C, Hannaford B. Measurement and modeling of McKibben pneumatic artificial muscles. IEEE Transac Robot Autom. 1996;12(1):90–102.
[23] Daerden F, Lefeber D. Pneumatic artificial muscles: actuators for robotics and automation. Eur J Mech Environ Eng. 2002;47(1):11–21.
[24] Daerden F. Conception and realization of pleated pneumatic artificial muscles and their use as compliant actuation elements [PhD thesis]. Brussels, Belgium: Vrije Universiteit Brussel; 1999.
[25] Beyl P, Van Damme M, Van Ham R, Vanderborght B, Lefeber D. Pleated pneumatic artificial muscle-based actuator system as a torque source for compliant lower limb exoskeletons. IEEE/ASME Trans Mechatronics. 2014;19(3):1046–56.
[26] Villegas D, Van Damme M, Vanderborght B, Beyl P, Lefeber D. Third-generation pleated pneumatic artificial muscles for robotic applications: development and comparison with McKibben muscle. Advan Robot. 2012;26(11–12):1205–27.
[27] Peel LD, Molina EJ, Baur JW, Justice RS. Characterization and application of shape-changing panels with embedded rubber muscle actuators. Smart Mat Struct. 2013;22(9):1–11.
[28] Kurumaya S, Suzumori K, Nabae H, Wakimoto S. Musculoskeletal lower-limb robot driven by multifilament muscles. Robomech J. 2016;3:1–15.
[29] DeLaHunt SA, Pillsbury TE, Wereley NM. Variable recruitment in bundles of miniature pneumatic artificial muscles. Bioinspir Biomim. 2016;11(5):1–16.
[30] Sanan S, Lynn PS, Griffith ST. Pneumatic torsional actuators for inflatable robots. J Mech Robot. 2014;6(3):1–7.
[31] Veale AJ, Anderson IA, Xie SQ. The smart peano fluidic muscle: a low profile flexible orthosis actuator that feels pain. SPIE smart structures and materials/NDE. International Society for Optics and Photonics: San Diego, CA. 2015. p. 94351V-1–11.
[32] Veale AJ, Xie SQ, Anderson IA. Modeling the peano fluidic muscle and the effects of its material properties on its static and dynamic behavior. Smart Mater Struct. 2016;25(6):1–16.
[33] Niiyama R, Rus D, Kim S. Pouch motors: printable/inflatable soft actuators for robotics. IEEE international conference on robotics and automation. IEEE: Hong Kong; 2014. p. 6332–37.

[34] Veale AJ, Xie SQ, Anderson IA. Characterizing the peano fluidic muscle and the effects of its geometry properties on its behavior. Smart Mat Struct. 2016;25(6):1–14.
[35] Chang SY, Takashima K, Nishikawa S, *et al.* Design of small-size pouch motors for rat gait rehabilitation device. Proceedings of the annual international conference of the IEEE engineering in medicine and biology society. IEEE: Milan, Italy; 2015. p. 4578–81.
[36] Van Damme M, Beyl P, Vanderborght B, *et al.* Modeling hysteresis in pleated pneumatic artificial muscles. IEEE international conference on robotics, automation and mechatronics. IEEE: Chengdu, China; 2008. p. 471–6.
[37] Vo-Minh T, Tjahjowidodo T, Ramon H, Van Brussel H. A new approach to modeling hysteresis in a pneumatic artificial muscle using the maxwell-slip model. IEEE/ASME Trans Mechatronics. 2011;16(1):177–86.

Chapter 4
Design of the reactive Peano muscle

Current rehabilitation devices require many sensors to assess their user's physical ability, guide their user through precise movements and keep their user safe. In some rehabilitation applications, sensors can also be used to interpret the user's movement intention and maximise their involvement in the rehabilitation process. This improves the effectiveness of the rehabilitation. Unfortunately, these sensors add to rehabilitation devices' cost, complexity and bulk. In this chapter we present the design and characterisation of the reactive Peano muscle. Inspired by biological muscles' embedded sensors, the reactive Peano muscle measures its strain, pressure and force with novel dielectric elastomer (DE) sensors. These sensors are embedded into a Peano muscle in a manner that does not compromise its soft form or function. Thus, the reactive Peano muscle concept has the potential to not only actuate soft rehabilitation devices, but also to provide feedback on the physical ability and state of their users.

In this chapter we first explore how sensors are embedded into biological muscles and how researchers have mimicked this principle in various contractile fluid powered muscles. Next, we propose a method for sensing the physical state of the Peano muscle and describe how to fabricate these sensors and embed them into a Peano muscle. Finally, we characterise the resulting Peano muscle's actuation and sensing performance and demonstrate that embedded DE sensors do not compromise its capabilities as a soft actuator for rehabilitation.

4.1 Actuators that sense

Sensors in rehabilitation devices, such as exoskeletons, have different roles depending on the type of rehabilitation therapy. One way to classify rehabilitation exercises is based on the amount of effort provided by the person undergoing rehabilitation [1]. On the one hand, the person can put in no effort and allow themselves to be moved by external forces. This is passive rehabilitation. If, however, the person contributes effort to the rehabilitation movements, the therapy becomes active rehabilitation. In both types of rehabilitation, one role of an exoskeleton's sensors is to provide feedback for controlling the movement of the exoskeleton and its user [2]. As the exoskeleton moves its user, forces develop between the two. In some cases, sensors may be used to regulate these interaction forces [3]. Another use of force and movement measurements is to ensure the exoskeleton does not harm its user. If a joint is moved too far or too fast, or a large enough torque is applied to it, the exoskeleton can be shutdown [3–5]. This helps keep the user and people around them safe. A further use of sensing force and movement in an exoskeleton is to assess the physical ability of its wearer and hence quantitatively track their rehabilitation progress [6–8]. Exoskeleton impairment assessment is relevant to passive and active rehabilitation. In active rehabilitation, sensors may also be used to gauge the movement the exoskeleton's user wants to make. This allows the exoskeleton to track the voluntary movements of its user, as they try to complete a rehabilitation exercise, without getting in their way [3,5]. If the exoskeleton's user has trouble completing the desired movement, the exoskeleton can provide the minimum amount of assistance required to finish the rehabilitation exercise [9]. The advantage of this assistance-as-needed (AAN) approach is that it maximises the user's involvement in the rehabilitation process, which is beneficial for the therapy of people with stroke [10].

Evidently, sensors are important to the safety and effectiveness of rehabilitation devices, but how can their effect on the devices' affordability, portability and size be minimised? Every sensor that is added onto an exoskeleton's actuator increases its cost, complexity, size and weight. One place this problem has already been solved is in the design of biological actuators: muscles.

Biological muscles have proprioceptive organs embedded into their tissue that sense their physical state without compromising their form or function. Figure 4.1 shows that muscle contractile strain and motion are measured by spindle organs arranged throughout the muscle. As a muscle changes length, so do its spindle organs, generating electrical signals that are sent to the brain. Also sending information to the brain are a muscle's Golgi organs. Golgi organs are connected in series between a muscle's fibres and the tendons that connect them to bones. These organs measure muscle force. Together the spindle and Golgi organs provide feedback for intelligent control and pain sensing essential to accurate and safe muscle movements [11]. As the organs are small and soft they do not affect the size or performance of the muscle.

4.1.1 Prior art in embedded sensors for linear fluid powered muscles

Researchers have realised that embedding sensors directly into actuators has its advantages and have done so in many different ways. Here we focus on sensors embedded into linear contractile fluid powered muscles because these techniques are most relevant to the Peano muscle discussed in the previous chapter. Sensors in the literature have been used to measure fluid powered muscle strain, pressure and force, with varying impact on muscle performance and form. These sensors have relied on capacitive, resistive, piezoelectric, optical, ultrasonic, magnetic or inductive effects.

Goulbourne *et al.* [12,13] first suggested DE-based capacitive strain sensing of fluid powered muscles. DE sensors respond quickly and are soft, solid state and have good repeatability. Nakamoto *et al.* [14] validated the use of a DE strain sensor to

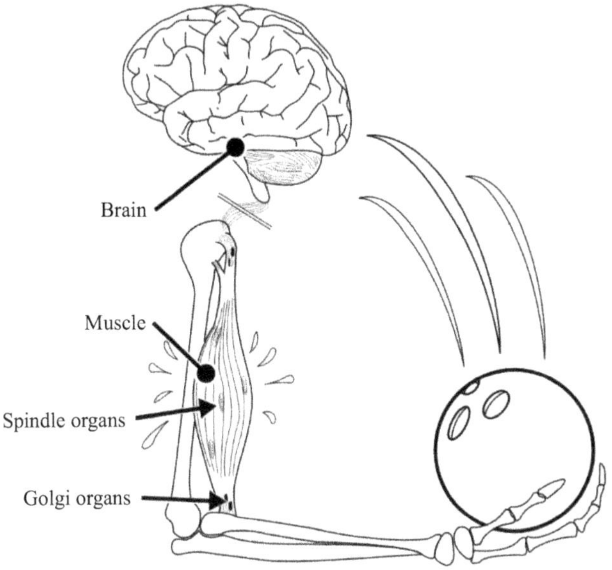

Figure 4.1 Biological muscles have natural sensors embedded into them that measure their motion and force. Muscle motion is measured by spindle organs coupled in parallel with a muscle's fibres. Muscle force is measured by Golgi organs connected in series with a muscle's fibres and its tendons. Both spindle and Golgi organs produce electrical signals that report the physical state of a muscle to the brain

measure the length of McKibben pneumatic artificial muscles (PAMs). Their sensor had an accuracy of 1.5 mm over a 60 mm stroke at a speed of 114.5 mm s^{-1}. However, the sensor was not an integral part of the muscle structure. Miron and Plante [15] did integrate their DE strain sensor into an extending-contracting PAM, and validated its accuracy at 0.14% over the PAM's length. Although these examples demonstrated the accuracy of a DE sensor, they did not show its versatility. Apart from strain, DE sensors also have the ability to measure pressures and forces, but this has not yet been done in a fluid powered muscle.

One method of making a resistive strain sensor is to coat a rubber substrate in a layer of conductive ink. Wakimoto *et al.* [16] made such a sensor for a PAM and found it to be very sensitive and flexible, but with a slow, viscoelastic response. Wakimoto *et al.* [17] also made a resistive pressure sensor by wrapping a conductive fibre into the braid of a McKibben PAM. As the PAM was pressurised, the conductive fibre was compressed between the PAM's bladder and other fibres in the braid, altering the conductive fibre's resistance. The sensing fibre was completely integrated into the PAM's structure, but had a low sensitivity and was specific to the PAM's geometry.

Another resistive sensor integrated into the walls of a PAM was Park and Wood's [18] resistive strain sensor. They first moulded helical microchannels into a PAM's rubber walls. Then they filled the channels with eutectic Gallium Indium (eGaln), a liquid conductor. Changes in the PAM's length altered the channels' dimensions, which corresponded to a highly linear and low hysteresis change in the eGaln's resistance. Park and Wood additionally proposed that extra eGaln micro-channels could be moulded into the PAM's wall to measure its force. Although the accuracy of this technique is promising, its disadvantages are that the moulded microchannels reduce the PAM's wall strength and if punctured, the eGaln will leak out and the sensor will stop working.

Yamamoto *et al.* [19] measured PAM strain with an electroded piezoelectric paste bonded to a urethane rubber strip. However, it had large hysteresis and some noise.

Akagi *et al.* [20] chose an optical sensing technique: photoreflectors were mounted inside a McKibben PAM and used to measure its inner diameter and hence estimate its length.

Shimooka *et al.* [21] placed ultrasonic transmitter and receivers inside opposing ends of a McKibben PAM. Both sensing methods were low cost, but reduced McKibben PAM flexibility.

Shin *et al.* [22] measured the angle of a magnet embedded into the outside of a McKibben PAM using a magnetic sensor mounted in the PAM's centre. By correlating the magnet's angle to the PAM's length, they estimated the PAM's strain from the magnetic sensor's output. They also measured the PAM's force with a miniature load cell attached to the end of the McKibben PAM. These sensing approaches used readily available hardware, but the magnetic sensing method presumed the PAM was straight, and the load cell was rigid and significantly increased the PAM's cost.

A good example of embedded force and strain sensing in a PAM is Felt and Remy's smart braid McKibben PAM [23,24]. They made their PAM's braid from insulated copper wire and measured its inductance and resistance to estimate the length and force of a McKibben PAM to 0.5 mm and 5 N resolution [23]. However, compared to standard PAM braid materials, copper wire is less flexible and more susceptible to fatigue. This technique is also not directly applicable to fluid powered muscles with other geometries.

From the literature, it can be seen that while some embedded sensing techniques have potential, there is not yet a definitive solution for the embedding of strain, pressure and force sensing capabilities into fluidic muscles. Of the techniques summarised, those that affected the physical form and behaviour of the PAM the least were those that integrated the sensor into the PAM's structure. These techniques required the sensing element to be made from similar materials to the PAM. For example, Felt and Remy [23,24] used the braid of the McKibben PAM to sense its force and length by substituting this normally passive structural element with a conductive braid that was used as a sensor. Similarly, in biological muscle the spindle and Golgi organs are made of comparable stiffness and flexibility materials to the adjacent muscle fibres. As such, these organs are directly integrated into the structure of the muscle rather than being 'bolted on.' We used the same principle to develop a completely soft and flexible Peano muscle with embedded strain, pressure and force sensors. This muscle is called the reactive Peano muscle because its sensors enable it to react to its environment. As the muscle was made from rubber and fabric, these too were the materials of choice for the sensors. Sensing techniques relevant to these materials are DE, resistive and piezoelectric sensors. DE sensors were selected because they do not have the large hysteresis of piezoelectric sensors, have a fast response compared to Wakimoto *et al.*'s [16] conductive ink resistive sensors and are solid state compared to Park and Wood's [18] liquid metal filled microchannel resistive sensors.

4.2 The reactive Peano muscle

Before describing the fabrication of the reactive Peano muscle, we explain how it works. The muscle functions as described in the previous chapter. It measures its strain, pressure and force with custom made capacitive DE sensors. The strain and pressure DE sensors operate in stretch mode and the force sensor in compression mode.

4.2.1 DE sensors

A DE sensor is a deformable capacitor. As shown in Figure 4.2(a), it is made from a DE or insulating rubber, sandwiched between stretchable electrodes. The DE sensor has a capacitance C_{DE} that depends on the insulating properties of its dielectric layer as described by the relative permittivity ε_r, the overlapping area of its electrodes A_{DE} and the thickness of its dielectric layer t_{DE}, as in equation (4.1).

$$C_{\mathrm{DE}} = \varepsilon_0 \varepsilon_r \frac{A_{\mathrm{DE}}}{t_{\mathrm{DE}}}, \tag{4.1}$$

where ε_0 is the permittivity of free space, $1/(36\pi \times 10^9)$, and ε_r is between two and five for commonly used dielectric rubbers [25,26]. Figure 4.2(b) shows compression

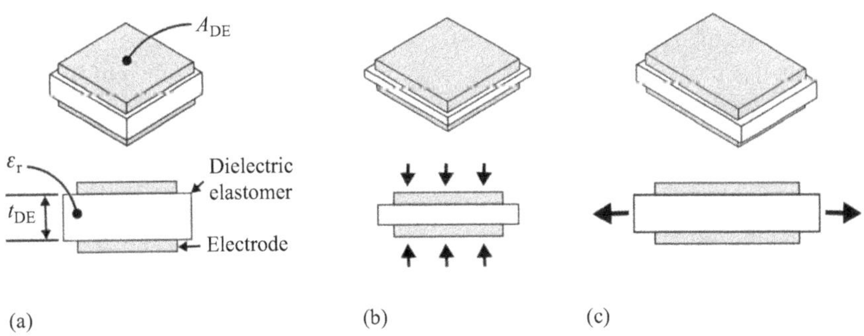

Figure 4.2 A DE sensor is a rubber capacitor with a dielectric elastomer of thickness t_{DE} sandwiched between stretchable electrodes with overlapping area A_{DE} and relative permittivity ε_r (a). If the sensor is used in compression mode (b), a reduction in its thickness is measured as an increase in its capacitance C_{DE}. It can also be used in stretch mode (c), where in-plane stretching of the sensor also increases C_{DE}

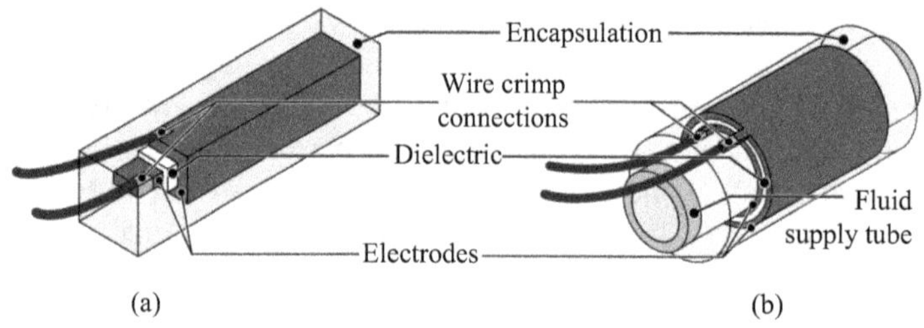

Figure 4.3 Construction of the DE strain (a) and pressure (b) sensors embedded into the reactive Peano muscle (adapted from Figures 1 and 3 in [27])

mode sensing where the DE sensor is squashed out-of-plane, directly decreasing t_{DE} and increasing A_{DE} by Poisson's effect. In stretch mode (Figure 4.2(c)), the DE sensor is stretched in-plane with its dielectric layer, directly increasing A_{DE} and decreasing t_{DE} by Poisson's effect. In both cases C_{DE} increases, allowing the length or thickness change in the DE sensor to be estimated by its measured capacitance.

After the technique of Goulbourne *et al.* [12] the reactive Peano muscle's strain sensor is a DE sensor like that in Figure 4.3(a) that is integrated along the length of a Peano muscle and operates in stretch mode. The sensor is initially pre-stretched when the muscle is deflated so that as the muscle contracts the sensor relaxes and its capacitance reduces. Notably, the sensor is made with conductive stretch fabric electrodes that increase the sensor's size and stiffness but make it easier to fabricate.

Both the pressure and force DE sensors were inspired by mechanisms found in nature. In our bodies, fluid pressure in the stomach and bladder is indicated by stretch sensitive mechanoreceptors embedded within their walls [28]. Our DE pressure sensor shown in Figure 4.3(b) uses a similar principle. It wraps a DE sensor around the stretchable tube supplying fluid to the Peano muscle. When the Peano muscle is pressurised the tube expands, stretching the DE sensor and increasing its capacitance by an amount that can be adjusted by selecting an appropriate tube stiffness and geometry. Since we first proposed this pressure sensing concept [29], Chavanne *et al.* [30] suggested a similar DE pressure sensor concept along with analytical and finite element models. Elsewhere, the closest sensing concept is the cuff-like mechanism Cong *et al.* [31] used with a rigid Microelectromechanical (MEMs) pressure sensor to measure the blood pressure of rodents. Hence, we believe we are the first to have used DE sensors to measure fluid pressure with this bioinspired technique.

The mechanism of the force sensor is also bioinspired. It is similar to the way Golgi tendon sensory nerves are compressed by stretched loops of collagen fibres in biological muscles. Figure 4.4 shows how the tensile load of the Peano muscle can be converted into a compressive force by placing a DE sensor within a tight-fitting fabric loop. The fabric loop is then placed in series between the muscle and its load. This way, significant increases in the sensor capacitance with increasing muscle force can be obtained without compromising the stiffness of the muscle–load coupling. Although we have used the basic DE sensor geometry of Figure 4.3(a), higher

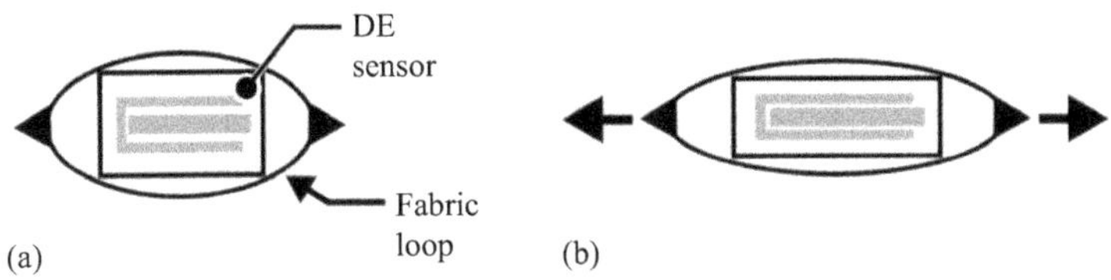

Figure 4.4 *A side cross-section of the DE force sensor. The sensor is made of a DE sensing element like that shown in Figure 4.3(a) that is inserted into a fabric loop (a). When a load is applied to either side of the fabric loop it compresses the DE sensor, increasing the sensor's capacitance (b). Note that deformation is exaggerated for clarity; in the prototype sensor the stiffness of the sensor element is relatively high so it does not reduce the reactive Peano muscle's tensile stiffness by too much*

sensitivity DE sensors for measuring compressive forces have been made with profiled electrodes, microscale patterned dielectrics and foam dielectrics by Böse *et al.* [32], Mannsfeld *et al.* [33] and Vandeparre *et al.* [34], respectively. The disadvantage of these sensors is the specialised fabrication techniques they require. Now we have seen how the reactive Peano muscle and its sensors work, we look at how they are fabricated.

4.3 Fabrication of the reactive Peano muscle

The reactive Peano muscle and its sensors are fabricated using sheets of composite materials built up in a layerwise fashion. The layer-based fabrication technique enables the muscles to be simply made and scaled and lends to automated processes. Composite materials allow for the advantages of different materials to be combined into a monolithic structure. For example, in the muscles, impregnating a fabric with a rubber yields a flexible, soft, impermeable and stiff material. The use of composites in the DE sensors creates soft, stretchable and reliable devices that are readily embedded into the structure of the Peano muscle.

As shown by the three-dimensional (3D) cross-section in Figure 4.5, the muscle is made of two triple-layer sheets of a woven fabric and rubber. These sheets are connected by rubber seam blocks that go around the periphery of the muscle and separate it into tubes. The seam blocks form a passage for fluid to flow through the muscle and seal the fluid passage from stitching that connects the top and bottom sheets. As shown earlier in Figure 4.3, sensors in the muscle are made from layers of insulating rubber sandwiched between fabric electrodes. Wires are crimped onto the electrodes and the whole assembly is encapsulated in a rubber block. The stiffness of both the muscle and sensor can be altered significantly depending on the orientation of the fabric weave. For example, orienting the textile fibres at an angle to the muscle tube's longitudinal axis, such as the 45° weave in Figure 4.5, results in a stretchy type of Peano muscle called the slanted weave (SW)

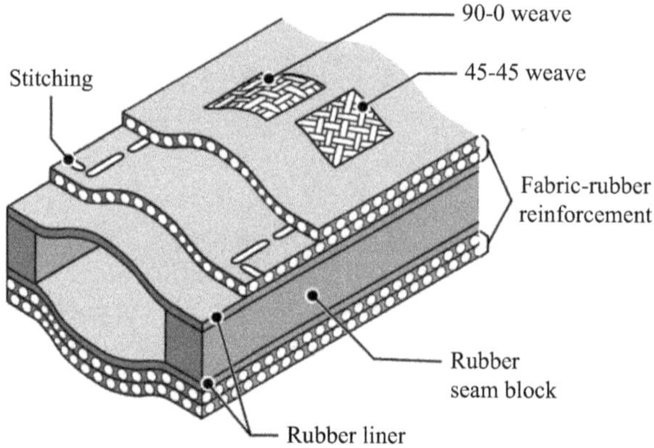

Figure 4.5 A 3D cross-section of one of the reactive Peano muscle's tubes. The sides of the muscle's tubes are formed by rubber seam blocks. The tops of the muscle's tubes are sealed with a triple-layer composite of an internal rubber liner and two sheets of rubberised fabric. The assembly is bonded together with rubber and stitching. Depending on the orientation of the reinforcing fabric weave the Peano muscle can be made as a stiff (90-0 weave) Peano muscle or a stretchable (45-45 weave) SW Peano muscle. Adapted from [35]. © IOP Publishing. Reproduced with permission. All rights reserved

Peano muscle. More on the differences in behaviour between stretchable and unstretchable Peano muscles can be found in [35].

The completely soft reactive Peano muscle prototype with embedded strain, pressure and force sensors is shown in Figure 4.6. The reactive Peano muscle's fabrication process is summarised by the sequence of images in Figures 4.7 and 4.8. First, the sensors are fabricated, and then the muscle, with the sensors embedded during the process. The strain and force sensors are identical, with a double layer dielectric, whereas the pressure sensor has a single layer dielectric wrapped around a silicone tube.

Fabrication of the DE sensors involves the steps outlined in Figure 4.7. Electrodes are cut from a conductive stretch fabric (Less EMF Inc., NY) with tabs for crimping wires onto (a). The tabs should be aligned in the least stretchy direction of the fabric for maximum connection robustness. Although the fabric electrodes are thick (0.55 mm) compared to the commonly used carbon black and silicone electrodes, they have the advantages of robustness, a low series resistance (less than 100 Ω), being easier to work with and being able to be crimped to a wire. Next, miniature crimps (0500798000, Molex Inc., Lisle, IL) with pre-soldered wires are crimped to the electrode tabs (b). The sensors have a 0.1 mm thick silicone (PlatSil Gel-10, Polytek Development Corp., Easton, PA) dielectric cast with an adjustable doctor blade. Platsil Gel-10 is used throughout the sensor fabrication as it is a soft silicone (Shore 10 A) that minimises the sensor stiffness and hence

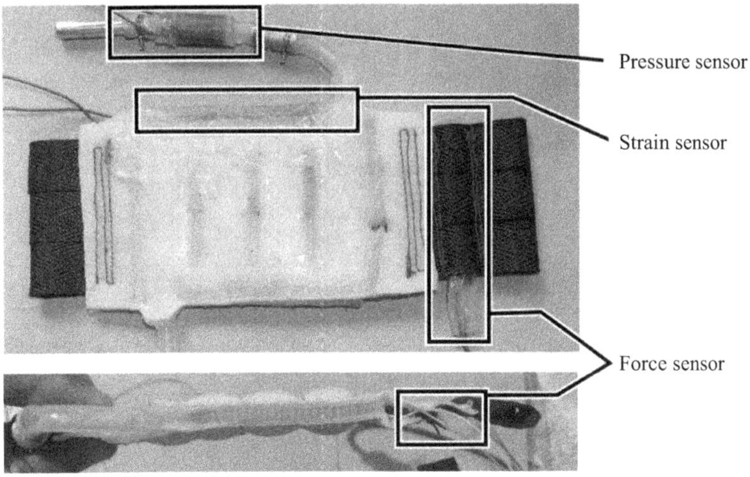

Figure 4.6 *Top and side views of the reactive Peano muscle prototype. Its DE sensors can be seen with the pressure sensor embedded into its fluid supply tube, its strain sensor along its side and its force sensor in the mounting straps that connect the muscle to its load (top view adapted version of Figure 5(b) in [27])*

influence on the characteristics of the muscle it is embedded into. It is also used in the muscle for its fast curing time and flexibility.

In the strain and force sensors, the dielectric is wrapped around the inner electrode and the outer electrode around the dielectric, as shown in (c). These sensors use Platsil Gel-10 silicone to adhere these layers with an insulating 0.3 mm thick silicone block between the outer electrode crimp and dielectric.

A 6 mm outside diameter (OD), 4 mm inside diameter (ID) silicone tube forms the base of the pressure sensor. Around it the inner electrode is wrapped and cured, then the dielectric and finally the outer electrode (c). A stiffer silicone (RS 692–542, RS Components Ltd., Northants, UK) was used to adhere the pressure sensor electrode and dielectric layers for its better adhesion to the relatively stiff tube. Finally, the strain or force sensing layer assembly is encapsulated in Platsil Gel-10 silicone by casting it in a foam sheet (d). After casting, the foam is broken away and the silicone trimmed to size. The foam has a cut-out for the sensor and slits for its wires. The top and bottom of the encapsulation are formed by films of Platsil Gel-10 silicone. The pressure sensor is encapsulated by wrapping it in a 0.25 mm thick film of Platsil Gel-10 with the dimensions shown, and curing it in place with RS 692–542 silicone (d). The two sensor geometries are shown in 3D in Figure 4.3.

Muscle fabrication presumes strain, force and pressure sensors have already been fabricated and follows the sequence in Figure 4.8. First, a plain woven fabric is rubberised with Platsil Gel-10 silicone (a), forming the muscle membrane. This involves impregnating the fabric with the silicone, allowing it to cure and then casting a 0.3 mm thick Platsil Gel-10 silicone coating on top. It must be ensured

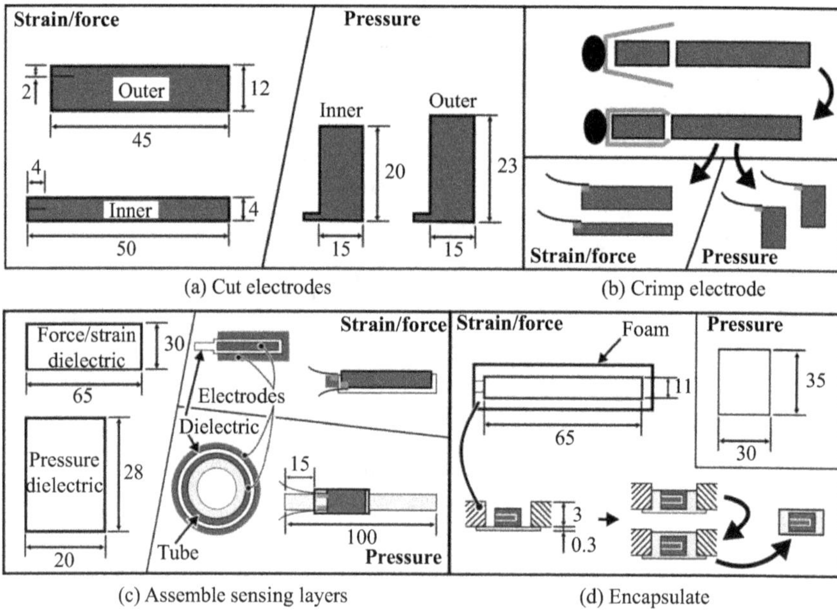

Figure 4.7 Fabrication of a DE strain, pressure or force sensor follows the sequence of cutting out fabric electrodes (a); crimping wires to them (b); layering the inner and outer electrodes with a dielectric in between (c); and casting a dielectric encapsulation layer (d) around the whole assembly. All dimensions are in millimetres, drawings are not necessarily to scale and refer to the main text for further details

that the stiffest direction of the fabric is aligned with the length of the muscle (for a non-stretchable Peano muscle). The fabric used in the prototype muscle was a generic 100 g m^{-2} polycotton (65% polyester, 35% cotton). Then a sacrificial foam core is cut (using a laser cutter, for example). This core is used to cast vertical walls called seam blocks that separate the top and bottom membranes of the muscle. Before casting the seam blocks, a membrane is placed below the foam core (coated side up). Platsil Gel-10 is cast into the foam cut-outs, cured and a top membrane adhered coated side down (c).

Next, the top and bottom membranes are stitched together through the seam blocks. It is important that the stitching passes through the seam blocks 1 mm within the outside edge of the blocks (d). The stitching should not penetrate the foam or the muscle may leak. A strong thread that adheres well to the silicone is recommended, such as the cotton wrapped polyester Glace used in the prototype. At this point, an optional membrane layer can be added for redundancy against leakage, as shown in Figure 4.5. The prototype used such a layer with the same polycotton fabric rubberised with a high tear-strength Dragon Skin® 20 silicone (Smooth-On Inc., Macungie, PA) to help prevent delamination.

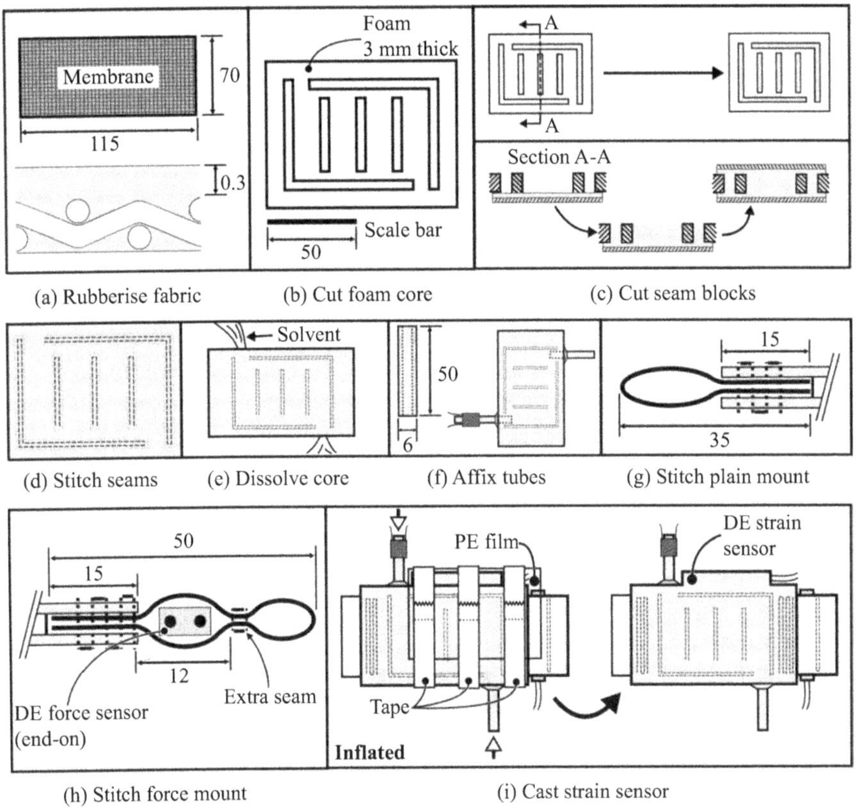

Figure 4.8 Fabrication of the reactive Peano muscle is a layer-based process. First, muscle membranes are made from rubberising a fabric (a). These form the top and the bottom of the muscle. The muscle walls, or seam blocks, are cast between the membranes with the aid of a sacrificial foam core (b)–(c). The membranes are then stitched together (d); the foam dissolved (e); a plain tube, a pressure sensing tube (f) and mounting straps attached (g)–(h); the force sensor inserted (h); and the strain sensor cast onto the muscle (i). All dimensions are in millimetres, drawings are not necessarily to scale and refer to the main text for further details

Following the sequence of steps (e)–(h), the foam core is dissolved in a solvent such as petrol, plain and pressure sensing silicone tubes attached, nylon webbing mounting straps stitched on and the force sensor inserted. The plain tube is a 50 mm length of 6 mm OD, 4 mm ID silicone tube and the pressure sensing tube, the segment from Figure 4.7. They should be cleaned with a solvent (mineral turpentine, for example) and attached with a relatively stiff silicone (RS 692–542). Lastly, the strain sensor is cast along the muscle edge with Platsil Gel-10 silicone (i). For this step, the muscle must be inflated so that when the muscle is deflated the sensor will be stretched out. Silicone is contained during this process by wrapping the muscle side tightly in a polyethylene (PE) film. This also serves to further pre-compress the sensor, increasing the muscle strain range it can measure. After the silicone cures, the PE film is removed and the reactive Peano muscle is ready for use. Next, we investigate how the reactive Peano muscle and its sensors performed.

4.4 Characterising the reactive Peano muscle

There were three steps to characterising the performance of the reactive Peano muscle. First, we compared its performance with that of the sensorless Peano muscle from the previous chapter. Second, we measured the repeatability and sensitivity of the reactive Peano muscle's sensors' capacitance changes and fitted their characteristics to simple regression models. Third, we validated the accuracy of these models to predict the reactive Peano muscle's strain, pressure and force under arbitrary motion, pressurisation and load conditions.

4.4.1 Methods

As with the Peano muscle, the reactive Peano muscle prototype shown in Figure 4.6 was characterised in the tensile testing rig described in [36]. It was hydraulically pressurised and quasi-statically unloaded to its free-strain and loaded back to its starting length. This process was repeated three times for each of the test pressures of 0, 50, 100 and 200 kPa. We also conducted an additional experiment for validation of the DE sensor models' accuracies. In this experiment the pressure and load applied to the muscle were slowly varied in a random manner over a period of 30 s.

During all of these experiments, the DE sensors' capacitances were measured with the StretchSense capacitive sensing module (SCSM, StretchSense Ltd., Auckland, New Zealand) at a rate of 100 Hz and filtered over a moving window of 128 samples. This filter removed noise in the measured capacitance. The SCSM was chosen because it is specifically designed for DE sensors' high and variable equivalent electrode series resistances. It also has a simple interface, suitable capacitance range, compact size and supports five input channels [37].

4.4.2 Muscle performance results and discussion

Figure 4.9 shows the reactive Peano muscle produced a blocking force of 70 N at 200 kPa and had a free-strain of 14%. In its 0 kPa experiment it had an average stiffness of 0.69 kN m^{-1} from 0% to 10% extension. In comparison, the Peano muscle from the previous chapter, which had similar muscle tube dimensions, had a blocking force of 170 N and a free-strain of 16%. It had an average stiffness of 4.3 kN m^{-1} from 0% to 6% extension in its 0 kPa experiment.

The completely soft reactive Peano muscle produced significantly less force and contracted slightly less than the Peano muscle with metal components. The lower blocking force of the reactive Peano muscle is simply explained by its relatively compliant connection to the tensile testing rig with fabric mounting straps.

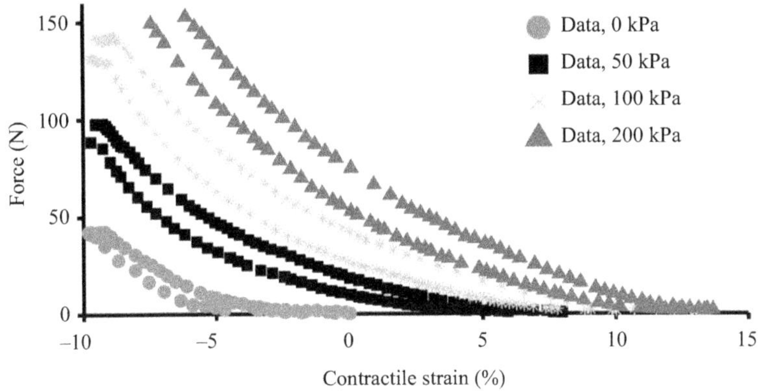

Figure 4.9 Force-strain loading and unloading curves of the reactive Peano muscle at various pressures (adapted from Figure 6(a) in [27])

These could be seen to noticeably stretch as the muscle was pressurised. The portion of the mounting straps wrapped around the DE force sensor did not significantly stretch. Instead, stretching occurred where the mounting straps were sewn onto the muscle body. This indicated a reduced muscle tensile stiffness, as demonstrated by the average stiffness in the 0 kPa experiment, and hence a reduced blocking force at a given pressure. The Peano muscle with metal components had rigid metal mounts connecting the muscle to the testing rig, increasing its tensile stiffness and blocking force. This muscle also did not have the third fabric layer of the reactive Peano muscle, which reduced the bending stiffness of reactive muscle's tubes and slightly decreased its free-strain.

Another performance difference between the muscles was their maximum operating pressures: the Peano muscle was tested at up to 500 kPa and the reactive Peano muscle at up to 200 kPa. The reactive Peano muscle could not reliably hold higher pressures without leaking. This was a fabrication issue. We discovered that at higher pressures voids in the silicone seam blocks allowed fluid to leak out of the muscle via the stitching. In future muscles we plan to fix this problem by degassing the silicone before it cures. Amongst all these observations the most important thing to note is that the reactive Peano muscle's sensors did not noticeably affect its performance. Rather, its performance was affected by its wholly soft nature and could be improved with stiffer muscle mounts and degassing of silicone during the muscle's fabrication.

4.4.3 Sensor performance results and discussion

The results of the characterisation experiments are plotted in Figure 4.10 along with the simple regression models listed in Table 4.1.

The embedded strain sensor had an average sensitivity of 7.9% pF^{-1}, the pressure sensor, 54 kPa pF^{-1} and the force sensor, 7.4 N pF^{-1}. All sensors exhibited good repeatability and significant hysteresis, which was greatest in the pressure

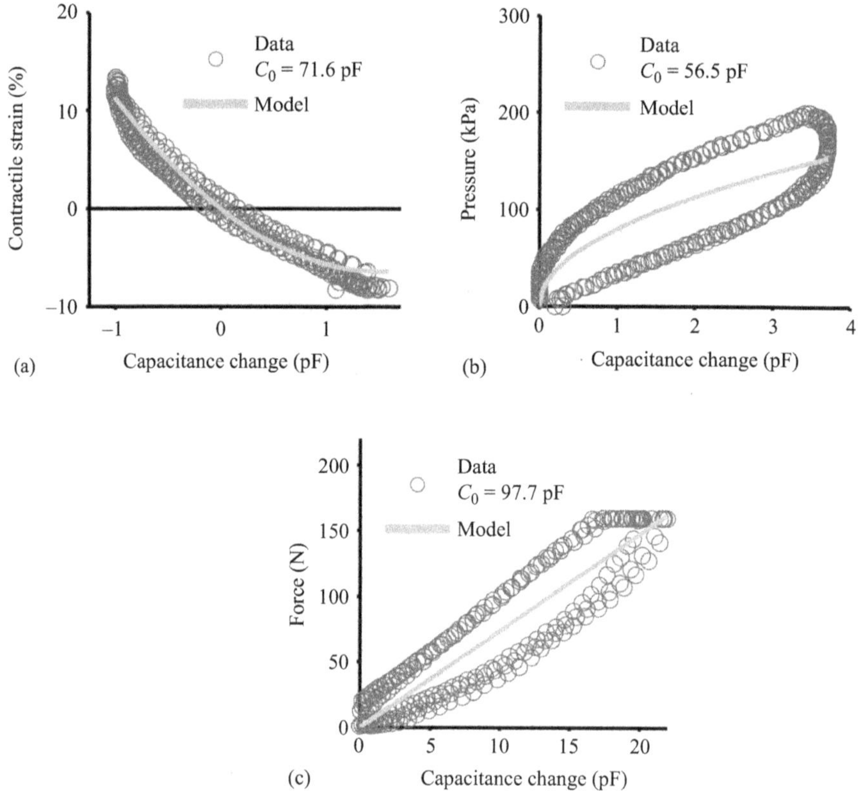

Figure 4.10 Characterisation curves of the DE strain (a), pressure (b) and force sensors (c). Initial, zero strain, pressure and force capacitances are noted as C_0 *((a) adapted from Figure 2 in [27])*

Table 4.1 DE sensor regression models

Sensor	**Model**
Strain (%)	$\varepsilon(\Delta C) = 2.8\Delta C^2 - 8.4\Delta C$
Pressure (Pa)	$P(\Delta C) = 8.0 \times 10^4 \sqrt{\Delta C}$
Force (N)	$F_s(\Delta C) = 7.4\Delta C$

sensor. Although strain clearly was quadratically related to capacitance change, the large hysteresis of the pressure sensor made the form of its regression model ambiguous. Here a squareroot model was chosen, but a linear model may also be appropriate. A linear model was suitable for modelling the force sensor characteristic. Next, the accuracy of these models was validated.

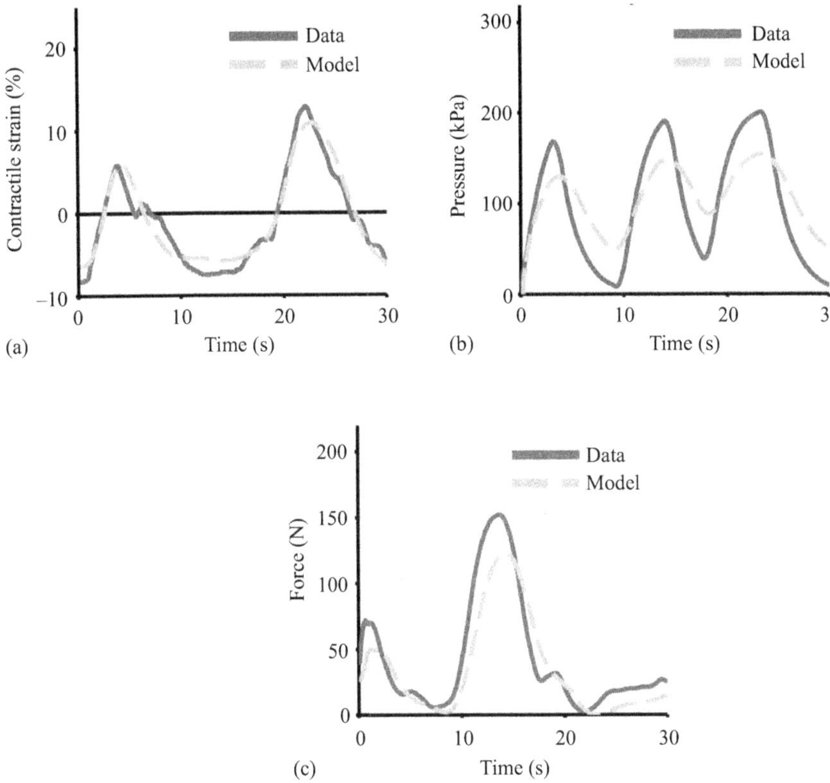

Figure 4.11 Validation of the models for the embedded DE strain (a), pressure (b) and force sensors (c). Each plot compares the value of one of these quantities as measured by test rig mounted sensors (Data) with that measured from embedded DE sensors (Model). The sensor capacitance changes used in these models were calculated with initial, zero strain, pressure and force capacitances (C_0) of 71.3, 55.1 and 97.1 pF ((a) adapted from Figure 7(a) in [27])

Validation results (Figure 4.11) of the embedded sensors' accuracies revealed reasonable performance for sensing of forces and strains with normalised root mean square errors (NRMSEs) of 12.1% and 11.4% respectively. The pressure sensor tracked the general trend in pressure changes reasonably, but underestimated pressure changes when the sign of the rate of change of pressure reversed. It had an NRMSE of 18.7%. This error was caused by the sensor's hysteresis, which was not captured by the simple linear model, but is clearly observable in Figure 4.11(b). Error due to hysteresis was also seen in the validation of the strain and force sensors, but to a lesser extent. These latter two sensors notably produced a smoother output compared to the test rig measured muscle strain and force. Furthermore, comparing the sensors' initial zero strain, pressure or force capacitances with those observed in the characterisation experiments we noted a significant shift of up to 1.5 pF, which was seen in the pressure sensor.

Considering the validation results highlights that the reactive Peano muscle's DE sensors' accuracies were limited by their potentially large hysteresis. All of the sensors' models could be improved with the addition of a hysteretic operator such as in the Preisach or virgin curve models [38,39]. Alternatively, their hysteresis could possibly be reduced through a different choice of sensor materials. A popular and low hysteresis DE electrode is that made from carbon black and silicone. In the case of the pressure sensor, the silicone tube may be a significant contributor to sensor hysteresis and alternative elastomers should be tried. Hence, future development of these sensors would consider low material hysteresis as a key design requirement.

The validation results also showed the strain and force DE sensors had a smoother output than that measured by the test rig. This could be because these sensors' outputs were filtered whereas the test rig's measurements were not. Another possibility is that the test rig measured additional higher frequency force and movement dynamics introduced by the couplings between the test rig and muscle. These dynamics would not have been measured by the DE sensors because of their filtering as well as their direct mounting on the reactive Peano muscle. If these hypotheses are correct, future results could be improved by directly mounting the test rig strain sensor on the Peano muscle and reducing the size of the SCSM filtering window.

In spite of the sensors repeatability in the characterisation experiments (Figure 4.10), there was a significant change in the sensors' initial capacitances, C_0. Reasons for these capacitance shifts included the sensitivity of the sensors to the position of their wires, and the sensors' sensitivities to loads independent of the quantity the sensors were designed to measure. This was particularly an issue in the pressure sensor because its initial capacitance was influenced by the position of its fluid inlet tube. Flexing of the tube deformed the sensor, altering its initial capacitance. The initial capacitance of the force sensor was also affected by its lateral position in its fabric loop. Possible solutions to these sources of sensor error are adding stress relief to the sensors' wires, directly embedding the pressure sensor into the Peano muscle and adhering the force sensor to its fabric loop with silicone. Implementing these solutions could further cement success of the embedded strain, pressure and force sensing concept demonstrated in the reactive Peano muscle.

Although the present accuracy of the reactive Peano muscle's sensors may not be enough for control of most rehabilitation devices, it does have immediate applications. For example, the reactive Peano muscle can be used to measure the approximate physical state of an exoskeleton's user. This information is useful for interpreting the user's movement intent, perhaps for interfacing with motivational electronic games that make the rehabilitation process more enjoyable. The sensor measurements can also be used as redundant information on the interaction between the exoskeleton and its user, providing a fail-safe indication of whether the forces and movements applied to the user are safe. Compared to traditional 'bolted on' sensors, those in the reactive Peano muscle can provide these extra rehabilitation device functions without affecting its actuators' form or operation. This achievement is all the more significant when its actuators are completely soft yet produce significant force and motion, as is the case with the reactive Peano muscle.

4.5 Summary

Soft actuators for rehabilitation devices can use sensors to control their movement and force, and monitor the safety and movement intention of their user. The reactive Peano muscle is a soft fluid powered actuator with embedded sensors. Embedding nature inspired DE sensors into the Peano muscle's structure transforms it into a reactive yet soft actuator that can sense its interaction with the real world. This is analogous to how, for example, the muscles of a human continuously detect the loading and motion of the joints they move. Making this possible in the reactive Peano muscle are DE strain, pressure and force sensors with average sensitivities of 7.9% pF^{-1}, 54 kPa pF^{-1} and 7.4 N pF^{-1} respectively. Unlike previous fluid powered muscles with embedded sensors, the reactive Peano muscle is completely soft, and the similarly soft nature of its DE sensors did not significantly affect either its behaviour or unobtrusive form. However, the muscle was limited by its maximum inflation pressure and the embedded sensors were limited by their hysteresis, filtering and sensitivity to quantities other than that being measured. Improvements could be made through degassing silicone during the muscle's fabrication; adding a hysteresis component to the sensors' models; reducing the size of the sensors' filtering windows and improving sensor integration and wire stress relief.

The next step is to investigate the qualities of soft rehabilitation devices, starting with a study on a device for the wrist that is presented in the following chapter.

References

[1] Hu XL, Tong KY, Song R, Zheng XJ, Leung WW. A comparison between electromyography-driven robot and passive motion device on wrist rehabilitation for chronic stroke. Neurorehabil Neural Repair. 2009;23(8):837–46.

[2] Nef T, Mihelj M, Kiefer G, Perndl C, Müller R, Riener R. ARMin-exoskeleton for arm therapy in stroke patients. IEEE 10th international conference on rehabilitation robotics. IEEE: Noordwijk, Netherlands; 2007. p. 68–74.

[3] Banala SK, Agrawal SK, Kim SH, Scholz JP. Novel gait adaptation and neuromotor training results using an active leg exoskeleton. IEEE Trans Mechatronics. 2010;15(2):216–25.

[4] Nef T, Guidali M, Riener R. ARMin III – arm therapy exoskeleton with an ergonomic shoulder actuation. App Bion Biomech. 2009;6(2):127–42.

[5] Meuleman J, van Asseldonk E, van Oort G, Rietman H, van der Kooij H. LOPES II—design and evaluation of an admittance controlled gait training

robot with shadow-leg approach. IEEE Trans Neural Syst Rehabil Eng. 2016;24(3):352–63.
[6] Balasubramanian S, Colombo R, Sterpi I, Sanguineti V, Burdet E. Robotic assessment of upper limb motor function after stroke. Am J Phys Med Rehabil. 2012;91(11):S255–S269.
[7] Guidali M, Schmiedeskamp M, Klamroth V, Riener R. Assessment and training of synergies with an arm rehabilitation robot. IEEE 11th international conference on rehabilitation robotics. IEEE: Kyoto, Japan 2009. p. 772–6.
[8] Pisano F, Miscio G, Del Conte C, Pianca D, Candeloro E, Colombo R. Quantitative measures of spasticity in post-stroke patients. Clin Neurophysiol. 2000;111(6):1015–22.
[9] Wolbrecht ET, Chan V, Reinkensmeyer DJ, Bobrow JE. Optimizing compliant, model-based robotic assistance to promote neurorehabilitation. IEEE Transac Neural Syst Rehabil Eng. 2008;16(3):286–97.
[10] Srivastava S, Kao P, Kim SH, *et al.* Assist-as-needed robot-aided gait training improves walking function in individuals following stroke. IEEE Trans Neural Syst Rehabil Eng. 2015;23(6):956–63.
[11] Mileusnic MP, Loeb GE. Force estimation from ensembles of golgi tendon organs. J Neural Eng. 2009;6(3):1–15.
[12] Goulbourne NC, Son S. Numerical and experimental analysis of McKibben actuators and dielectric elastomer sensors. Proceedings of the ASME international mechanical engineering congress and exposition. ASME: Seattle, WA; 2007. p. 175–86.
[13] Goulbourne NC, Son S, Fox JW. Self-sensing McKibben actuators using dielectric elastomer sensors. SPIE Smart Structures and Materials/NDE. International Society for Optics and Photonics: San Diego, CA; 2007. p. 1–12.
[14] Nakamoto H, Oida S, Ootaka H, *et al.* Design and response performance of capacitance meter for stretchable strain sensor. IEEE/RSJ international conference on intelligent robots and systems. IEEE: Hamburg, Germany; 2015. p. 2348–53.
[15] Miron G, Plante J. Design of a durable air-muscle with integrated sensor for soft robotics. International design engineering technical conferences and computers and information in engineering conference. ASME: Boston, MA; 2015. p. 1–9.
[16] Wakimoto S, Suzumori K, Kanda T. Development of intelligent McKibben actuator with built-in soft conductive rubber sensor. International conference on solid state sensors and actuators and microsystems. IEEE: Seoul, South Korea; 2005. p. 745–8.
[17] Wakimoto S, Misumi J, Suzumori K. New concept and fundamental experiments of a smart pneumatic artificial muscle with a conductive fiber. Sens Actuators A Phys. 2016;250:48–54.
[18] Park YL, Wood RJ. Smart pneumatic artificial muscle actuator with embedded microfluidic sensing. IEEE sensors. IEEE: Baltimore, MD; 2013. p. 1–4.

[19] Yamamoto Y, Kure K, Iwa T, Kanda T, Suzumoru K. Flexible displacement sensor using piezoelectric polymer for intelligent FMA. IEEE international conference on intelligent robots and systems. IEEE: San Diego, CA; 2007. p. 765–70.

[20] Akagi T, Dohta S, Kenmotsu Y, Zhao F, Yoneda M. Development of smart inner diameter sensor for position control of Mckibben artificial muscle. Procedia engineering. Elsevier: Kuching, Malaysia; 2012. p. 105–12.

[21] Shimooka S, Dohta S, Akagi T, Moriwake Y. Position control of rubber artificial muscle using built-in ultrasonic sensor and quasi-servo valve. Intl J Mech Eng Robot Res. 2015;4(4):304–08.

[22] Shin H, Saitoh H, Kawakami T, Yamanishi S, Ikemoto S, Hosoda K. Development of an embedded sensor system for pneumatic artificial muscle proprioceptors. Artif Life Robot. 2016;21(4):486–92.

[23] Felt W, Remy CD. Smart braid: air muscles that measure force and displacement. IEEE international conference on intelligent robots and systems. IEEE: Chicago, IL; 2014. p. 2821–26.

[24] Felt W, Chin KY, Remy CD. Contraction sensing with smart braid McKibben muscles. IEEE Trans Mechatronics. 2016;21(3):1201–09.

[25] McKay TG, Calius E, Anderson IA. The dielectric constant of 3M VHB: a parameter in dispute. SPIE smart structures and materials/NDE. International Society for Optics and Photonics: San Diego, CA; 2009. p. 72870P-1–10.

[26] Typical Properties for RS692–542. RS Components: Corby, UK; 2007.

[27] Veale AJ, Anderson IA, Xie SQ. Dielectric elastomer strain and pressure sensing enable reactive fluidic artificial muscles. SPIE smart structures and materials/NDE. International Society for Optics and Photonics: Las Vegas, NV; 2016. p. 97982A-1–8.

[28] Freberg LA. Nonvisual sensation and perception in discovering behavioral neuroscience: an introduction to biological psychology. Cengage Learning: Boston, MA; 2016. p. 215–52.

[29] Veale AJ, Anderson IA, Xie SQ. The smart peano fluidic muscle: a low profile flexible orthosis actuator that feels pain. SPIE smart structures and materials/NDE. International Society for Optics and Photonics: San Diego, CA; 2015. p. 94351V-1–11.

[30] Chavanne J, Civet Y, Perriard Y. Modelling of a dielectric electroactive polymer tubular shape sensor for pressure measurements. IEEE International conference on advanced intelligent mechatronics. IEEE: Banff, Canada; 2016. p. 810–15.

[31] Cong P, Ko WH, Young DJ. Wireless batteryless implantable blood pressure monitoring microsystem for small laboratory animals. IEEE Sens J. 2010; 10(2):243–54.

[32] Böse H, Fuß E, Lux P. Influence of design and material properties on the performance of dielectric elastomer compression sensors. SPIE smart structures and materials/NDE. International Society for Optics and Photonics: San Diego, CA; 2015. p. 943029-1–12

[33] Mannsfeld SCB, Tee BCK, Stoltenberg RM, *et al.* Highly sensitive flexible pressure sensors with microstructured rubber dielectric layers. Nat Mater. 2010;9(10):859–64 .

[34] Vandeparre H, Watson D, Lacour SP. Extremely robust and conformable capacitive pressure sensors based on flexible polyurethane foams and stretchable metallization. Appl Phys Lett. 2013;103(20):1–4.

[35] Veale AJ, Xie SQ, Anderson IA. Modeling the peano fluidic muscle and the effects of its material properties on its static and dynamic behavior. Smart Mater Struct. 2016;25(6):1–16.

[36] Veale AJ, Xie SQ, Anderson IA. Characterizing the peano fluidic muscle and the effects of its geometry properties on its behavior. Smart Mater Struct. 2016;25(6):1–14.

[37] StretchSense Capacitive Sensor Module (SCSM) Information Sheet – Rev. A. Auckland, New Zealand: StretchSense Ltd.; 2013.

[38] Van Damme M, Beyl P, Vanderborght B, *et al.* Modeling hysteresis in pleated pneumatic artificial muscles. IEEE international conference on robotics, automation and mechatronics. IEEE: Chengdu, China 2008. p. 471–76.

[39] Vo-Minh T, Tjahjowidodo T, Ramon H, Van Brussel H. A new approach to modeling hysteresis in a pneumatic artificial muscle using the Maxwell-slip model. IEEE/ASME Trans Mechatronics. 2011;16(1):177–86.

Chapter 5
Soft wrist rehabilitation robot

Ageing society in many countries has led to an increasing number of stroke and cerebral palsy patients who require rehabilitation therapy. Affected wrist joints often show an increased spasticity and stiffness, caused by impairments of the surrounding muscles and tendons. However, the medical devices for wrist joint assessment and rehabilitation are lacking. The goal of this chapter is to develop and control a robotic orthosis to assist the patient's wrist to perform rehabilitation exercise in a compliant way. A one-degree of freedom (DOF) robotic device with parallel mechanism was designed for the wrist joint by utilising pneumatic artificial muscles (PAMs) that are compliant and lightweight. Mechanical design of the wrist orthosis and the corresponding development of pneumatic control system were presented. A model-based pressure close-loop control strategy was implemented for the PAMs in order to track the trajectory in high-performance. Experiments on the orthosis demonstrated that the robot could assist the hand to move along a torque-sensitive trajectory with small errors and the differential forces were also kept stable.

5.1 Introduction

Paralysis is a loss of muscle functionality which is usually caused by damage to the nervous system of the human body, rather than damage to the muscle itself. Common causes of paralysis are stroke, head injuries, spinal cord injuries, multiple sclerosis or cerebral palsy [1]. Being impaired or completely unable to perform motor and sensor tasks, paralysis is likely to have a huge impact on a patient's life.

Rehabilitation is inevitable to maintain the flexibility of the locomotor system and to regain motor abilities. The method of rehabilitation needs to be adapted to the patient's capability to move and the extent of the initial injury. While 'active' exercises involve the patient moving a limb on his own, 'passive' exercises require the support of a therapist, who moves the limb carefully. The lack of motion in a joint can lead to the contracture of the attached muscles, thereby increasing the stiffness of the joint and reducing its range of motion. Through kinesitherapy, this impairment can be gradually resolved. Joint stiffness is hence a plausible indicator for the therapy's progress [2].

The number of patients with paralysis is expected to grow over the next years, since most of the industrial countries are facing demographic changes towards an ageing society. This is due to the fact that the triggering diseases, first and foremost stroke, are most common among older people [3]. While 22% of people experiencing stroke die in the first 30 days, almost 80% of the survivors require a rehabilitation therapy [4]. Since manual therapy requires a great deal of labour costs, industry has started seeking solutions for this problem. The field of rehabilitation robotics has thus seen a continuous growth over the last years. Huge effort has been expended in the field of soft robotics, in order to make robotic solutions safer, while interacting with humans. This involves not only the development of novel soft actuators, but also the utilisation of sensor systems for force or environmental monitoring in order to alleviate collisions or overusing joints [5].

Using robots for rehabilitation purposes offers several advantages. Human therapists tend to fatigue during the exercises, thus the number of patients to treat will be very limited. Highly accurate force and torque measurements allow robots to provide a minimum active movement support for a maximum training effect during the therapy. Furthermore, rehabilitation devices can be coupled with virtual reality environments in order to play games during the therapy, which increases fun and motivation for patients to practice more often [6]. Recent studies [7] have shown that patient participation is a key feature for a successful rehabilitation. Finally, these systems allow the recording of information about the patient's performance (torque, force, velocity, etc.) for eventual analysis and result comparison.

An increasingly deployed actuator in soft and rehabilitation robotics is the (McKibben) PAM, based on the working principle of the human muscle [8,9]. Consisting of a tube-like bladder, surrounded by a braided mesh shell, the muscle contracts when pressurised and thereby induces an axial force. The actuator has an outstanding power-to-weight ratio, offers natural compliance as well as other pneumatic related advantages, such as compactness, cleanliness and simplicity [10].

The control of these actuators, however, proves to be difficult, due to their highly non-linear behaviour. Nevertheless, significant progress in pneumatic components, such as high speed solenoid and servo valves, as well as novel control strategies lead to an increasing dissemination of the muscles. The purpose of this chapter is to describe the design of a measurement tool for the determination of joint stiffness using two PAMs in an antagonistic setup (this is required, as the muscles can only induce a pulling force). In this case, the flexion and extension of the wrist joint will be examined with the help of a one-DOF device. In the following section, the mechanical design will be illustrated. Afterwards, the control strategy will be explained in detail and results will be presented.

5.2 Device design

In this section, the basic mechanical design of the wrist orthosis, and later on, the force distribution over the pneumatic actuators and the mechanical parts are explained. The orthosis is designed to fit on the back of the patient's forearm, which is why the weight of the device is meant to be kept as low as possible. The PAMs used in this project are Festo Fluidic Muscles DMSP20 with an effective length of 90 mm. The mechanical hinge is placed coaxial with the biological joint,

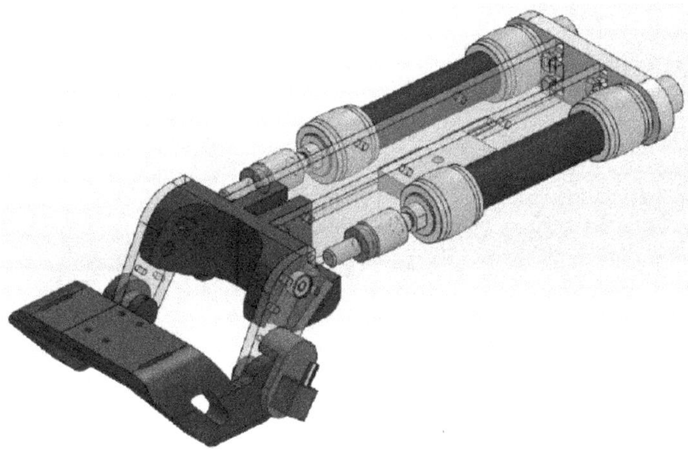

Figure 5.1 Mechanical design of the robotic wrist orthosis. © 2015 IEEE. Adapted from [11] with permission

which requires the connection of the muscles with the hinge pulleys through a redirected steel wire. Ball bearings are utilised to reduce friction in the hinge. Miniature in-line load cells are mounted on each muscle to measure the axial force. Using only 3D-printed plastic parts as well as laser-cut acrylic resin for the frame, the orthosis' weight is kept under 1,000 g. Figure 5.1 shows mechanical design of the wrist orthosis [11].

Two Festo Fluidic Muscles are used as antagonistic actuators and are placed on a plastic plate which is strapped on the back of the patients forearm. Both muscles are attached to a mechanical hinge through a steel wire. The wires are guided around the cylindrical hinge in a way, so that one PAM rotates it in a clockwise direction, and the other PAM in a counter clockwise direction when contracting. The hinge is located approximately 40 mm above the biological wrist joint. A hand rest is connected to it, rotating the hand during operation.

A compact load cell is placed in-line with the wire-connection for each muscle. The mechanical hinge, however, is split into two metal pulleys, placed on each side of the wrist. Those are fixed to the hand rest and rotate within ball bearings in order to avoid friction. Furthermore, a potentiometer is utilised as an angle sensor, placed on the outside of the hinge's left pulley. The materials used in the device's frame are either 3D printed plastic or laser-cut acrylic resin, which leads to a low overall weight of 1,086 g. The arm rest located under the frame has an adjustable position, allowing to customise the device for a patient's geometry. Any other electrical and pneumatic components are placed on a remote board. Experiment setup of the robotic wrist orthosis is presented in Figure 5.2.

The maximum displacement for the Festo PAMs is found to be 20% for non-loaded situations, which equals 18 mm for the provided muscles of 90 mm effective length. With the maximum angular displacement of the hand rest of 60° (due to

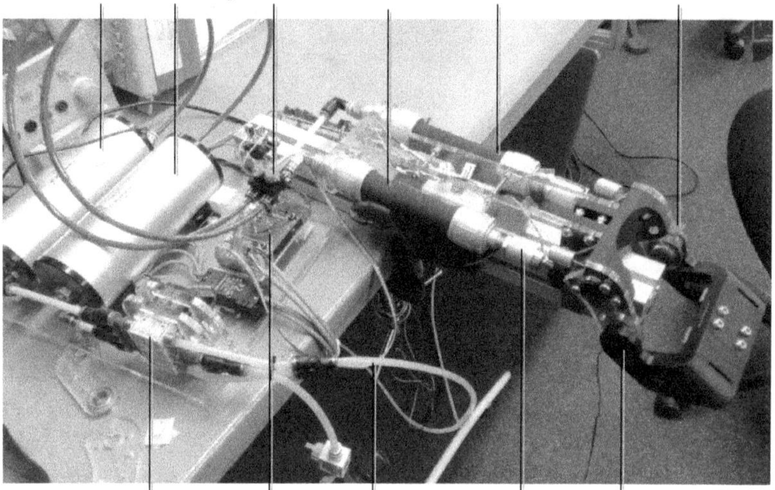

Figure 5.2 Setup of the robotic orthosis system. © 2015 IEEE. Adapted from [11] with permission

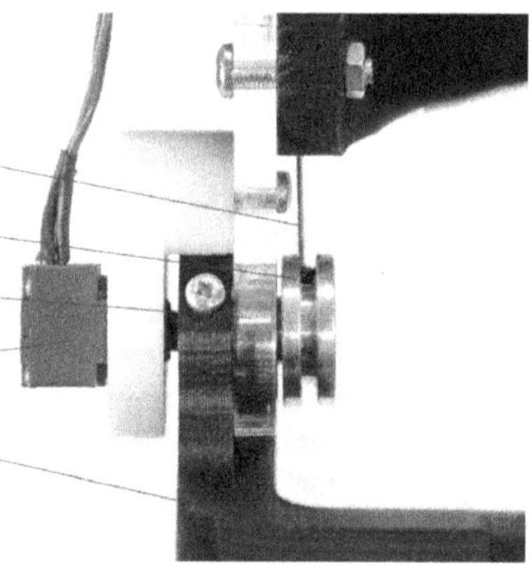

Figure 5.3 Angle measurement using a potentiometer

the mechanical design), the radius can be calculated to:

$$r_p = \frac{d_{max} \cdot 180}{\Theta_{max} \cdot \pi} \approx 8.6 \text{ mm} \tag{5.1}$$

In order to provide angle feedback, a simple linear rotational potentiometer is placed on the mechanical hinge of the device and connected to the microcontroller. The chosen package offers a total electrical angle of 240° and nominal mechanical impedance. The attachment of the potentiometer to the hinge is illustrated in Figure 5.3.

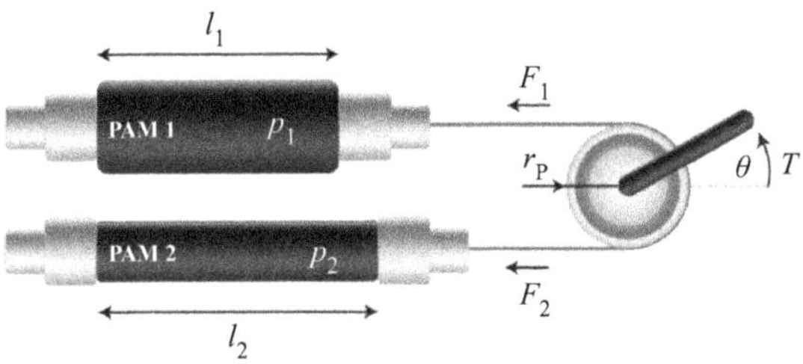

Figure 5.4 *Force distribution in the orthosis. © 2015 IEEE. Adapted from [11] with permission*

5.3 Force and torque distribution

In this section, the principles of force and torque distribution will be examined. Considering that both of the PAMs are fixed to the frame, the muscles, the wire-connections and the hinge pulleys create a closed system. In a first step, both muscles need to be pressurised, so that the wire connections are under tension (with the muscle lengths still being equal, $l_1 = l_2$). This offset point is desirably found to be $l_{offset} = l_{max}/2$, in order to achieve the same contraction/relaxation potential in each direction. For any further movements, the muscle lengths should follow this rule:

$$l_1 + l_2 = 2 \cdot l_{offset} = \text{Const} \tag{5.2}$$

Assuming that the double hinge of the hand rest can be considered as a single constant radius pulley, the basic force distribution illustrated in Figure 5.4 is agreeable. First, we have to make sure that the steel wire connection is always pulled taut, in order to guarantee the hand rest's angular displacement:

Given the constant radius of the pulley r_p, θ can be expressed as:

$$\theta_{deg} = \frac{l_0 - l_1}{2 \cdot \pi \cdot r_p} \cdot 360 \tag{5.3}$$

As long as no torque T is applied, the forces F_1 and F_2 are equal. For an attached load however, the distribution becomes:

$$F_1 + \frac{T}{r_p} - F_2 = 0 \tag{5.4}$$

which means that the torque T can be explained by the differential force $F_2 - F_1$, without the total force $F_1 + F_2$ having any influence on the torque measurement. As a consequence, any inaccuracies within the displacement control of the muscles do not affect the measurement.

5.4 Control strategies

In this section, the control strategy for the PAMs will be explained. Recent papers have shown different approaches to control similar actuators, using either expensive servo valves or a pair of fast switching on/off valves. Utilising digital valves only, a proper control strategy needs to be implemented. Pulse width modulation (PWM) has been proved to be superior to a simple bang–bang controller [12], thus being adopted in this project.

5.4.1 Pneumatic setup

The valves are energised through the supplied Festo MHJ9-KMH valve amplifier, which operates at 24 V DC. Accepting digital input signals down to 3 V, the valves can easily be controlled via a microcontroller unit without any further electrical components. Furthermore, a pressure sensor is connected in between the valves and the PAM, in order to provide pressure feedback for the control system.

Figure 5.5 illustrates the pneumatic setup for one PAM. Two digital high speed valves Festo MHJ9 [13] are utilised to control the air flow into and out of the muscle. The valves are operated via pulse width modulation, running at 50 Hz. The magnitude and direction of the air flow is obtained by altering the pulse widths for both valves. Since the actual flow rate depends equally on the pressure gradient across the valve, the relation between the pulse width and the flow rate needs to be linearised.

Goal of the PWM principle is to control the air flow rate in a linear manner. However, it is not enough to adjust the timing of the two valves, since the air flow rate additionally depends on the pressure gradient across the valve's ports. This interdependency can be resolved to a linear behaviour with the help of a suitable compensation algorithm. Goal of the actuator linearisation is to control the flow rate of the valve linearly, regardless of the pressure gradient across the valve. This will cause the plant to act as a single integral element, simplifying the controller design.

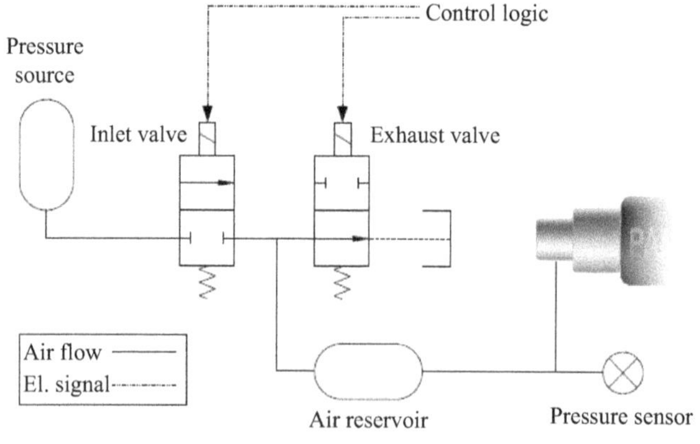

Figure 5.5 The pneumatic setup used for PAMs. © 2015 IEEE. Adapted from [11] with permission

Neglecting temperature effects, the flow rate Q through a valve is defined as:

$$Q = C_V \cdot \sqrt{\frac{\Delta p}{S_G}} \tag{5.5}$$

where C_V is the flow coefficient of the valve and S_G is the specific gravity of the gas. Both of these parameters are constant, thus being substituted to a_V. Given that the pressure gradient Δp and thus the flow rate Q becomes 0 when $pG = pS$ for the inlet and $pG = 0$ for the exhaust, a linearisation over the whole pressure range is not possible (pS is the supply pressure, pG is the gage pressure in the muscle). The pressure gradient Δp_i across the valve I differs for the inlet and the exhaust valve:

$$\Delta p_{inlet} = p_{source} - p_{muscle} \tag{5.6}$$

$$\Delta p_{exhaust} = p_{muscle} - 0 \tag{5.7}$$

The resulting air flow rate for each valve during PWM operation is a fractal of the nominal flow rate, depending on the adjusted duty cycle τ of the square-wave signal:

$$Q_i = \tau_i \cdot a_V \cdot \sqrt{p_i} \tag{5.8}$$

The total flow rate into/out of the muscle Q results is:

$$Q = a_V \cdot \left(\tau_{inlet} \cdot \sqrt{\Delta p_{inlet}} - \tau_{exhaust} \cdot \sqrt{\Delta p_{exhaust}}\right) \tag{5.9}$$

As has been outlined above, a major flaw of the presented pneumatic set-up is the high air flow rate of the valves, in combination with the small volume of the utilised PAMs. Small changes in the valve's differential duty cycle have a big impact on the pressure in the PAM. In addition, a mechanical vibration of the PAM has been observed in PWM operation, which is likely to be disturbing for the patient. For that reason, an additional air reservoir will be connected between the valves and the air muscle. The provided component has a volume of 0.5l, which will increase the existing muscle volume by 1600%.

5.4.2 Model-based control

As mentioned in the introduction of the pneumatic actuators, their relations between displacement, force and pressure are highly non-linear. This behaviour however, can be investigated in advance in order to look up or calculate the parameter to be determined, based on the measurement of the other parameters. In this case, it is always desired to obtain a certain displacement of the muscle, which can be achieved by controlling the pressure in it. The force induced by the muscle, is measured with the help of the load cell, allowing to be compensated for accurate displacement.

The generation of a model can be achieved in two different ways. A mathematical model can be created by establishing all relevant relations of the physical parameters involved in the system. This way is usually chosen for simple systems that are easy to describe with mathematical equations. For the McKibben PAM, this has been done in research papers such as [14]. The result shows that it is rather difficult to describe the actuator in a precise way, not least because their behaviour additionally changes over time.

For this reason, the model will be generated based on measurement data. Each utilised PAM will therefore be tested for a defined number of different pressure levels and loads. Measuring the resulting displacement will create a set of data points, which will be processed using the numerical computing environment MATLAB. With the help of this software, the data points are illustrated in a 3D-plot (see Figure 5.6). Furthermore, the acquired data is interpolated, using a 5 × 5 polynomial fitting tool, which creates the illustrated surface, based on an equation with 25 parameters. With the help of this model, any given pressure of the PAM can be calculated, based on the measurement of the muscles load, as well as the desired displacement.

The model based controller is fundamentally the implementation of an open loop displacement control with force feedback and an embedded closed-loop pressure control. The desired displacement, determined by the trajectory planning module, is used together with the force feedback to look up the required pressure. This again, is controlled in a closed-loop system, which will be illustrated in Figure 5.7.

There are numerous ways to design a closed-loop pressure control system, however a proportional-integral-derivative (PID) controller is the most commonly utilised one. In this case, the actuators have been linearised, which leads to a plant consisting of a single integrating element only. The resulting proportional-derivative (PD)-controller is thus capable of operation without any steady-state error (most commonly the main reason to add an integrating element to the controller). In detail, the desired pressure is compared with the measured value, leaving an error e. The unsaturated controller output S_U results from:

$$S_U = K_P \cdot e + K_D \cdot \frac{de}{dt} \tag{5.10}$$

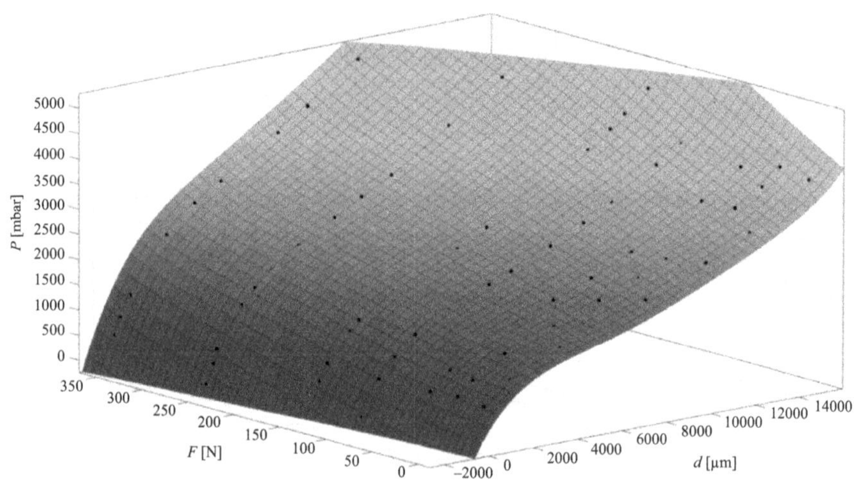

Figure 5.6 Measurement model of the PAM. © 2015 IEEE. Adapted from [11] with permission

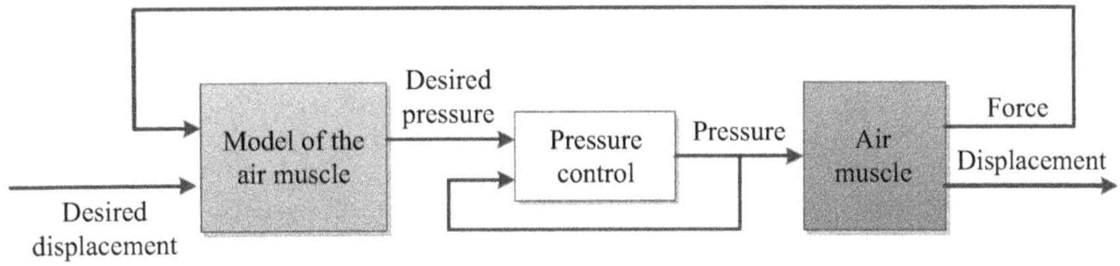

Figure 5.7 Block diagram of the implemented model-based controller. © 2015 IEEE. Adapted from [11] with permission

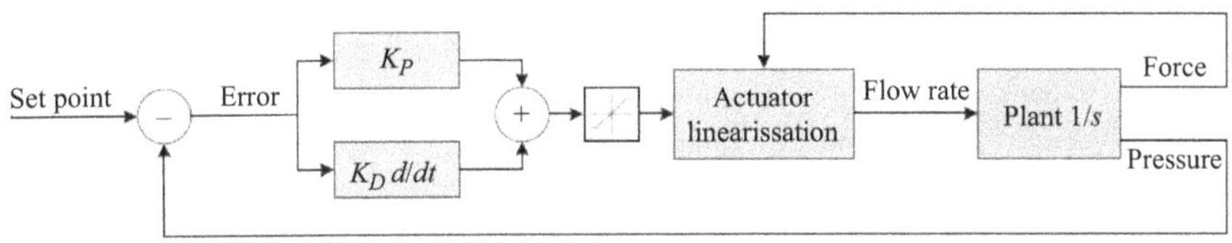

Figure 5.8 Block diagram of the closed-loop pressure control system. © 2015 IEEE. Adapted from [11] with permission

Afterwards, the controller output is saturated (*S*) in order not to exceed the actuator linearisation's input limits. The consequence is a linearly controlled air flow rate, which is integrated in the PAM, resulting in air pressure. This value again, is quantified using a pressure gauge and fed back in order to calculate the error. A block diagram of the controller is illustrated in Figure 5.8.

The final values for these parameters are $K_P = 2$ and $K_D = 1$, given that the control frequency is synchronised with the PWM frequency of the actuators ($f = 50$ Hz). For the validation of the closed loop pressure control, a sine wave trajectory is planned. The result of this experiment is illustrated in Figure 5.9. The magnitude of the pressure error does not exceed 25 mbar.

Although the result for the closed-loop pressure control is good, this does not imply similar results for the superior displacement control, which is open-loop controlled. Even though sine trajectory of the reference angle is smoothed and does not have any hard jumps, the measured angle is conspicuously delayed behind the reference. Regarding the simultaneous force measurement of the same trajectory movement, the distinct difference between the two force curves stands out.

5.4.3 Feedback-based control

The basic requirement for the trajectory is to move the wrist within an arbitrary angular limit. In a first step, the trajectory will be planned with the help of a simple sine curve. Its amplitude is set to a predefined angular limit max, and the maximum speed can be derived from the periodic time, which is set to 15 s. Since only one full period of movement is desired, the transmission between steady state and the sine curve does not have a continuous slope, and is thus being smoothed with the help of a digital filter. The start of the sine curve is initiated by pressing the user button on the microcontroller-board.

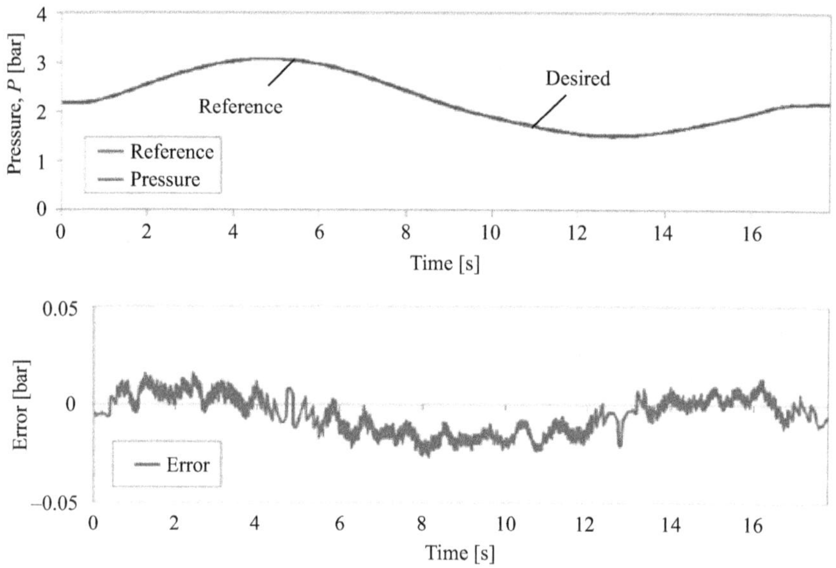

Figure 5.9 Top: pressure curve of the presented control system. Bottom: error of the curve above. 2015 IEEE. Adapted from [11] with permission

In a second step, the safe operation of the orthosis will be incorporated. That means that the trajectory planning module will be monitoring the applied torque, and prevent the orthosis to take on an angular displacement which is considered to be unsafe for the patient's wrist. Here, the desired angle will not be calculated by a predefined function, but by the integration of an adjustable speed. The maximum speed will be set to a similar amount like in the sine wave, however it will be dampened when it approaches either the angular or the torque limit. Upon reaching one of these limits, the algebraic sign of the speed will be inverted, and the maximum speed restored. The damping of the speed D is calculated by the following law:

$$D = \min\left(\frac{\Theta_{max} - \Theta}{k_A}, \frac{T_{max} - T}{k_T}\right) \tag{5.11}$$

$$v = \begin{cases} v_{max} \cdot D^{k_d} & D < 1 \\ v_{max} & D \geq 1 \end{cases} \tag{5.12}$$

Figure 5.10 illustrates the result of this algorithm. The emerging trajectory is similar to the previously discussed sine wave, if no torque is applied. The graph shows as well, that a rising torque (induced by the angular displacement of the wrist) will dampen the trajectory speed and finally result in its reversal when reaching the limit.

Utilising the force- and angle-feedback capabilities of the device, the antagonistic actuators can be treated as a black-box, making their behaviour model unnecessary. The embedded closed-loop pressure controller is superfluous as well, since the proposed system will not provide a desired pressure (due to the lack of a model). Instead, both feedback items will be treated in an individual controller,

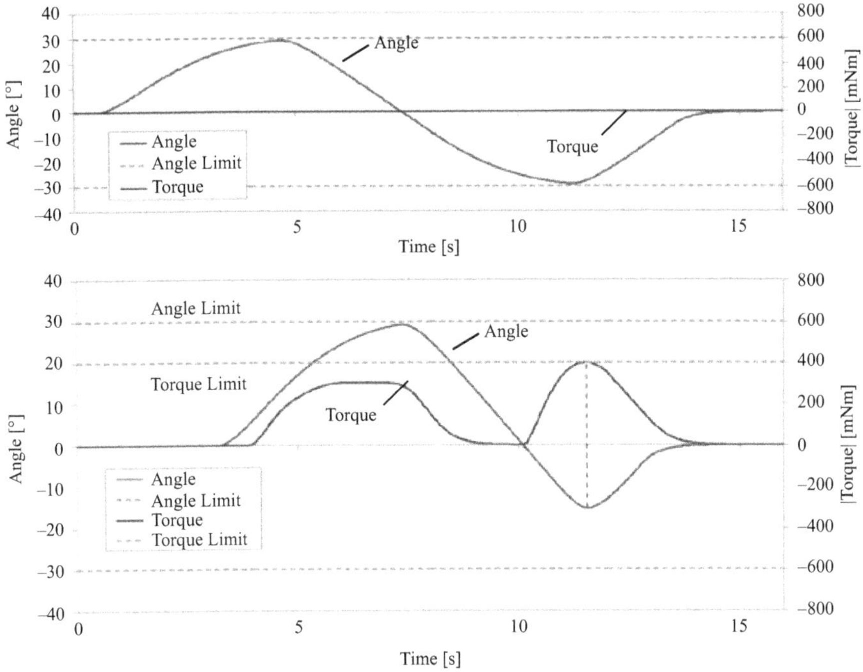

Figure 5.10 Safe trajectory planning. Top: movement within the angular limit, no torque applied. Bottom: if the applied torque exceeds the predefined limit, the trajectory's speed will slow down and finally reverse. *© 2015 IEEE. Adapted from [11] with permission*

affecting the pressure in the PAMs indirectly through a mix table. The main advantage of this approach is the closed-loop control of the angle as well as the total force, which will guarantee to keep these items at a desired value.

As mentioned above, two individual controllers for each of the feedback items are implemented in this approach. At first, a force controller is designed to keep the total force $F_T = F_1 + F_2$ constant. Its output is designated as S_{Force}. Second, an angle controller is implemented to keep the angle at the desired trajectory. This output again is designated as S_{Angle}. The key part of this system is the mix table, where the output signals of the independent controllers are mixed as follows:

$$\begin{aligned} S_1 &= S_{Force} - S_{Angle} \\ S_2 &= S_{Force} + S_{Angle} \end{aligned} \tag{5.13}$$

These equations can be explained by the fact that a lack of force in the system requires an increase of pressure in both of the PAMs, whereas an angular error requires the increase of pressure in only one of the PAMs and a decrease in the other. In other words, the output of the force control affects the flow rate into both muscles in a positive way, the angle control affects the flow rate in a differential way. In contrast to the previously presented pressure control system, the output of the controllers do not affect the force or the angle in a linear way, since the relations between pressure, force

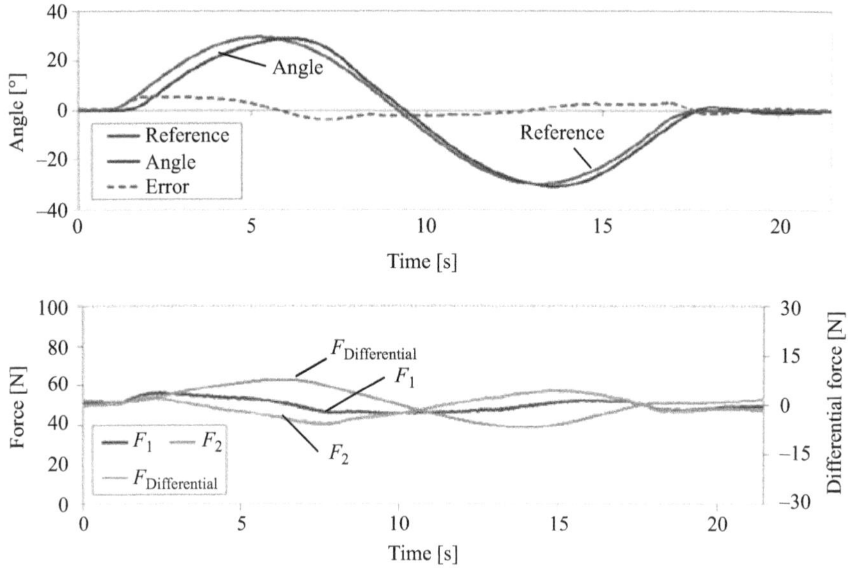

Figure 5.11 Top: result for the open-loop angle/displacement control, including an error graph. Bottom: result of the parallel force measurements. © 2015 IEEE. Adapted from [11] with permission

and displacement are highly non-linear. This may cause deviant behaviour, especially for large angles, where an inverted flow rate into both muscles will not cause a proportional change of displacement and thus increase or decrease the total force. That is why the adjustment of both controllers needs to be coordinated well. Again, the same trajectory as used for testing the model-based controller is now utilised for the test of the proposed feedback-based controller. The result of the angle control, as well as the parallel force measurement can be retrieved from Figure 5.11. Regarding the graph of the angle trajectory, a smaller error than in the previous control system can be observed throughout the whole sine period. In addition, the measured angle does reach the desired angle for the maximum as well as the minimum value. This was not achieved with the open-loop controller. The mean squared error of the angle control is 6.0, which is considerably lower. The measured forces F_1 and F_2 have less variance than in the previous experiment, given that they are closed-loop controlled, with a desired total force of 50 N. The shape of the curves show a similar behaviour, but with a smaller amplitude, resulting in a more consistent differential force.

5.4.4 Design comparison

In this section, the two presented control systems will be compared, in order to find the more suitable solution for the proposed orthosis. The first is a model-based open-loop displacement control. The behaviour of the actuators has been investigated beforehand, resulting in a look-up table which characterises the relations between the crucial actuator parameters. An embedded closed-loop pressure control system has been implemented, in order to set the pressure in the muscle to the corresponding desired value. In a second step, a closed-loop angle and force control system has been implemented. Hereby, the model of the actuators is discarded, instead both relevant feedback items (angle and force) are used for the control. The same sample trajectory has been used for both systems, to test their performance. The resulting angle curve has been presented as well as their parallel force measurements.

Regarding the first controller, the measured angle was notably delayed behind the trajectory curve. In addition, the desired maximum angle has not been reached. Given, that the embedded pressure control was validated beforehand, and the results were fine (maximum error of < 0.025 bar), the occurring error in the angle control is likely to be caused by the utilised actuator model. The presented model is based on the static behaviour of the muscle, and does not include any dynamic characteristics, such as deviant behaviour for deflating and inflating the PAM. Subsequent research on this matter shows, that a hysteresis behaviour of the utilised PAMs has been ascertained in [15]. It is demonstrated that the tube's rubber shell does not only deform elastically, but also plastically. That means that the tube's displacement upon pressurisation is shorter than the displacement for the same pressure-/force-pair upon deflation. This circumstance can only be described within a mathematical model, which assumingly requires long computation time on the real-time controller. The lack of this knowledge in the present model leads to inaccurate displacement behaviour, since the two PAMs always act in a different direction (inflation/deflation) due to the antagonistic setup. The notable delay between measured angle and trajectory can only be introduced by the compliance of the actuators, since the actual pressure is evidently undelayed. Even more crucial is the fact, that the desired maximum angle was not achieved with the given control strategy. Since this phenomenon has likewise been observed for smaller maximum angles, the lack of reachability with the actuator's possible displacements can be excluded as a reason. It is more likely, that the observed differences of the muscle's behaviour is responsible for the circumstance, however this assumption could not have been approved.

Considering the results for the feedback-based control system, the previously identified problems of the model-based control have been improved significantly. The delay between the measured angle and the trajectory and thus the control-error was reduced. The desired maximum angle has been reached as well. Both of these issues have been resolved, by adding the angle feedback to the system and abandoning the model of the actuators, which has been identified as inapplicable due to the missing hysteresis characteristics. In this way, the system becomes a closed-loop control, which is able to react to the angular error, by inflating/deflating the respective PAMs additionally. The fact that the relation between the specific controller outputs S_{Force} and S_{Angle} and their respective process variables are not linear any more, has not affected the performance, since the well balanced controllers have compensated that issue.

Regarding the parallel force measurements for both of the controllers, it is also obvious that the force-controlled system is able to keep both of the forces F_1 and F_2 at a constant level. The open-loop controller only uses the force feedback for the calculation of the desired pressure, but not to correct the force itself. Thus the variance of these forces is higher. Irrespectively of the course of the individual forces,

$F_{Differential}$ is not zero. The reason for this is to be seen in friction occurring in several parts of the mechanical wiring system. Especially the pulleys of the hinge, which are mounted in ball bearings, are likely to cause static and dynamic friction. The redirection of the wires from the muscles towards the pulleys will induce an additional force to the system. In the end, the feedback-based controller offers less undesired torque, based on the more consistent force curves of the individual muscles.

5.5 System integration and experiments

5.5.1 Software architecture

For the pressure control of one PAM, two valves need to be interconnected. With one being the inlet valve, allowing air to travel from the pressure source into the muscle, the second valve works as an exhaust, allowing to deflate the muscle. In order to set a specific pressure in the PAM, the opening times of both valves need to be controlled.

The main control task of the system is undertaken by a microcontroller-board Texas Instruments LM4–F120XL. Containing a fast operating 32 bit microprocessor and various peripherals such as analogue-to-digital (AD)-converter, universal asynchronous receiver and transmitter (UART)-interface and timer modules, the board is suitable for the present control tasks. It is mounted on a distributor printed circuit board (PCB), which contains connection sockets as well as the signal conditioning for all the components. The valve's amplifiers are connected to the digital output pins of a 32 bit timer, capable of fast PWM operation. The load cell's amplifiers as well as the potentiometer are routed to the microcontroller's analogue–digital converter. A serial data transmission to a remote PC can be established through the UART-interface provided. The chip is programmed though the on-board debugging interface via universal serial bus (USB) using the Texas Instruments integrated development environment (IDE) Code Composer Studio.

The measurement of the pressure in the PAMs is an inevitable step for a closed-loop pressure control. The Freescale MPX5700 is capable of measuring absolute pressure up to 700 kPa = 7 bar. The supply voltage is 5 V DC and the analogue output voltage is proportional to the measured pressure. The maximum response time is rated 1 ms, which allows fast operation. The tensile force on the two PAMs needs to be measured. Therefore, two compact in-line load cells Omega LC201 are connected between the PAMs and their respective wire guide. Being capable of measuring forces up to 1334 N (3001 b), their output voltage is rated 2 mV = V with a nominal 10 V DC bridge excitation. The energisation and signal amplification of the load cells is undertaken by two linear DC amplifiers.

Concept of the electronics is shown in Figure 5.12. This involves basically two parts, with the microcontroller software being the first one, and the PC software for the data-evaluation being the second one. The interface between these two parts is the serial data transmission. The software running on the microcontroller is responsible for the main control task. This includes the communication with the established hardware (the orthosis), as well as the communication with the PC for the transmission of the measured data. The PC software on the other side, is designed to receive this data, evaluate it and finally visualise it.

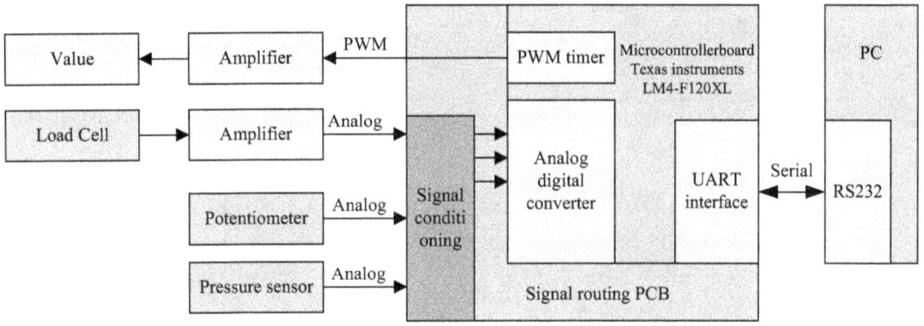

Figure 5.12 Concept of the electronics: a microcontroller undertakes the main control task, sensors are connected through a signal routing PCB

The microcontroller software is running independently and implements the main control task. Besides the calculation of the control algorithm itself, precedent and subsequent hardware interaction is essential to get the sensor feedback as well as to energise the valves. In addition, the transmission of the measured data to the PC is required.

The first step of the actual control loop, is the acquisition of the feedback data. The integrated analogue–digital converter is configured to sample the analogue signals from the sensors and store the resulting values in a volatile array, based on a periodical interrupt. In the next stage, the actual control algorithm, established in the previous chapter, is computed. Additionally, controller output values are transformed into an according duty cycle for the PWM operation. In the next step, the determined values are converted and stored into a buffer array. Each time, the PWM-timer finishes a period an interrupt occurs and the cached values are written into the match register. This procedure prevents the duty cycle to be changed during the period, possibly resulting in undesired behaviour. The final step is the serial data transmission.

In order to transmit the measured data from the device to the PC-system, a serial connection via USB is established. The microcontroller board has a built-in debug interface, which is capable of data conversion between the UART- and the USB-protocol. Sending data through the UART-interface of the controller will thus result in data transmission via the USB-connection to the remote PC, where a virtual COM-port is ready to receive the data.

The PC Interface is designed to illustrate the data measured by the device, in order to allow the assessment of the joint stiffness by the therapist. A screen-shot of the interface is shown in Figure 5.13. If the software is running in the 'receive'-mode, incoming serial data will evoke an interrupt, and the data will be read from the buffer and stored into an organisable list. Located on the left side of the interface, this is where the information about the latest data package is displayed. The individual forces F_1 and F_2, the total force F_T as well as the calculated torque T are illustrated with the help of a bar graph. Underneath, the desired and the actual angle are drawn as a line.

5.5.2 Experiments

At first, measurements without any load will be discussed, afterwards a spring-test will be utilised to simulate elastic behaviour. In order to simulate an analogical

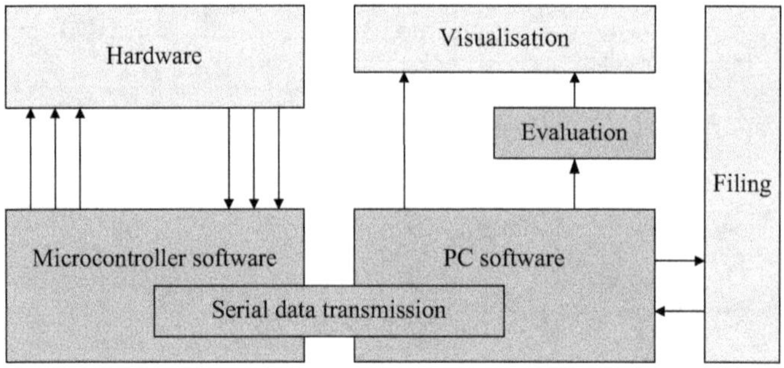

Figure 5.13 Schematic of the developed software architecture, including the hardware-based microcontroller software, serial data transmission and PC software

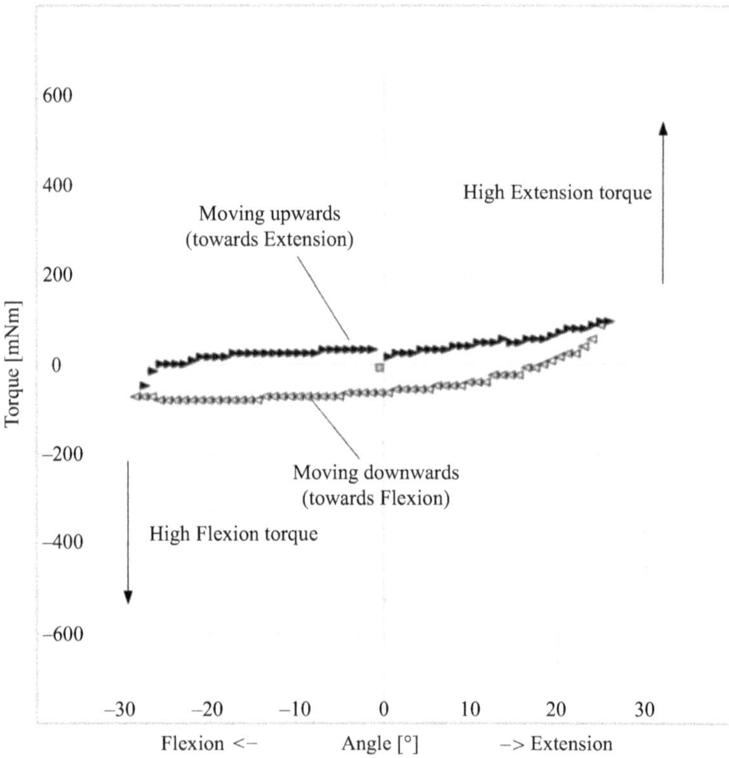

Figure 5.14 Experimental result: reference run without any load attached to the device

behaviour, the device is tested on a healthy wrist, with an impairment being pretended. In a first experiment, the device is tested without being attached to a human wrist. Figure 5.14 shows the processed stiffness graph of this measurement. Similar to the previous result, the measured intrinsic torque of the device shows a maximum

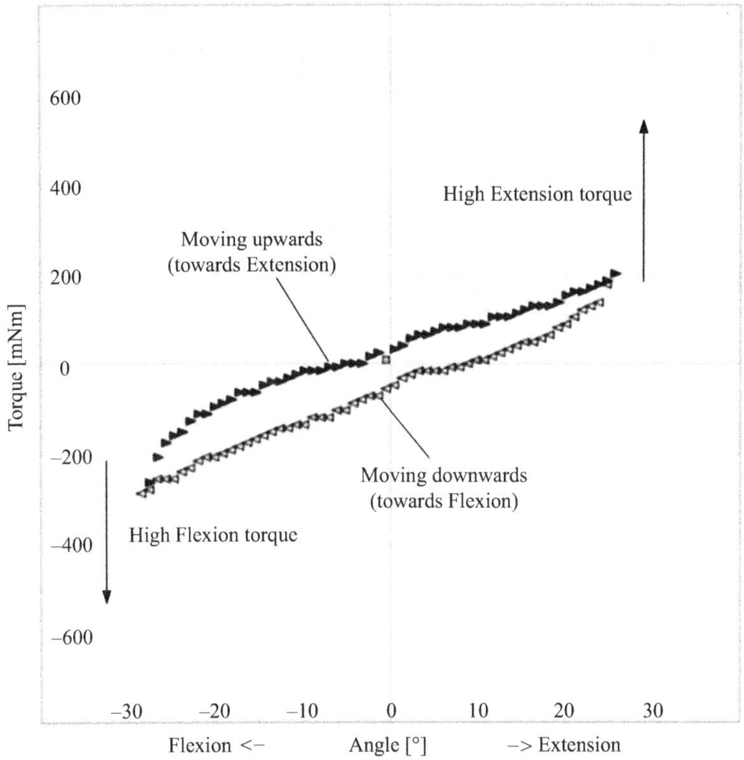

Figure 5.15 Experiment result: a spring attached to the hand rest applies a linear torque to the system

of 0.104 Nm for extension and 0.08 Nm for flexion. The reason for this undesired value is identified as mechanical friction in the device.

Before the device is tested on a human wrist, a spring is utilised to deliver a linear torque to the system. With this method, a purely elastic behaviour can be guaranteed. The device itself is mounted on an aluminium profile, with the spring attached to the end. The point, where the spring is fixed to the profile, is in the centre of the orthosis' rotational axis. The other end of the spring is fixed to the device's hand rest. Located in the neutral position, no torque will be applied to the system. Any given angular displacement, however, will bend the spring and apply a torque, approximately proportional to the angle. The plotted stiffness graph for this experiment can be found in Figure 5.15.

The amount of plastic stiffness (the torque difference between flexion and extension) did not increase notably compared to the reference run, however elastic stiffness was increased. Especially the distal movements for both directions show almost linear behaviour with an estimated stiffness of 6.84 mNm deg^{-1} in extension and 8.54 mNm deg^{-1} in flexion. During proximal movement (towards the centre/ neutral position), the graph shows a similar behaviour to the reference run. This result was expected, since the utilised spring offers elastic behaviour and does not deform plastically. Without the undesirable friction in the mechanical parts, the graph would have the characteristics of a straight line, subtending the origin, with a slope proportional to the spring's suspension rate. The resulting graph for this experiment is thus the superposition of this expected line and the graph of the reference run.

Finally, the device was tested upon interaction with a human wrist. An experiment with an impaired wrist could not have been arranged, thus a healthy wrist is incorporated and the impairment/stiffness is pretended. For this purpose the hand is stretched out and the forearm muscles are tensed up. The result of this experiment is illustrated in Figure 5.16. The graph shows that almost constant stiffness could have been simulated for both movements. The average stiffness for distal extension is 27 mNm deg^{-1}, and the average stiffness for distal flexion is 14 mNm deg^{-1}. If only one of the wrist's antagonists is impaired, or their impairment is not symmetrical, the neutral position of the wrist will shift away from the healthy muscle. Likewise, the measurable stiffness will differ for flexion and extension.

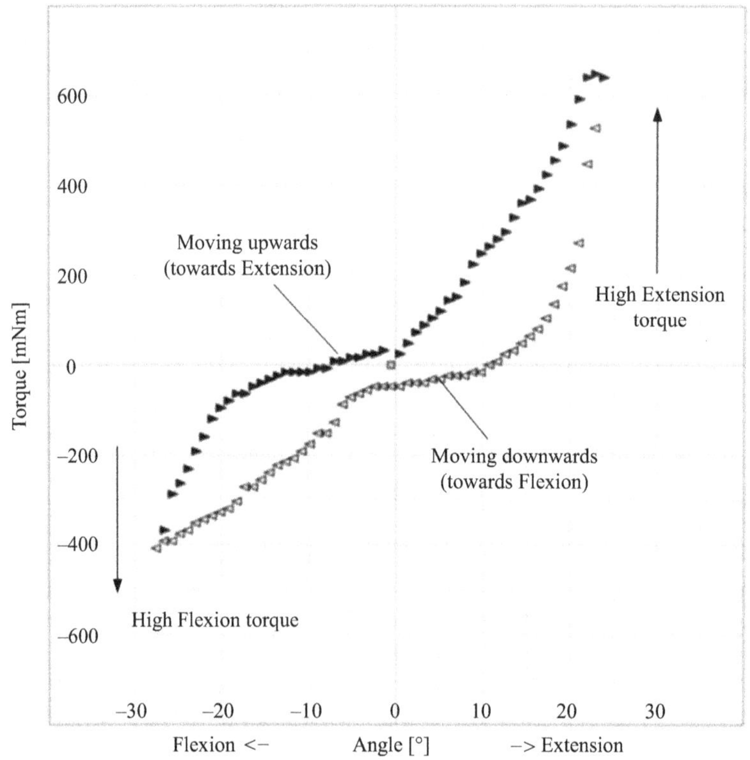

Figure 5.16 Experiment result: a simulated two-sided impairment

5.6 Summary

Within this chapter, the development of a robotic wrist orthosis for the assessment of joint stiffness has been presented. Before a mechanical prototype, incorporating an antagonistic setup of PAMs was developed. One of the main tasks of this research was the investigation of a suitable control system for the proposed actuators. For this reason, two different strategies have been implemented and compared. Finally, a feedback-based closed-loop angle and force controller were chosen to suit the desired system best. Furthermore, the development of a PC interface was demonstrated, designed to illustrate the measured data for further analysis. Experiments have been conducted on the presented system, showing that the desired measurement functionalities could have been achieved. Regarding future works, the most promising update to the present device can be seen in the incorporation of additional degrees of freedom. If it was possible to reduce the friction to a neglectable amount, the measurement accuracy would be improved significantly. Considering the control-part of this project, additional approaches can be investigated in future. There are numerous control strategies that can be adapted to the present antagonistic setup.

References

[1] Krebs HI, Hogan N, Aisen ML, Volpe BT. Robot-aided neurorehabilitation. IEEE Trans Rehabil Eng. 1998;6(1):75–87.

[2] Maciejasz P, Eschweiler J, Gerlach-Hahn K, *et al.* A survey on robotic devices for upper limb rehabilitation. J Neuroeng Rehabil. 2014;11(3).

[3] Wright V, Johns RJ. Quantitative and qualitative analysis of joint stiffness in normal subjects and in patients with connective tissue diseases. Ann Rheum Dis. 1961;20:36–46.

[4] Krebs HI, Palazzolo JJ, Dipietro L, *et al.* Rehabilitation robotics: performance-based progressive robot-assisted therapy. Auton Robots. 2003;15(1):7–20.

[5] Rogers JA. A clear advance in soft actuators. Science. 2013;341(6149):968–69.

[6] Kiguchi K, Iwami K, Yasuda M, Watanabe K, Fukuda T. An exoskeletal robot for human shoulder joint motion assist. IEEE/ASME Trans Mechatronics. 2003;8(1):125–35.

[7] Mirelman A, Bonato P, Deutsch JE. Effects of training with a robot-virtual reality system compared with a robot alone on the gait of individuals after stroke. Stroke. 2009;40(1):169–74.

[8] Lenze EJ, Munin MC, Quear T, *et al.* Significance of poor patient participation in physical and occupational therapy for functional outcome and length of stay. Arch Phys Med Rehabil. 2004;85(10):1599–601.

[9] Rohrer B1, Fasoli S, Krebs HI, *et al.* Movement smoothness changes during stroke recovery. J Neurosci. 2002;22(18):8297–304.

[10] Chou CP, Hannaford B. Measurement and modeling of McKibben pneumatic artificial muscles. IEEE Trans Robot. 1996;12(1):90–102.

[11] Tondu B, Lopez P. Modeling and control of McKibben artificial muscle robot actuators. IEEE Control Syst. 2000;20(2):15–38.

[12] Situm Z, Herceg S. Design and control of a manipulator arm driven by pneumatic muscle actuators. ASME dynamic systems and control conference. ASME: Minneapolis, MN; 2008.

[13] Merkmale. (2013). Fluidic muscle dmsp/mas. [online] Available from https://www.festo.com/cat/de_de/data/doc_de/PDF/DE/DMSP-MAS_DE.PDF. [Assessed May 2017].

[14] Festo AG. (2014). Festo fluidic muscle. [Online]. Available from http://www.festo.com/cms/en_corp/9790.htm. [Assessed May 2017].

[15] Damme MV, Beyl P, Vanderborght B, *et al.* Modeling hysteresis in pleated pneumatic artificial muscles: robotics. IEEE conference on automation and mechatronics. IEEE. Vrije Universiteit Brussel: Brussels, Belgium; 2008. p. 471–76.

Chapter 6

Development of a soft ankle rehabilitation robot

Traditionally ankle injuries are rehabilitated via physiotherapy and however evidence suggests that without sufficient rehabilitation: 44% of people will have future problems [1,2]; ambulation is markedly compromised; re-injury prevalence is high and approximately 38% of people will have recurrent activity limitations affecting their function [3]. Furthermore, during a rehabilitation treatment, cooperative and intensive efforts of therapists and patients are required especially over prolonged sessions [4]. Robotics technology can provide an overdue transformation of rehabilitation clinics from labour-intensive operations to technology-assisted operations as well as a rich stream of data that can facilitate patient diagnosis, customisation of the therapy and maintenance of patient records (at the clinic and at home) [5].

Robot-assisted rehabilitation techniques have been demonstrated to be effective for the treatment of a variety of ankle disabilities [6]. Zhang *et al.* [6] concluded that an optimal ankle rehabilitation robot should be characterised by multiple degrees of freedom (DOFs), compliant actuation, appropriate workspace and actuation torque, aligned rotation centre between the robot and the ankle joint, and the integration of real-time ankle assessment. Zhang *et al.* [7] also proposed suitable assessment techniques that can be well integrated with ankle rehabilitation robots. In this chapter, a new soft ankle rehabilitation robot (SARR) was proposed and developed based on two critical reviews [6,7].

The SARR has three rotational DOFs for ankle dorsiflexion and plantarflexion (DP), inversion and eversion (IE), and adduction and abduction (AA), respectively. These DOFs are actuated by four compliant Festo Fluidic Muscles (FFMs) in parallel. The function of real-time ankle assessment is achieved using some built-in sensors (three magnetic rotary sensors for measuring the position of the end effector and a six-axis load cell for measuring patient–robot interaction). This chapter begins with the structural description of the ankle complex and an overview of existing ankle rehabilitation robots. The design requirements of an ankle rehabilitation robot are then summarised. Following it, the conceptual design of the SARR, kinematics and dynamics are successively presented. Lastly, the construction of the SARR is presented, including the robot structure and its control box.

6.1 Ankle complex

The ankle complex contributes significantly to the function of the lower extremity, and is fundamental to balance, support and propulsion [8,9]. However, it is particularly susceptible to musculoskeletal or neurological injuries. Ankle sprains are very common and mainly involve the overstretching or tearing of tendons and ligaments. There are over 23,000 cases estimated to occur in the United States everyday [10]. In New Zealand, 230,288 new claims and 278,657 active claims related to musculoskeletal ankle injuries were made to the Accident Compensation Corporation from July of 2009 to June of 2014 [11]. Neurological injuries may also cause the ankle to operate inefficiently – a typical example is drop foot following stroke. Based on a report from the American Heart Association, approximately 795,000 people experience stroke in the United States each year [12]. There are an estimated 60,000 stroke survivors living in New Zealand, and many of them have mobility impairments [13].

The ankle complex mainly consists of tibia, fibula, talus and calcaneus [9], as shown in Figure 6.1(a). The tibia and fibula are considered as a unit to simplify the motions of the ankle complex. The ankle joint is the articulation between the tibia-fibula unit and the talus [9]. The sub-talar joint, also known as the talocalcaneal joint, locates between the talus and the calcaneus [9]. The term 'ankle' encompasses both the ankle and sub-talar joints, is primarily rotational and is often described by rotations on three mutually perpendicular anatomical planes. The plane which distinguishes the left and right sides of the body is termed the sagittal plane, where ankle plantarflexion and dorsiflexion exist and occur about the *X*-axis. Ankle IE exist and occur about the *Y*-axis in the frontal plane that divides the body into front and back halves. The transverse plane is perpendicular to the sagittal and the frontal planes, and divides the body into top and bottom

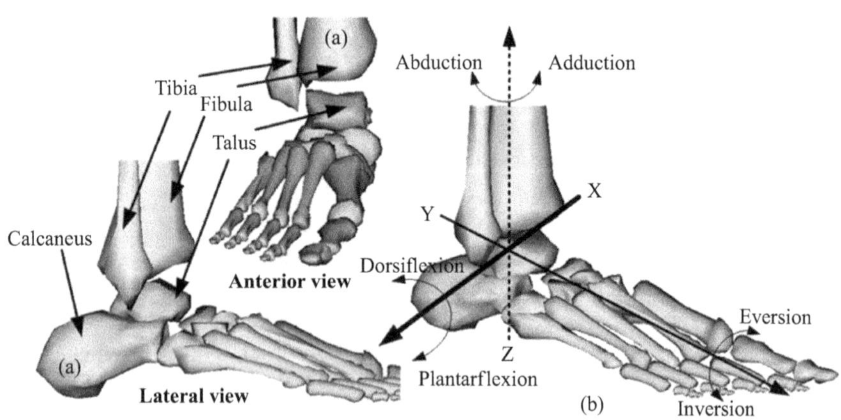

Figure 6.1 (a) Anatomy of the human ankle complex. (b) Rotational motions of the human ankle complex as a three-DOF revolute joint

portions, where ankle AA exist and occur about the *Z*-axis. Rotational motion of the foot in the sagittal plane is termed plantarflexion when the toes are pushed further away from the head and dorsiflexion in the opposing direction. Inversion is used to describe the rotation of the foot on the frontal plane where the inner or medial side of the foot is raised upwards, with eversion being its complementary motion. Adduction is used to describe rotational motion on the transverse plane which moves the toes towards the centre of the body while movement in the contrary direction is termed abduction. These ankle motions are also presented in Figure 6.1(b). In this chapter, as Wu *et al.* [14] recommended, ankle dorsiflexion, adduction and inversion are defined as positive while plantarflexion, abduction and eversion as negative.

6.2 Existing ankle rehabilitation robots

A general rehabilitation program for musculoskeletal ankle injuries involves an acute phase treatment by immobilisation and a sub-acute phase with passive and active range of motion (ROM) and muscle strengthening exercises. Neurological rehabilitation usually includes repetitive, intensive and task-specific movement training to promote motor recovery [15]. However, rehabilitation exercises for both musculoskeletal and neurological ankle disabilities usually require cooperative and intensive efforts from therapists and patients over prolonged sessions [4].

Robot-assisted ankle rehabilitation solutions, as therapeutic adjuncts to facilitate clinical practice, have been actively researched during the past few decades. There are two types of ankle rehabilitation devices. In one group are the wearable exoskeletons aimed at ankle rehabilitation during gait training, such as the MIT Anklebot developed by Roy *et al.* [16]. The other group consists of platform-based robots that conduct pure ankle training [17–21]. Platform-based ankle robots can be further divided into single- DOF and multi-DOF devices. The single-DOF device is mostly actuated by a rotating motor [21], while multi-DOF robots are usually based on parallel mechanisms.

Further and most significantly, parallel ankle rehabilitation robots can be classified in terms of the mechanical structure. Robots actuated from below [19,20] require synergic movement of the lower limb from the patient during the training due to the fact that the rotation centre of the robot does not coincide with the ankle joint. In contrast, the patient can keep his/her lower limb stationary and fully relaxed on devices actuated from above [17,18]. From this point of view, the parallel manipulator wherein the rotation centre of the robot coincides with the ankle joint is more suitable for ankle rehabilitation. To distinguish the structural differences, the actuated-from-below parallel ankle robot is named B-PAR, and the actuated-from-above parallel ankle robot as A-PAR. A hierarchy chart is also presented in Figure 6.2 on the classification of existing ankle rehabilitation robots, and examples are provided in Figure 6.3. This chapter introduces the development of a novel ankle rehabilitation robot based on the A-PAR.

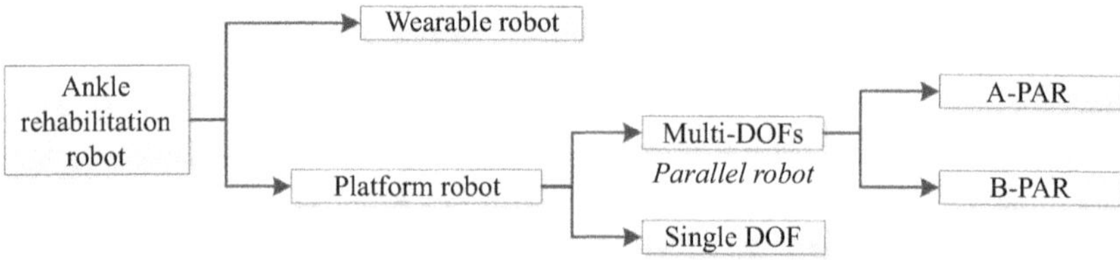

Figure 6.2 Hierarchy chart of existing ankle rehabilitation robots

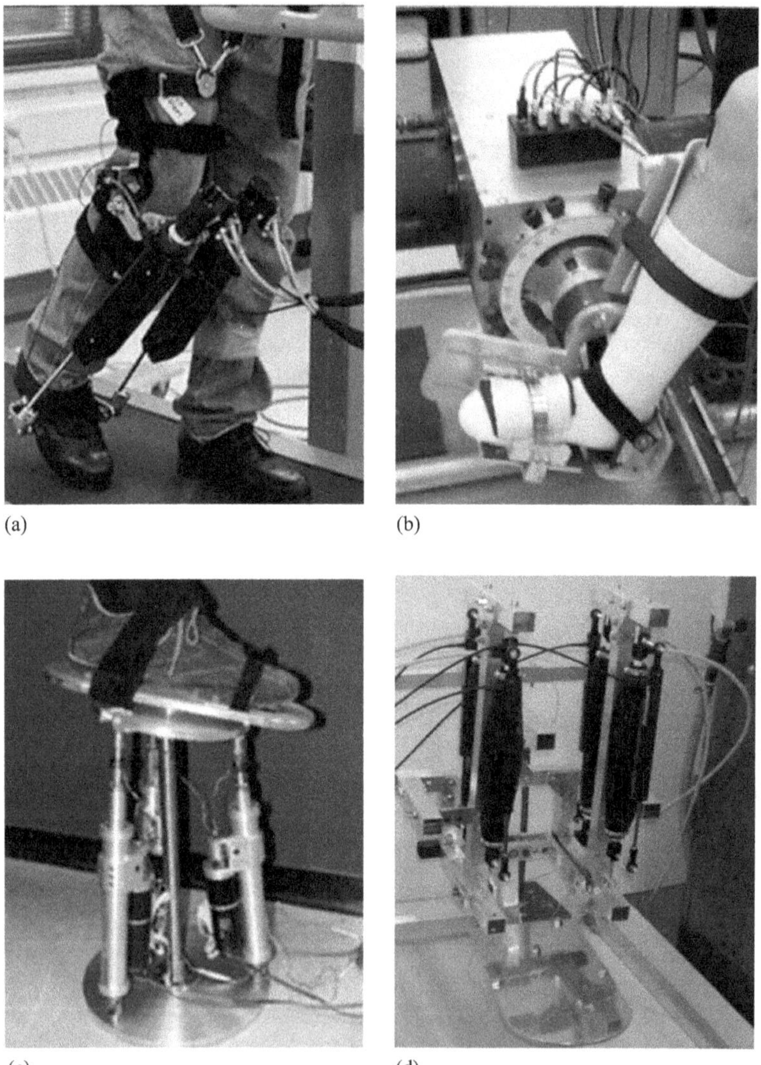

Figure 6.3 Existing ankle rehabilitation robots. (a) The MIT Anklebot [21], (b) an intelligent single-DOF ankle stretching device [16], (c) the B-PAR [19] and (d) the A-PAR [17]

6.3 Design requirements of ankle rehabilitation robots

6.3.1 Ankle range of motion and torque

Ankle ROMs suggested by Siegler *et al.* [8] would be considered as references in designing the workspace of the SARR, as summarised in Table 6.1. It can be seen that the ROMs in different directions are quite different, with around −45° to 25° in the sagittal plane, −15° to 20° in the frontal plane, and −20° to 25° in the transverse plane. However, since the robot is designed to cater for both the left and right ankles, different motion limits in ankle IE and AA will be inverted in the robot coordinate frame when a foot from the different side of the body is placed on the robot. The limits of the required robot workspace on the frontal and transverse planes are therefore symmetric.

Ankle torque also has to be considered on the design of the SARR and play a significant role in the control of the robot, especially for active training strategies. The maximum passive ankle torques obtained from 32 fresh human lower legs are summarised in Table 6.1 [22]. Results from a study [23] with 15 subjects have shown that the required torque to drive an ankle from maximum plantarflexion to maximum dorsiflexion can reach up to 71.7 Nm. This study also evaluated the torques produced by maximum voluntary contraction of the subjects and the corresponding values for DP are 54.4 Nm and 126.0 Nm, respectively. Unfortunately, the maximum torque for ankle adduction/abduction is not available from the above studies. The SARR to be developed in this research was therefore designed by assuming that the maximum AA rotation torques are similar in magnitude to the IE torques. In general, the torque requirements of the SARR are set at 120 Nm for ankle DP, and 60 Nm for ankle IE and AA to meet the general use of human users.

6.3.2 Robot flexibility

An optimal robot for ankle rehabilitation should be able to deliver a subject-specific training with a suitable robotic ROM and torque capacity for a given patient. As can be seen from the systematic review of the effectiveness of

Table 6.1 Typical ROM [8] and maximum passive torque [22] of the human ankles

Type of motion	Ankle motions			Maximum PAT (Nm)
	ROM (deg)	Mean (deg)	SD (deg)	
Dorsiflexion	20.3–29.8	24.68	3.25	34.1 ± 14.5
Plantarflexion	37.6–45.75	40.92	4.32	48.1 ± 12.2
Inversion	14.5–22	16.29	3.88	33.1 ± 16.5
Eversion	10–17	15.87	4.45	40.1 ± 9.2
Adduction	22–36	29.83	7.56	NA
Abduction	15.4 25.9	22.03	5.99	NA

PAT: Passive ankle torque; SD: Standard deviation; NA: Not available.

existing ankle rehabilitation robots in Chapter 2, the robotic training can be passive, active-assist and active ROM exercises, as well as muscle strengthening schemes. Passive ROM exercises involve the robot guiding the patient's foot through the predefined training trajectory when the patient's foot remains relaxed. A relaxed ankle means that the participant does not actively engage with the robot. Active-assist ROM exercises on the other hand require the robot to cooperate with the patient to perform the predefined motion, providing certain assistance based on real-time ankle assessment. Active ROM exercises are conducted completely depending on the patient's intention and ankle disability level, with the robot providing minimal interaction forces and torques. For muscle strength training exercises, the robot should be able to provide certain resistance to the foot according to the joint position and capacity to challenge the patient over time. Taking all into consideration, an optimal ankle rehabilitation robot should be adjustable in providing certain robotic ROM and driven torque to meet a variety of training purposes. It should be noted here that the training mode is categorised on the basis of whether it is conducted under passive or active conditions. It is passive training if without any active contribution from the participant, active training if without any assistance from the robot, or training in a passive-active mode where the robot provides certain assistance but not enough for the training.

6.4 Conceptual design of the soft ankle rehabilitation robot

As what has been discussed in Chapter 1, an actuated-from-A-PAR can be considered as the most suitable mechanism for ankle rehabilitation. The major benefit of such a structure design is that the robotic training can be delivered without requiring synergic movement of the lower limb of the patient due to compatible rotation centres of the robot and the ankle joint. The A-PAR mechanism, considered as a general parallel platform, has several advantages over their serial counterparts. First, the parallel robot has high positioning accuracy since errors in the actuated joints no longer accumulate as in the case of serial robots. Secondly, the robotic end effector is supported by multiple actuators, which allows for a higher load capacity of the mechanism. Lastly, as actuators of a parallel robot are located at the fixed platform instead of the moving links, the total load driven by the robot is also minimised. Taking all into consideration, an A-PAR mechanism will be adopted in this research for ankle rehabilitation.

The proposed A-PAR for ankle therapy is expected to provide three rotational DOFs of ankle training for a variety of rehabilitation applications, and thus actuated in parallel by four FFMs that are intrinsically compliant and lightweight with superb force/weight ratio. The reason why the proposed ankle robot is redundantly actuated is that the FFM can only pull and cannot push, which means that $n+1$ actuators are required to achieve n-DOF motion [24]. Moreover, it was found that few ankle rehabilitation devices can conduct real-time ankle assessment to facilitate the robot control [6]. A variety of assessment techniques have also been reviewed by Zhang *et al.* [7] for use in robot-assisted ankle therapy. To incorporate the function of real-time ankle assessment into the proposed A-PAR, in this research, three magnetic rotary encoders are employed for the position measurement of the robotic end effector and a six-axis load cell for measuring patient–robot interaction. From the viewpoint of functionality, the proposed A-PAR is named the SARR.

A preliminary concept design of the SARR is presented in Figure 6.4. Specifically, the robot consists of an upper platform and a lower platform that are both fixed with respect to the ground. These two platforms are connected with the sliding rail that is further connected with the support leg. Out from the lower platform, there is a three-link serial manipulator whose end is a moving platform. To allow for the measurement of patient–robot interaction, a six-axis load cell is mounted between the end effector/footplate and the moving platform. The SARR can also be adjusted for use on different patients, as shown in Figure 6.5.

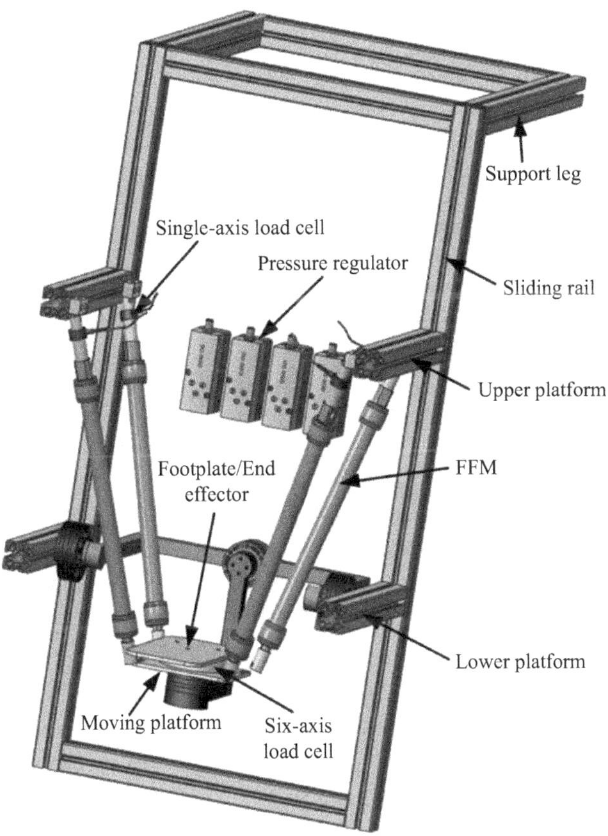

Figure 6.4 The concept design of the proposed SARR

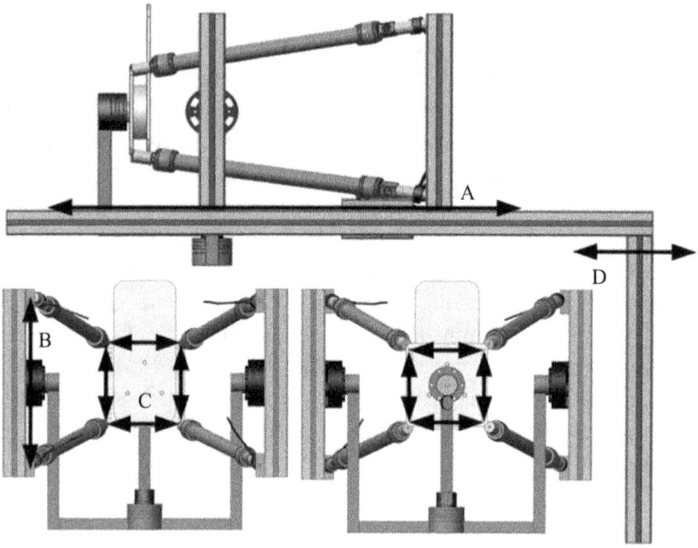

Figure 6.5 The adjustments of the SARR to allow for its use on different patients. (A: the robot body can be horizontally adjusted along the sliding rail to adapt the length of the lower limb of the patient; B and C: the adjustments of the connection location of the FFMs to change the robotic ROM and driven torque; D: the horizontal adjustment of the supporting leg can change the inclination angle of the robot)

6.5 Kinematics of the soft ankle rehabilitation robot

The inverse kinematics of the proposed SARR is easy to be implemented and provides a unique solution of the length of the FFM for a give end effector pose. The kinematic geometry of the proposed SARR is presented in Figure 6.6, where the upper platform is fixed while the lower platform is a moving one that is rigidly attached on a three-DOF serial manipulator. The fixed coordinate frame for the fixed platform is denoted as O_f and the moving one as O_m. Connection points on the fixed and moving platforms are denoted as P_i^f and P_i^m, respectively. Their position vectors P_i^f and P_i^m are defined in (6.1) as well as the position vector $\overrightarrow{O_f O_m}$, where H refers to the distance between the origins of the fixed and moving coordinate frames, h is the Z-axis coordinate of P_i^m in O_m. The position vectors L_i^f of the actuators are described in (6.2), where the rotation transformation matrix of the end effector with respect to the fixed platform using a fixed axis rotation sequence of its

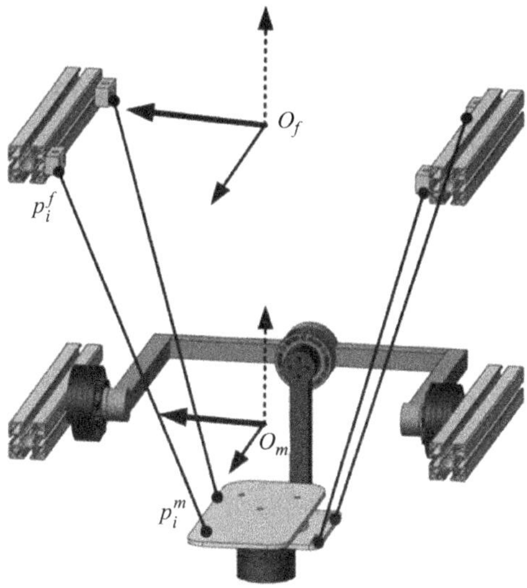

Figure 6.6 Kinematic geometry of the SARR (the heavy lines, fine lines and dotted lines are denoted as x-, y-, and z-axes, respectively, representing the rotation axes of ankle DP, IE and AA)

orientation θ_x, θ_y, θ_z is denoted as R_m^f in (6.3), and R_{12}, R_{13}, R_{22}, and R_{23} are defined in (6.4).

$$\begin{cases} P_i^f = \begin{bmatrix} x_i^f & y_i^f & 0 \end{bmatrix}^T \\ P_i^m = \begin{bmatrix} x_i^m & y_i^m & -h \end{bmatrix}^T \\ O = \overrightarrow{O_f O_m} = \begin{bmatrix} 0 & 0 & -H \end{bmatrix}^T \end{cases} \tag{6.1}$$

$$L_i^f = O + R_m^f P_i^m - P_i^f \tag{6.2}$$

$$R_m^f = \begin{bmatrix} \cos\theta_z \cos\theta_y & R_{12} & R_{13} \\ \sin\theta_z \cos\theta_y & R_{22} & R_{23} \\ -\sin\theta_y & \cos\theta_y \sin\theta_x & \cos\theta_y \cos\theta_x \end{bmatrix} \tag{6.3}$$

$$\begin{cases} R_{12} = -\sin\theta_z \cos\theta_x + \cos\theta_z \sin\theta_y \sin\theta_x \\ R_{13} = \sin\theta_z \sin\theta_x + \cos\theta_z \sin\theta_y \cos\theta_x \\ R_{22} = \cos\theta_z \cos\theta_x + \sin\theta_z \sin\theta_y \sin\theta_x \\ R_{23} = -\cos\theta_z \sin\theta_x + \sin\theta_z \sin\theta_y \cos\theta_x \end{cases} \tag{6.4}$$

The Jacobian matrix is further derived in (6.5), where l_i^f represents the length of the ith actuator [4]. This matrix relates the link velocities and the twist of the end effector, and is extensively used for kinematics and dynamic analysis.

$$J_i = \left(P_i^f \times \frac{L_i^f}{l_i^f}\right)^T \tag{6.5}$$

Note that for any type of Euler angles, the angular velocity is not equal to the rate of change of the Euler angles. The angular velocity relates to the rate of change of the Euler angles as in (6.6), where $\mathrm{E}(\theta_x, \theta_y, \theta_z)$ is defined in (6.7) and its inverse matrix in (6.8) [25]. For later use, (6.6) can be also expressed in (6.9) and its differentiation in (6.10).

$$\omega = E(\theta_x, \theta_y, \theta_z)\begin{bmatrix}\dot{\theta}_x & \dot{\theta}_y & \dot{\theta}_z\end{bmatrix}^T \tag{6.6}$$

$$E(\theta_x, \theta_y, \theta_z) = \begin{bmatrix} \cos\theta_y \cos\theta_z & -\sin\theta_z & 0 \\ \cos\theta_y \sin\theta_z & \cos\theta_z & 0 \\ -\sin\theta_y & 0 & 1 \end{bmatrix} \tag{6.7}$$

$$E^{-1}(\theta_x, \theta_y, \theta_z) = \frac{1}{\cos\theta_y}\begin{bmatrix} \cos\theta_z & \sin\theta_z & 0 \\ -\cos\theta_y \sin\theta_z & \cos\theta_y \cos\theta_z & 0 \\ \sin\theta_y \cos\theta_z & \sin\theta_y \sin\theta_z & \cos\theta_y \end{bmatrix} \tag{6.8}$$

$$\omega = E(\theta)\dot{\theta} \tag{6.9}$$

$$\dot{\omega} = E(\theta)\ddot{\theta} + \dot{E}(\theta)\dot{\theta} \tag{6.10}$$

The kinematic configuration of the SARR used for experiments in this research is summarised in Table 6.2, by which the robotic ROM respectively for ankle dorsiflexion, plantarflexion, inversion, eversion, AA can reach 36°. By considering normal

Table 6.2 The kinematic configuration of the SARR

Robot kinematic configuration	**Absolute values of coordinates (mm)**	
	X	*Y*
Distance between the UP and the LP	445	445
Upper connection points of the FFMs	202.5	140
Lower connection points of the FFMs	65	60

UP: Upper platform; LP: Lower platform; The upper connection points of the FFMs are located at the UP and the lower connection points of the FFMs are located at the moving platform.

ankle ROM presented in Table 6.1, it is found that the SARR provides enough workspace for the training of ankle IE and AA, not for DP. Fortunately, the SARR can generate varying robotic ROMs by changing the connection location of the FFMs. For example, the robotic ROM can reach up to 45° for both ankle DP if the absolute value of the Y coordinates of the lower connection points of the FFMs is changed to 40 mm. Other configurations regarding the adjustment of the posture of the SARR were set to make the robot suitable for a subject with the height of 170 cm.

6.6 Dynamics of the soft ankle rehabilitation robot

The dynamics of the SARR can be described by (6.11) in task space, where $I(\theta)$ is the inertial matrix of the robot, $G(\theta)$ represents the gravity term, $C_f(\theta,\dot{\theta})\dot{\theta}$ is the friction term, $d(\theta,\dot{\theta},\ddot{\theta},t)$ is all other forces acting at the joints, T_r is the torque generated by the robot, and T_a is the ankle torque from the patient or the patient-robot interaction torque.

$$I(\theta)\dot{\omega} + \omega \times I(\theta)\omega + C_f(\theta,\dot{\theta})\dot{\theta} + G(\theta) + d(\theta,\dot{\theta},\ddot{\theta},t) = T_r + T_a \qquad (6.11)$$

Substitute (6.9) and (6.10) into (6.11), as in (6.12), (6.13) can be obtained, where $M(\theta) = I(\theta)E(\theta)$, $C(\theta,\dot{\theta}) = I(\theta)E(\theta) + \tilde{\omega}I(\theta)E(\theta)$, $\tilde{\omega}$ is the skew symmetric matrix of ω. The friction term $C_f(\theta,\dot{\theta})\dot{\theta}$ and other force interventions $d(\theta,\dot{\theta},\ddot{\theta},t)$ are considered very small and ignored in this research, thus the dynamic equation can be simplified into (6.14).

$$\begin{aligned} &I(\theta)\left(E(\theta)\ddot{\theta} + \dot{E}(\theta)\dot{\theta}\right) + \tilde{\omega}I(\theta)E(\theta)\dot{\theta} + C_f(\theta,\dot{\theta})\dot{\theta} + G(\theta) + d(\theta,\dot{\theta},\ddot{\theta},t) \\ &= I(\theta)E(\theta)\ddot{\theta} + \left(I(\theta)\dot{E}(\theta) + \tilde{\omega}I(\theta)E(\theta)\right)\dot{\theta} + C_f(\theta,\dot{\theta})\dot{\theta} + G(\theta) + d(\theta,\dot{\theta},\ddot{\theta},t) \\ &= T_r + T_a \end{aligned} \qquad (6.12)$$

$$M(\theta)\ddot{\theta} + C(\theta,\dot{\theta})\dot{\theta} + C_f(\theta,\dot{\theta})\dot{\theta} + G(\theta) = T_r + T_a \qquad (6.13)$$

$$M(\theta)\ddot{\theta} + C(\theta,\dot{\theta})\dot{\theta} + G(\theta) = T_r + T_a \qquad (6.14)$$

6.6.1 *Ankle force and torque*

Ankle forces and torques denoted as frame a can be computed by transforming the forces and torques measured from a six-axis load cell denoted as frame slc using a force/torque transformation [25], where a and slc represent the 'ankle' and the 'six-axis load cell', respectively. Specifically, ankle forces and torques can be calculated using (6.15) and (6.16), where ${}^{a}_{slc}R$ is a 3×3 rotation matrix from frame a to frame slc, $P^{a}_{slc} \times {}^{a}_{slc}R$ is a 3×3 skew matrix from frame a to frame slc.

$$\begin{bmatrix} F_a^{3\times1} \\ T_a^{3\times1} \end{bmatrix} = \begin{pmatrix} {}^{a}_{slc}R & 0_{3\times3} \\ P^{a}_{slc} \times {}^{a}_{slc}R & {}^{a}_{slc}R \end{pmatrix} \begin{bmatrix} F_{slc}^{3\times1} \\ T_{slc}^{3\times1} \end{bmatrix} \qquad (6.15)$$

Table 6.3 Inertial parameters of the three-link moving platform

No.	Link	Mass (kg)	COM (mm)	IT at CS_i (Tonne mm^2)
1	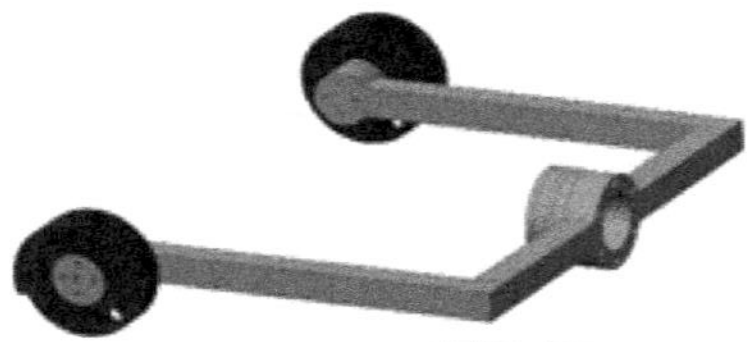	1.61	(0,0,–122)	$\begin{bmatrix} 74.8 & 0 & 0 \\ 0 & 41.5 & 0 \\ 0 & 0 & 33.7 \end{bmatrix}$
2	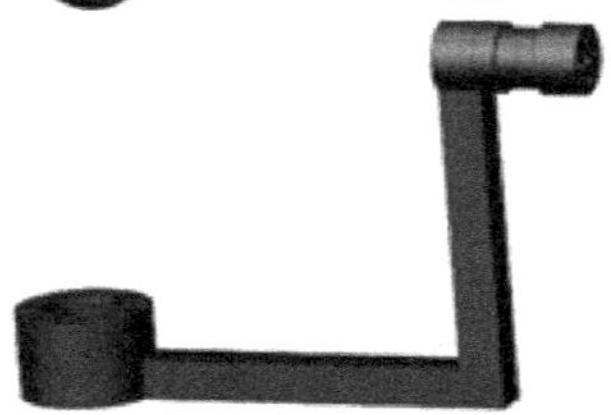	1.01	(0,–133,–88)	$\begin{bmatrix} 40.7 & 0 & 0 \\ 0 & 13.7 & -6.1 \\ 0 & -6.1 & 27.3 \end{bmatrix}$
3	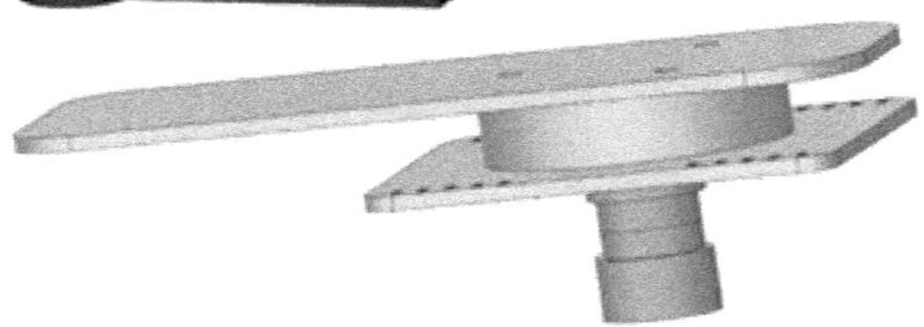	1.76	(0,10.5,–119)	$\begin{bmatrix} 29.4 & 0 & 0 \\ 0 & 27 & 1.8 \\ 0 & 1.8 & 5 \end{bmatrix}$

COM: Centre of mass; IT: Inertia tensor; CS_i: The coordinate system used in the Creo model of the ith link.

$$P_{slc}^{a} = \begin{bmatrix} 0 & -p_z & p_y \\ p_z & 0 & -p_x \\ -p_y & p_x & 0 \end{bmatrix} \tag{6.16}$$

6.6.2 Inertial property of the moving unit

The knowledge of the inertial property of the moving unit is crucial to the motion control of the SARR. As shown in Figure 6.4, the moving unit consists of the three-link manipulator, the six-axis load cell and the end effector, of which the three-link serial manipulator are for ankle DP, IE and AA, respectively. These inertial parameters of the moving unit mainly include the mass, centre of mass (COM) and inertia tensor for each link. They were obtained from the Creo model presented in Figure 4.1 and summarised in Table 6.3. The global inertial tensor and gravitational effect of the moving unit can be calculated using (6.17) and (6.18), respectively, where I is the global inertial tensor, I_i is the inertial tensor of the ith link, R_i is the rotation matrix that relates the ith link coordinate frame to the global frame, O_i^{com} represents the coordinate of the COM of the ith link, and m_i is the mass of the ith link. The global coordinate system is located at the rotation centre of the end effector with the X-axis pointing to the right, the Y-axis pointing forwards and the Z-axis pointing upwards with respect to patients.

$$I(\theta_x, \theta_y, \theta_z) = \sum_{i=1}^{3} I_i = R_i I_i R_i^T \tag{6.17}$$

$$G(\theta_x, \theta_y, \theta_z) = \sum_{i=1}^{3} G_i = R_i O_i^{com} m_i \tag{6.18}$$

To derive the global inertia and gravitational effect of the moving unit, the Denavit–Hartenberg transformation matrix A_i^{i-1} has to be obtained as in (6.19) to relate the ith coordinate system to the $(i-1)$th one. Since only rotations exist for the moving unit, $A_i^{i\;1}$ can be simplified into R_i^{i-1}, as expressed in (6.20). However, four parameters α_i, a_i, d_i, and θ_i have to be identified before deriving the rotation matrix R_i^{i-1}, which requires $(n+1)$ coordinate systems to be defined for an n-DOF manipulator [25]. Although the origins of the coordinate systems of link 0, link 1, link 2, link 3 and the global frame intersect at the centre of rotation of the end effector, they are placed separately in Figure 6.7 to facilitate the description of defined coordinate frames. The specific values of the four parameters are presented in Table 6.4.

$$A_i^{i-1} = \begin{bmatrix} \cos\theta_i & -\cos\alpha_i \sin\theta_i & \sin\alpha_i \sin\theta_i & a_i \cos\theta_i \\ \sin\theta_i & \cos\alpha_i \cos\theta_i & -\sin\alpha_i \cos\theta_i & a_i \sin\theta_i \\ 0 & \sin\alpha_i & \cos\alpha_i & d_i \\ 0 & 0 & 0 & 1 \end{bmatrix} \tag{6.19}$$

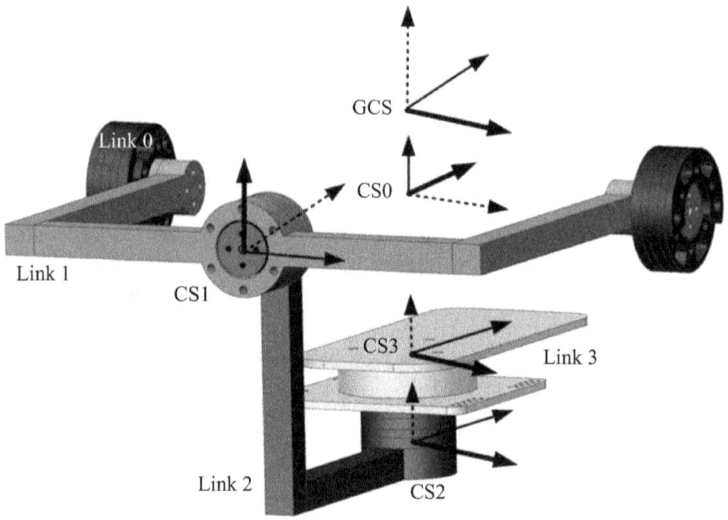

Figure 6.7 Coordinate systems of the moving unit of the SARR (the heavy lines, fine lines and dotted lines represent X-, Y-, and Z-axes, respectively)

Table 6.4 Four parameters used to relate different coordinate systems

Coordinate system	α_i	a_i	d_i	θ_i
Global	$\pi/2$	0	0	$\pi/2$
1	$\pi/2$	0	0	$\frac{\pi}{2}+\theta_x$
2	$\pi/2$	0	0	$\frac{\pi}{2}+\theta_y$
3	0	0	0	θ_z

$$R_i^{i-1} = \begin{bmatrix} \cos\theta_i & -\cos\alpha_i \sin\theta_i & \sin\alpha_i \sin\theta_i \\ \sin\theta_i & \cos\alpha_i \cos\theta_i & -\sin\alpha_i \cos\theta_i \\ 0 & \sin\alpha_i & \cos\alpha_i \end{bmatrix} \tag{6.20}$$

6.6.3 Force distribution

Cable-driven robots may lose controllability if certain cables are not in tension during the robotic operation [26]. The SARR employs four FFMs that work similar to cables along an actuator, and thus the determination of feasible force distribution of this SARR is required for a given robot driven torque T_r. In this study, two potential force distribution methods are compared and analysed.

Pott *et al.* [27] proposed a closed-form force distribution scheme that is shown in (6.21), where $A = J^T$, $A^+ = A^T(AA^T)^{-1}$, T_r represents the robot torque in task space generated by four FFMs, f is the mean feasible force distribution and can be defined according to specific applications. The distributed forces are continuous along trajectories and differentiable at most of the points, and the computational efforts are also strictly bounded and small even for large numbers of wires.

$$F = f - A^+(T_r + Af) \tag{6.21}$$

The other method is an analytic-iterative force distribution technique proposed by Taghirad *et al.* [28]. This method is formulated into an optimisation problem (6.22), where $B = I - A^+A$, and then handled by the Karush-Kuhn-Tucker theorem to draw an analytic-iterative solution.

$$\begin{cases} \min\ f(y) = (F_o + By)^T(F_o + By) \\ \text{Subject to } F_{min} - (F_o + By) \leq 0 \end{cases} \tag{6.22}$$

Since this approach adopted an optimisation search algorithm, the absolute sum of link forces can be smaller than that of the closed-form method, which means that the robot implemented using the analytic-iterative method can achieve a predefined motion with less energy consumption.

The closed-form method and the analytic-iterative one are evaluated by simulation in MATLAB. Both methods are applied to the developed SARR to achieve the same robot-driven torque. To compare the force distribution performance of these two methods, three cases with different angular trajectories and torques are analysed for each method. Case 1: the angular trajectory in task space is defined as: $\theta_x = 0.3\sin(2\pi ft), \theta_y = 0, \theta_z = 0$, and the defined interaction torque is defined as: $M_x = 10$ Nm, $M_y = 0, M_z = 0$; Case 2: the angular trajectory in task space is defined as: $\theta_x = 0.3\sin(2\pi ft), \theta_y = 0.2\sin(2\pi ft), \theta_z = 0$, and the defined interaction torque is defined as: $M_x = 10$ Nm, $M_y = 0, M_z = 0$; Case 3: the angular trajectory in task space is defined as: $\theta_x = 0.3\sin(2\pi ft), \theta_y = 0.2\sin(2\pi ft), \theta_z = 0$ and the defined interaction torque is defined as: $M_x = t$ Nm, $M_y = 0, M_z = 0$.

The calculated force results of each link are presented in Figure 6.8. It is found that both methods can achieve satisfied force distribution results with appropriate link force levels for a given interaction torque along a predefined angular trajectory. However, these two methods present significantly different force distributions due to their inherent characteristics. For the closed-form method, the force results largely depend on the predefined mean force parameter f (set at 70 N in the simulation). With the increase of the required torque in task space, the force distributed to each link increased significantly and even result in large negative force for links 3 and 4 (Case 3), which is undesired for cable-driven robots. For the analytic-iterative approach, however, the link forces are generated based on the predefined minimal force $f_{\min}$ (set at 10 N in the simulation). Thus, all the forces are positive and every cable can be kept in tension, which is very important for cable-driven manipulators. Meanwhile, as the analytic-iterative approach is developed with an optimisation search algorithm,

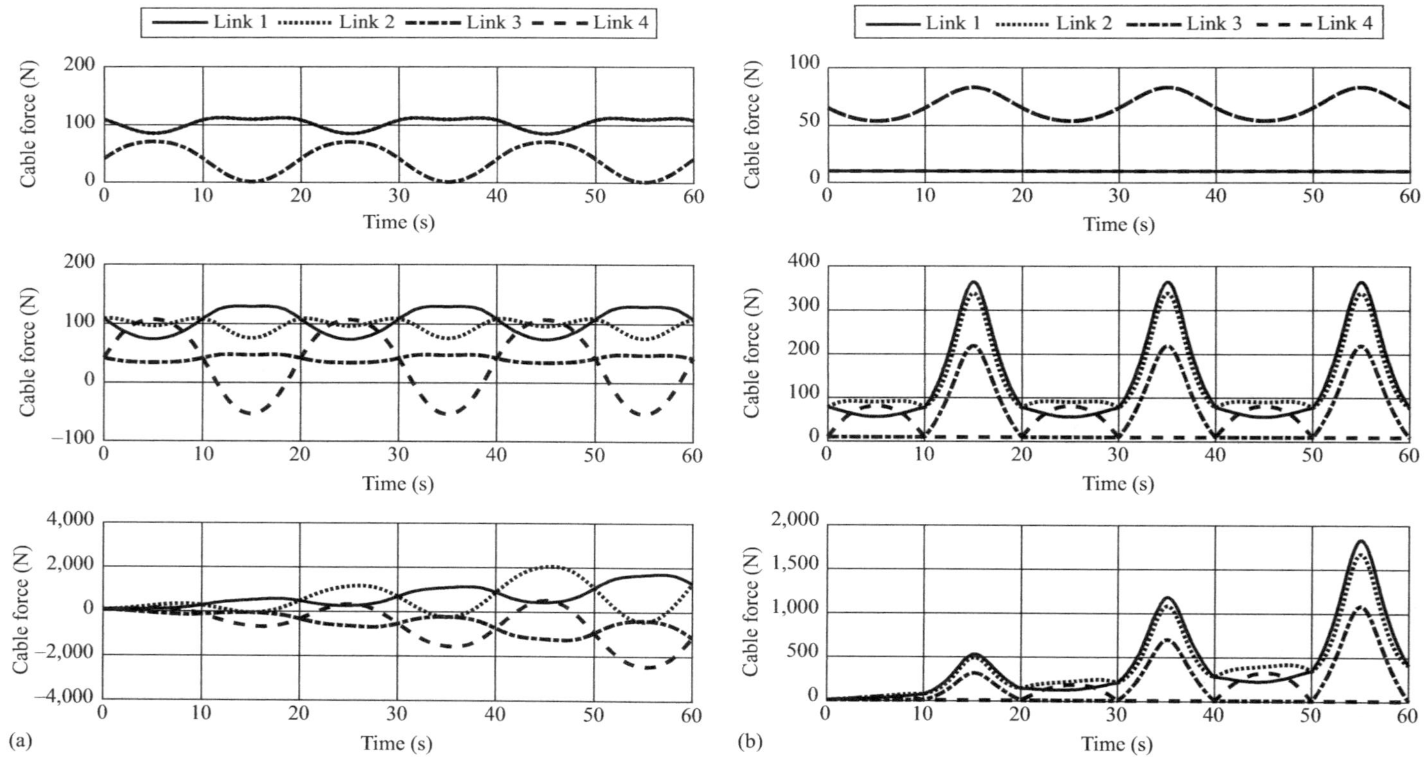

Figure 6.8 *Force distribution results of (a) the closed-form method $F_{min} = 50$ N, $F_{max} = 100$ N and (b) the analytic-iterative method $F_{min} = 10$ N. For each figure, the three plots from top to bottom represent the results of Cases 1, 2 and 3, respectively*

the absolute sum of link forces is much smaller than that of closed-form results, which means the robot controlled by analytic-iterative method is able to reach the required movement with much less energy consumption. On the other hand, the closed-form approach has less computation burden and numerical efforts compared to analytic-iterative approach. The calculation time of the closed-form method for 3,000 samples is 0.1926, 0.1905 and 0.1875 s for Cases 1, 2 and 3, respectively, while the counterparts of the analytic-iterative method are 1.1647, 1.3198 and 1.3274 s. Hence, the closed-form method is more suitable for robots with strict time bound. It should be noted in the analytic-iterative method that the time for each sample is less than 0.0005 s indicating that this scheme can meet the real-time calculation requirement for the control of SARR (the control loop operates with a period of 0.02 s).

Three cases were compared and analysed with different angular positions and drive torques. These include (a) closed-form method, (b) analytic-iterative method. Figure 6.8 shows the results where both methods calculate continuous force distribution. These two schemes also meet the real-time requirement in the control system of the SARR, although the analytic-iterative method has a higher computation burden due to a maximum of 16 iterations. In the simulation of Figure 6.8(b), the computation time for 3,000 samples in Cases 1, 2 and 3 is 1.1647, 1.3198, and 1.3274 s respectively. The time for each sample is less than 0.0005 s indicating that the analytic-iterative scheme can meet the real-time requirement (because the control loop operates with a period of 0.02 s). However, these two methods have significant differences that may affect the robotic training safety. For the closed-form method, the calculated force largely depends on the predefined mean force determined by the desired joint torque. As the desired torque increases, the force distributed to each actuator increases accordingly and can result in negative values, potentially reducing robot controllability (Figure 6.8(a)). For the analytic-iterative method, the actuator forces are generated based on a predefined minimal force, so that all distributed forces are positive with their sum optimised to a minimum. Therefore, the analytic-iterative force distribution scheme was adopted.

6.6.4 Festo fluidic muscle modelling

During the past few decades, there has been an increasing use of PAMs in the industrial and medical areas due to their advantages such as low power-to-weight ratio, high strength and lightweight [29]. The demand for a simple but physically meaningful model for control purposes is rising [30]. Based on the summary by Tri *et al.* [30], available models are mostly approximations and no model has achieved accurate contraction force prediction, which was also stated by Inoue [31] ‘it is nearly impossible to create a precise mathematic model’.

A recent survey conducted by Kelasidi *et al.* [32] summarised geometrical models of PAMs and demonstrated that Chou and Hannaford [33] model and Tondu and Lopez [34] model have been widely used for control applications. Chou and Hannaford [33] method is a static model based on trigonometric analysis but with assumptions like cylindrical shape and frictionless contact. Tondu and Lopez [34] added a dry friction term to the contraction force to improve the modelling response, however, which is limited to the assumption that hysteresis is caused by only the thread-on-thread dry friction between cords. Davis and Caldwell [35] developed a mathematical model to capture hysteresis due to friction between braid strands during muscle operation and verified it experimentally. However, these models give rise to complex problems in terms of control, since some parameters are difficult to be quantified. Some more complex models have been also developed recently. Andrikopoulos *et al.* [36] developed a dynamic model of PAMs based on a switch system approach. Xing *et al.* [37] proposed an Echo State Network as a basis to implement PAMs' modelling and control, and demonstrated that the proposed procedure has better dynamic performance and stronger robustness over other classical approaches.

The above-mentioned models were developed based on McKibben PAMs. In addition to conventional advantages (lightweight and intrinsically compliant behaviour) of McKibben PAMs, FFMs can generate a larger contraction force with the same size and contraction length, which makes them increasingly popular in robotic devices. FFMs follow well with the McKibben principle, and consists of a flexible cylindrical isotropic rubber tube with two fixed connection flanges at its ends. In between the rubber tube is a shell of non-contractive fibres. When the muscle is inflated with compressed air, it widens and a contraction force arises as well as a contraction movement in the longitudinal direction. The muscle can only generate contraction forces with its maximum at the beginning of the contraction and decreases as the contraction increases. Similar to McKibben PAMs, the FFM is highly nonlinear and its modelling is required for control purposes. Kerscher *et al.* [38] developed a dynamic model of fluidic muscles based on Tondu and Lopez [34] model and their own experience, but this method predicts less force in lower pressure range (≤ 2.5 bar). Hosovsky and Balara [39] modelled Festo MAS-20 using an adaptive neuro-fuzzy inference system with data points extracted from the characteristic supplied by the manufacturer. Szepe [40] conducted 340 measurements on a testbed using the Festo DMSP-20-400 type artificial muscle and modelled its static contraction force using an exponential function with six unknown parameters with low root-mean-square error (RMSE) in the whole operating range. The benefit of using this function is that only six unknown parameters result in fast and reliable parameter search. Furthermore, its inverse function is capable of expressing the pressure required to maintain a given contraction length and a force. This property of the function is necessary in an open-loop control system or generally, when it is not possible to take direct measurements of all three variables (pressure, length/strain and force), one of them can be expressed from the others. With reduced number of parameters, another approximation of the generated force of the FFM (Festo DMSP-20-400) was obtained by Sarosi [41] with the hysteresis considered.

Robot-assisted ankle rehabilitation exercises are considered to be slow and in quasi-static environment. Therefore, the function approximation proposed by Sarosi [41] is adopted in this research to derive the FFM contraction force based on

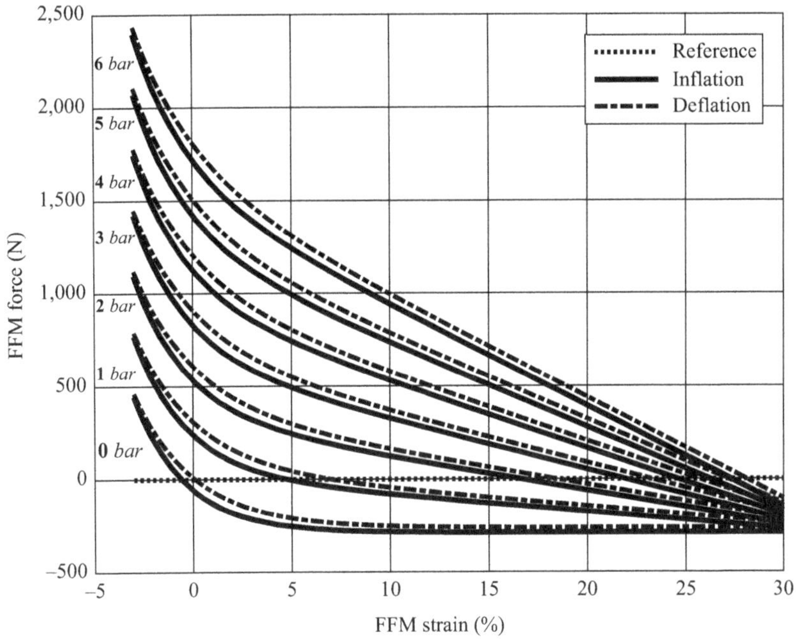

*Figure 6.9 Static model of the FFM (DMSP-20-400N-RM-RM) for certain separate pressure values (FFM strain = 100*FFM contraction length/400)*

its pressure and contraction strain, as shown in (6.23). These five parameters were experimentally obtained by changing the muscle length when the contraction force and pressure were recorded. Specifically, for the inflation process of the DMSP-20-400-RM-RM $a = 232.89$, $b = -38.32$, $c = -904.01$, $d = 294.86$ and $e = -289.06$, while for deflation $a = 272.70$, $b = -32.58$, $c = -908.24$, $d = 298.83$ and $e = -262.85$. The FFM strain is expressed as the ratio of the contraction length to the initial length. To facilitate its use in this research, a modified expression (6.24) is derived to calculate the desired FFM pressure based on the measured force and the desired strain. The specific relation among these three variables (force, pressure and strain) is also plotted in Figure 6.9 for certain discrete pressure values. With the hysteresis loop neglected, the corresponding relation for continuous pressure is shown in Figure 6.10.

$$F(p,k) = (p + a)e^{bk} + cpk + dp + e \tag{6.23}$$

$$p(k,F) = \frac{F - ae^{bk} - e}{e^{bk} + ck + d} \tag{6.24}$$

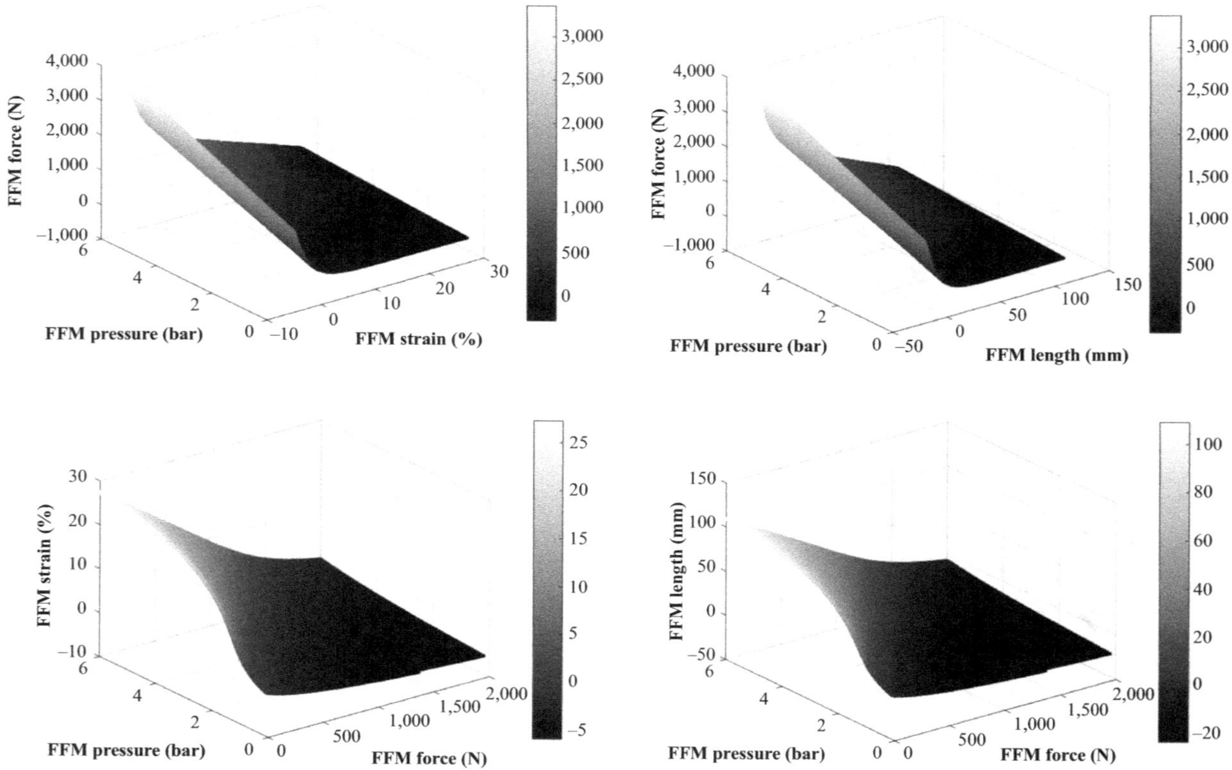

Figure 6.10 Static model of the FFM (DMSP-20-400N-RM-RM) for continuous pressure (FFM length = FFM strain × 400)

6.7 Construction of the soft ankle rehabilitation robot

The physical picture of the developed SARR is presented in Figure 6.11. The bill of materials needed for this SARR can be found in Appendix A. The SARR, as discussed earlier in this chapter, has three rotational DOFs that are actuated in parallel by four FFMs (Festo DMSP-20-400N). These three DOFs are for ankle DP, IE and AA. This robotic design makes the SARR have bio-inspired design by mimicking the configuration and actuation of the ankle joint by natural muscles.

The control box of the SARR is shown in Figure 6.13 with all hardware included. To actuate the SARR, four proportional pressure regulators (Festo VPPM-6L-L-1-G18-0L6H) are used to control the pressure of the FFMs. The sensing components include three magnetic rotary encoders (ams AS5048A) for measuring angular positions of the robotic end effector, four single-axis load cells (Futek LCM 300) together with four amplifiers (Futek CSG110) for measuring contraction forces of FFMs and a six-axis load cell (SRI M3715C) for measuring robot–patient interaction torque.

These electronic components including the actuation system and the sensing unit communicate with the embedded controller (NI Compact RIO-9022) through three independent modules (NI 9401, NI 9205 and NI 9263) for digital input/output (DI/O), analogue input (AI) and analogue output (AO), respectively. The six-axis load cell communicates with the controller through the RS232 port using a customised interface box (SRI M8125). The control box is presented in Figure 6.13 and the connection block diagram in Figure 6.12. To ensure the training safety of the patient, an emergency stop button is also set to prevent any further movement of the FFMs.

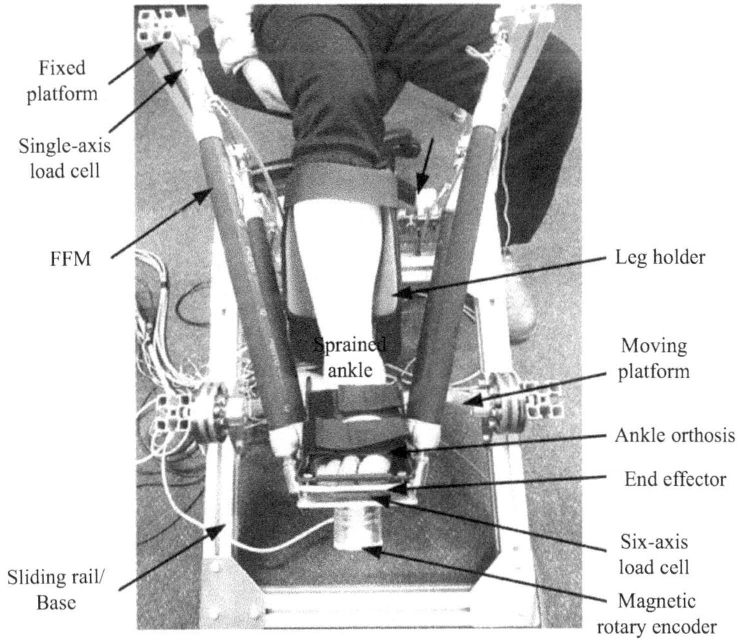

Figure 6.11 The intrinsically compliant SARR

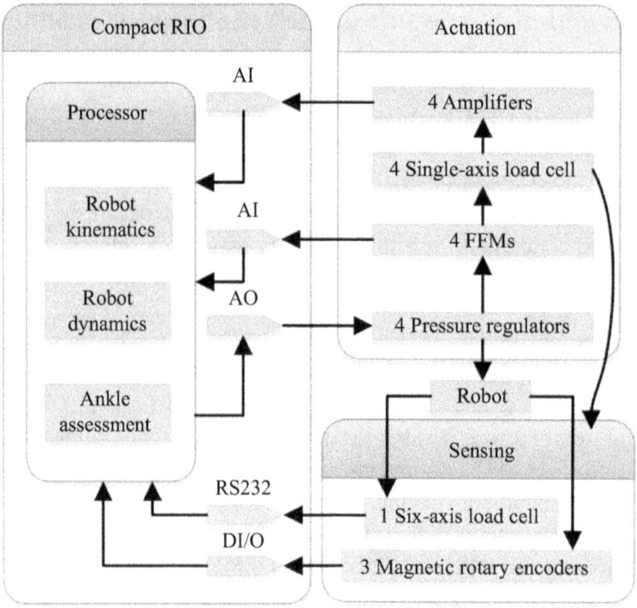

Figure 6.12 The connection block diagram of the control box of the SARR

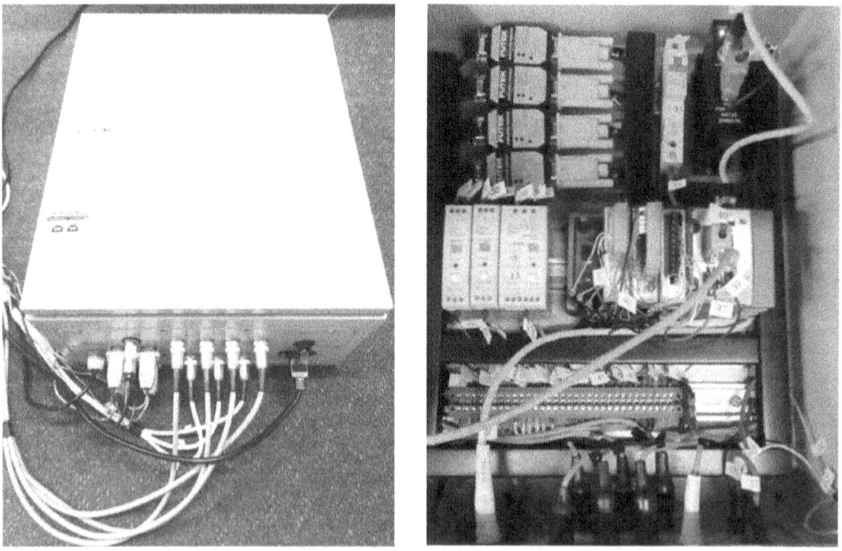

(a) (b)

Figure 6.13 The control box of the SARR. (a) The physical picture of the outside of the control box and (b) the physical picture of the inside of the control box

6.8 Summary

This chapter presents the development of an intrinsically compliant SARR. Specifically, it involves the robot kinematics and dynamics, the FFM modelling, the force distribution that distributes a given robot torque of the task space into individual FFM force of the joint space, the calculation of ankle forces and torques, and the construction of the SARR. These provide the basis for the implementation of advanced interactive training schemes.

In general, the SARR devised from two literature reviews has advantages over other rehabilitation devices, including intrinsically compliant actuation system, compatible robot structure with aligned rotation centre between the robot and the human ankle, three DOFs for three-dimensional rehabilitation exercises, and the integration of real-time ankle assessment. By using the SARR, robot-assisted ankle rehabilitation can be safer, more comprehensive and effective.

Appendix A Bill of materials

Materials including mechanical parts and electronic components for the SARR came from many sources. Some of mechanical parts were fabricated in the Machine Shop in the Department of Mechanical Engineering, University of Auckland; some of them were made using 3D printer. Following is the list of main electronic components that are for actuation, position/force sensing, and data communication/acquisition, respectively.

Functionality	Parts		Specification	Quantity
Actuation	Fluidic muscle		FESTO DMSP-20-400N-RM-CM	4
	Pressure regulator		FESTO VPPM-6L-L-1-G18-0L6H	4
Position sensing	Rotary encoder		AS5048A	3
Force sensing	Single-axis	Load cell	Futck LCM 300 250lb	4
		Amplifier	Futek CSG110	4
	Six-axis	Load cell	SRI M3715C	1
		Interface box	SRI M8125	1
Control	Real-time controller		NI Compact RIO-9022	1
	Digital input/output module		NI-9401	1
	Analogue input module		NI-9205	1
	Analogue output module		NI-9263	1

References

[1] Dettori J, Basmania C. Early ankle mobilization, part II: a one-year follow-up of acute, lateral ankle sprains (a randomized clinical trial). Mil Med. 1994;159(1):15–20.

[2] Trevino S, Davis P, Hecht P. Management of acute and chronic lateral ligament injuries of the ankle. Orthop Clin North Am. 1994;25(1):1–16.

[3] Braun BL. Effects of ankle sprain in a general clinic population 6 to 18 months after medical evaluation. Arch Fam Med. 1999;8(2):143–48.

[4] Jamwal PK. Design analysis and control of wearable ankle rehabilitation robot [PHD thesis]. Auckland, New Zealand: The University of Auckland; 2011.

[5] Krebs HI, Palazzolo JJ, Dipietro L, *et al.* Rehabilitation robotics: performance-based progressive robot-assisted therapy. Auton Robot. 2003;15(1):7–20.

[6] Zhang M, Davies TC, Xie S. Effectiveness of robot-assisted therapy on ankle rehabilitation – a systematic review. J Neuroeng Rehabil. 2013;10:30.

[7] Zhang M, Davies TC, Zhang Y, Xie S. Reviewing effectiveness of ankle assessment techniques for use in robot-assisted therapy. J Rehabil Res Dev. 2014;51(4):517–34.

[8] Siegler S, Chen J, Schneck CD. The three-dimensional kinematics and flexibility characteristics of the human ankle and subtalar joints—Part I: kinematics. J Biomech Eng. 1988;110(4):364–73.

[9] Sammarco GJ. Rehabilitation of the foot and ankle. Missouri, USA: Mosby-Year Book; 1995.

[10] Hertel J. Functional anatomy, pathomechanics, and pathophysiology of lateral ankle instability. J Athl Training. 2002;37(4):364–75.

[11] Injury Statistics Tool: Accident Compensation Corporation. Available from <http://www.acc.co.nz/about-acc/statistics/injury-statistics/index.htm#/>; 2014 [accessed 03.05.2017].

[12] Mozaffafian D, Benjamin EJ, Go AS, *et al.* Heart disease and stroke statistics—2015 Update. Circulation. 2015;131:e29–e322.

[13] Facts about stroke in New Zealand: Stroke Foundation of New Zealand; Available from <http://www.stroke.org.nz/stroke-facts-and-fallacies>; 2014 [accessed 03.05.2017].

[14] Wu G, Siegler S, Allard P, *et al.* ISB recommendation on definitions of joint coordinate system of various joints for the reporting of human joint motion—Part I: ankle, hip, and spine. J Biomech. 2002;35(4):543–48.

[15] Takeuchi N, Izumi SI. Rehabilitation with poststroke motor recovery: a review with a focus on neural plasticity. Stroke Res Treat. 2013;2013:128641.

[16] Roy A, Krebs HI, Williams DJ, *et al.* Robot-aided neurorehabilitation: a novel robot for ankle rehabilitation. IEEE Trans Robot. 2009;25(3): 569–82.

[17] Jamwal PK, Xie SQ, Hussain S, Parsons JG. An adaptive wearable parallel robot for ankle injury treatments. IEEE/ASME Trans Mechatronics. 2014; 19(1):64–75.

[18] Tsoi YH, Xie SQ, Graham AE. Design, modeling and control of an ankle rehabilitation robot. Stud Comput Intell. 2009;177:377–99.

[19] Saglia JA, Tsagarakis NG, Dai JS, Caldwell DG. A high-performance redundantly actuated parallel mechanism for ankle rehabilitation. Int J Robot Res. 2009;28(9):1216–27.

[20] Girone M, Burdea G, Bouzit M, Popescu V, Deutsch JE. A stewart platform-based system for ankle telerehabilitation. Auton Robot. 2001;10(2):203–12.

[21] Zhang L-Q, Chung SG, Bai Z, *et al.* Intelligent stretching of ankle joints with contracture spasticity. IEEE Trans Neural Syst Rehabil. 2002;10(3): 149–57.

[22] Parenteau CS, Viano DC, Petit PY. Biomechanical properties of human cadaveric ankle-subtalar joints in quasi-static loading. J Biomech Eng. 1998;120(1):105–11.

[23] Kearney RE, Weiss PL, Marie R. System identification of human ankle dynamics-intersubjectvariability and intrasubjectreliability. Clin Biomech. 1990;5(4):205–17.

[24] Pusey J, Fattah A, Agrawal S, Messina E. Design and workspace analysis of a 6–6 cable-suspended parallel robot. Mech Mach Theory. 2004;39(7): 761–78.

[25] Craig JJ. Introduction to robotics: mechanics and control. 3rd ed. Philadelphia, PA: Prentice-Hall; 2005.

[26] Hassan M, Khajepour A. Analysis of bounded cable tensions in cable-actuated parallel manipulators. IEEE Trans Robot. 2011;27(5):891–900.

[27] Pott A, Bruckmann T, Mikelsons L. Closed-form force distribution for parallel wire robots. In: Kecskeméthy A, Müller A, editors. Computational kinematics. Berlin Heidelberg: Springer; 2009. pp. 25–34.

[28] Taghirad HD, Bedoustani YB. An analytic-iterative redundancy resolution scheme for cable-driven redundant parallel manipulators. IEEE Trans Robot. 2011;27(6):1137–43.

[29] Frank D, Dirk L. Pneumatic artificial muscles: actuators for robotics and automation. Eur J Mech Environ Eng. 2002;47(1):11–21.

[30] Tri VM, Tjahjowidodo T, Ramon H, Van Brussel H. A new approach to modeling hysteresis in a pneumatic artificial muscle using the Maxwell-Slip model. IEEE/ASME Trans Mechatronics. 2011;16(1):177–86.

[31] Inoue K. Rubbertuators and applications for robots. Proceedings of the 4th international symposium on robotics research. University of California, Santa Clara, CA, USA, MIT Press Cambridge, MA, USA. 1988. pp. 57–63.

[32] Kelasidi E, Andrikopoulos G, Nikolakopoulos G, Manesis S, editors. A survey on pneumatic muscle actuators modeling. IEEE international symposium on industrial electronics. 2011. Gdansk.

[33] Chou C-P, Hannaford B. Measurement and modeling of McKibben pneumatic artificial muscles. IEEE Trans Robot Autom. 1996;12(1):90–102.

[34] Tondu B, Lopez P. Modeling and control of McKibben artificial muscle robot actuators. IEEE: IEEE Control Syst. 2000;20(2):15–38.

[35] Davis S, Caldwell DG. Braid effects on contractile range and friction modeling in pneumatic muscle actuators. Int J Robot Res. 2006;25(4): 359–69.

[36] Andrikopoulos G, Arvanitakis J, Manesis S, Nikolakopoulos G. A switched system modeling approach for a Pneumatic Muscle Actuator. IEEE international conference on industrial technology. IEEE: Athens; 2012.

[37] Xing K, Wang Y, Zhu Q, Zhou H. Modeling and control of McKibben artificial muscle enhanced with echo state networks. Control Eng Pract. 2012;20(5):477–88.

[38] Kerscher T, Albiez J, Zollner JM, Dillmann R. Evaluation of the dynamic model of fluidic muscles using quick-release. The first IEEE/RAS-EMBS international conference on biomedical robotics and biomechatronics. IEEE: Pisa; 2006.

[39] Hosovsky A, Balara M. Pneumatic artificial muscle force function approximation using ANFIS. J Appl Sci Thermodyn Fluid Mech. 2009;3(1):1–6.

[40] Szepe T. Accurate force function approximation for pneumatic artificial muscles. 3rd IEEE international symposium on logistics and industrial informatics. IEEE: Budapest, Hungary; 2011.

[41] Sarosi J. New approximation algorithm for the force of Fluidic Muscles. 7th IEEE international symposium on applied computational intelligence and informatics. IEEE: Timisoara; 2012.

Chapter 7
Control of a soft ankle rehabilitation robot

Interaction control is crucial to the soft ankle rehabilitation robot (SARR). This is usually implemented on the basis of a position controller by which accurate trajectory tracking can be obtained to guarantee safe passive training and active training control to promote the patient's participation. The first half of this chapter is dedicated to the development of a cascade position controller with position loop and force loop, which aims to implement smooth and safe robotic passive training on the SARR. The second half of this chapter proposes the active training strategies of generating an adaptive predefined trajectory according to the movement intention of the patient. The proposed adaptive interaction training can be then implemented by integrating it into a virtual reality based video game to make the robotic training process more attractive to the patients.

7.1 Introduction

A variety of robot-assisted ankle training strategies have been implemented and evaluated [1]. For single-degree of freedom (DOF) ankle rehabilitation devices, a typical example is the intelligent stretching device developed by Zhang *et al.* [2] to treat the spastic/contractured ankle of neurologically impaired patients. Although clinical evidences using combined passive stretching and active movement on children with cerebral palsy [3] and stroke patients [4] have been demonstrated, its potential applications for ankle rehabilitation are limited since it does not allow for mixed robotic motions of dorsiflexion/plantarflexion (DP), inversion/eversion (IE), and abduction/adduction (AA). Platform-based parallel robots present a comparative advantage for ankle rehabilitation due to the characteristic of multiple-DOFs. Tsoi *et al.* [5] developed a parallel ankle rehabilitation robot using a computed torque impedance controller that regulates the relationship between the applied moments at the joint and the ankle rotary motion. Jamwal *et al.* [6] constructed a wearable ankle rehabilitation robot using four pneumatic artificial muscles (PAMs), and proposed an adaptive fuzzy-logic controller for smooth training. The proposed adaptation scheme, however, was for the control of PAMs rather than the robotic interaction with human users.

Patient-cooperative training strategies were defined by Riener *et al.* [7] as that the robotic system takes into account patients' intention and voluntary efforts rather than imposing predefined motions. This kind of cooperative robotic training is expected to improve the therapeutic outcome compared to classical rehabilitation strategies by introducing a certain amount of robot compliance, and adapting robot behaviour to patients' motor abilities. Blaya and Herr [8] developed a variable-impedance ankle-foot orthosis, and clinical data suggested potential benefits for the treatment of drop-foot compared to conventional ankle-foot orthoses. In general, the patient-cooperative robot-assisted rehabilitation is feasible in clinical practice and enables patients to train in an active, variable and more natural way, which was also demonstrated by Duschau-Wicke *et al.* [9] on 11 patients with incomplete spinal cord injury. While many studies have demonstrated that training with different robotic control strategies reduces motor impairment as assessed with various outcome measures, only a few studies have found differential benefits of particular robotic control strategies with respect to other control strategies.

Passive and active training both play significant roles in the rehabilitation of injured ankles. Passive exercise is usually needed when the patient can hardly move his/her foot, and can be accomplished by a position control scheme that can guide the injured ankle to move along the pre-defined trajectory. Following passive exercises, active training is mostly conducted to make the patient fully regain his/her ankle range of motion (ROM) and strength, and can be implemented using an interaction controller based on impedance or admittance techniques. Ankle rehabilitation programmes usually involve ROM and muscle strengthening exercises which can be involved into a virtual game. Active assistance exercises are primarily aimed at neuro-motor training of patients suffering from neurological disorders, while resistive exercises are generally used for strength training of patients due to musculoskeletal disorders.

7.2 Passive training control

7.2.1 Force distribution based cascade control

The posture control of the SARR is the basis of a variety of robot-assisted rehabilitation exercises. This could be achieved by controlling individual Festo fluidic muscle (FFM) length in the workspace. Specifically, the required individual FFM length can be calculated by inverse kinematics based on the required posture of the end effector. The actual individual FFM length can be obtained from the measured posture of the end effector by inverse kinematics, although it cannot be directly measured. However, this method cannot guarantee all FFMs in tension and may not be safe for human users.

As FFMs can only generate pulling force, for a platform with n DOF, at least $m = n + 1$ FFMs are required to fully control the motion. However, this FFMs-driven PARR is over-determined for the forward kinematics and under-determined for force distributions in the FFMs. Cable-driven robots may lose controllability if certain cables are not in tension during the robotic operation [10]. The SARR employs four FFMs that work similar to cables along an actuator, and thus the determination of feasible force distribution of this SARR is required for a given robot driven torque T_r. In this section, we propose a force distribution-based cascade control scheme for the ankle rehabilitation robot to ensure its controllability.

Pott *et al.* [11] proposed a closed-form force distribution scheme that is shown in (7.1), where $A = J^T$, $A^+ = A^T(AA^T)^{-1}$, T_r represents the robot torque in task space generated by four FFMs, f is the mean feasible force distribution and can be defined according to specific applications. The distributed forces are continuous along trajectories and differentiable at most of the points, and the computational efforts are also strictly bounded and small even for large numbers of wires.

$$F = f - A^+(T_r + Af) \tag{7.1}$$

The other method is an analytic-iterative force distribution technique proposed by Taghirad *et al.* [12]. This method is formulated into an optimisation problem (7.2), where $B = I - A^+A$, and then handled by the Karush-Kuhn-Tucker theorem to draw an analytic-iterative solution. The redundancy resolution method is adopted here to achieve the minimum-norm actuator forces.

$$\begin{cases} \min f(y) = (F_o + By)^T(F_o + By) \\ \text{Subject to } F_{\min} - (F_o + By) \leq 0 \end{cases} \tag{7.2}$$

Since this approach adopted an optimisation search algorithm, the absolute sum of link forces can be smaller than that of the closed-form method by Pott *et al.* [11], which means that the robot implemented using the analytic-iterative method can achieve a predefined motion with less energy consumption.

This study proposes a cascade controller with measured posture as feedback in the outer loop, while the measured FFM forces as feedback in the inner loop, as shown in Figure 7.1. This method can guarantee not only trajectory tracking accuracy, but also ensure the FFMs are always in tension for safety. For the forward feedback controller, the individual FFM length can be calculated based on the

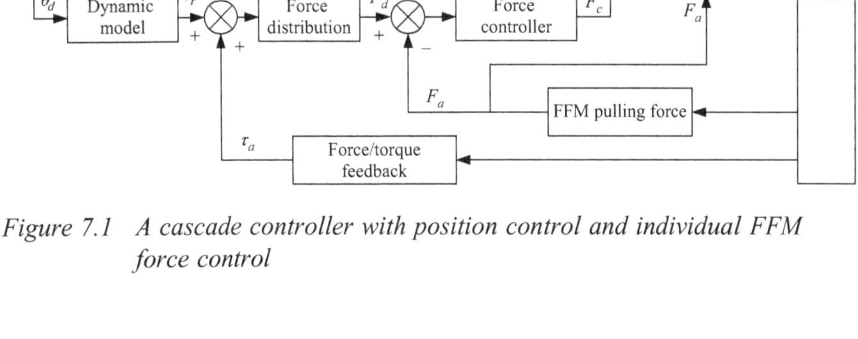

Figure 7.1 A cascade controller with position control and individual FFM force control

inverse kinematics. Specifically, suppose the desired motion trajectory of the robot end-effector is θ_d, the desired displacement of individual FFM in the joint space L_d can be obtained by inverse kinematics, and the actual displacement L_a is calculated from the sensor feedback. At the same time, according to the dynamic model of the robot, the desired output torque τ_d to achieve the desired movement can be calculated, and the active interaction torque applied by the patient is detected. In conjunction with the force distribution methods described above, the desired driving force for each FFM F_d can be calculated at the desired robot orientation, and the actual driving force F_a is obtained by the tension sensor. In this way, direct posture feedback in the task space and FFM forces feedback in the workspace are compensated to ensure both trajectory tracking accuracy and all FFMs in tension while in use.

The movement range of the robot in the *X*-direction is set to 0.2 rad, and the motion range in the *Y*-direction is 0.15 rad. The movement frequency is set to 0.05 Hz, that is, the motion period of the robot is 20 s. The target trajectory function is:

$$\begin{cases} \theta_x(t) = 0.2\sin(2\pi \cdot 0.05 \cdot t) \ (\text{rad}) \\ \theta_y(t) = 0.15\sin(2\pi \cdot 0.05 \cdot t) \ (\text{rad}) \end{cases} \tag{7.3}$$

Based on the experimental protocol, preliminary evaluations of the cascade controller implemented on the SARR are presented in Figures 7.2 and 7.3. Figure 7.2 plots the trajectory and FFM force tracking responses of the single-axis training, including *X* (Figure 7.2(a)) and *Y* (Figure 7.2(b)) motions. The trajectory and individual force tracking for the mixed-axis training is plotted in Figure 7.3, respectively, in which black line is the desired trajectory and grey line the actual one. From the results, we can conclude that the trajectory tracking accuracy of the single-axis training presents better than those of the mixed-axis training. Though the force tracking accuracy is not so high but is enough to keep all FFMs in tension. As we know, for rehabilitation devices, the posture control of the robotic effector is critical for both passive and active training. By contrast, the accurate control of the individual actuator force is not strictly required on condition that all cables are in tension.

7.2.2 IFT control for repetitive training

For rehabilitation recovery, clinical studies have shown that repetitive, intensive as well as task-specific rehabilitation programmes can contribute significantly to the effectiveness of treatment [13]. Traditionally, the rehabilitation exercises are performed using repetitive manual manipulation by the physiotherapist. When it comes to robot-assisted rehabilitation therapy, such a repetitive exercise principle is also necessary to mimic the actions of physiotherapists. The repetitive nature of robot-assisted therapy provides a good opportunity for iterative learning control (ILC) techniques [14]. ILC is able to learn from data recorded from the previous trials and updates the controller to optimise the performance [15]. As mentioned above, the controlled objective model of a PAM-driven parallel ankle rehabilitation robot is difficult to build. It indicates that a model-based ILC is not suitable, and a

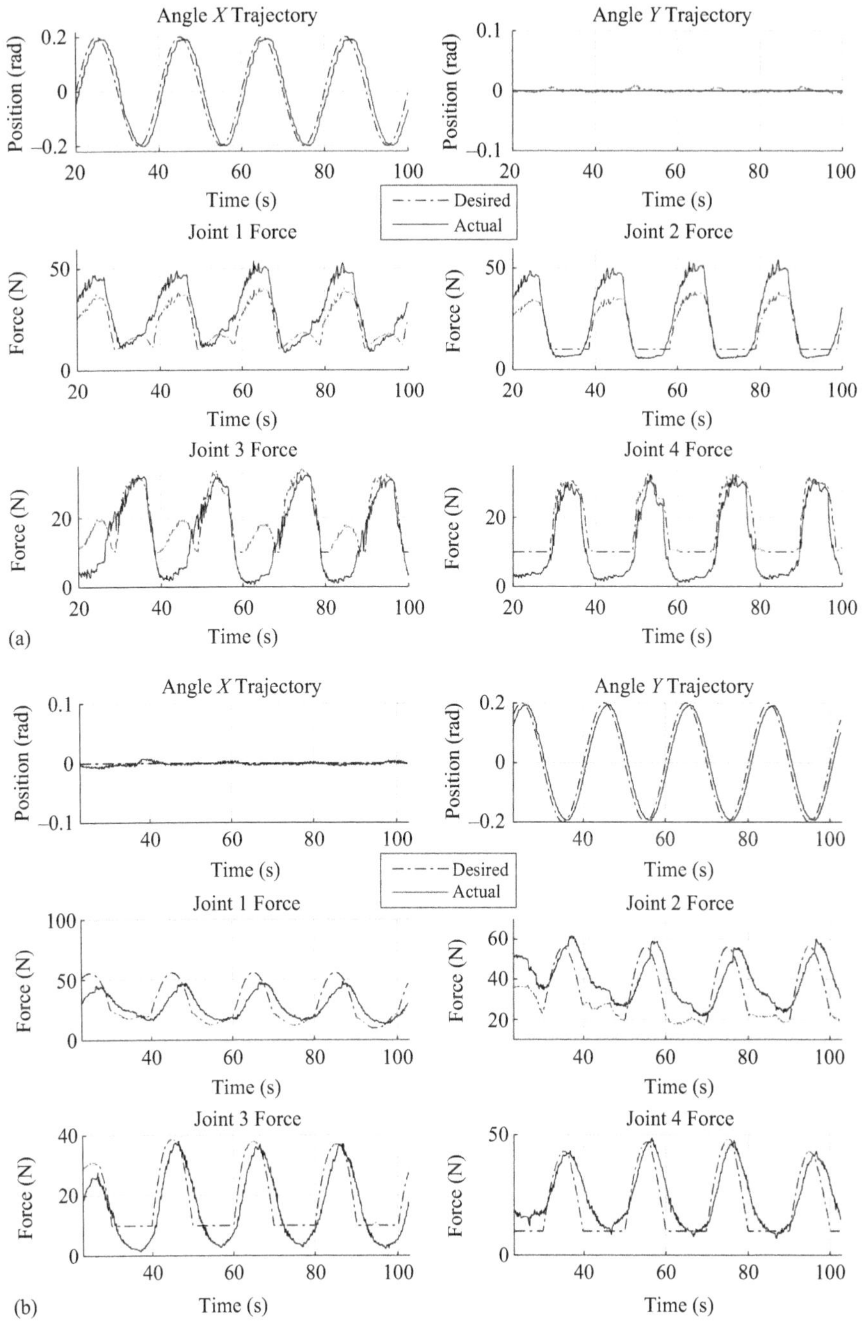

Figure 7.2 Trajectory and FFM force tracking responses of the single-axis training. (a) Trajectory and FFM force tracking responses of the X-axis motion. (b) Trajectory and FFM force tracking responses of the Y-axis motion

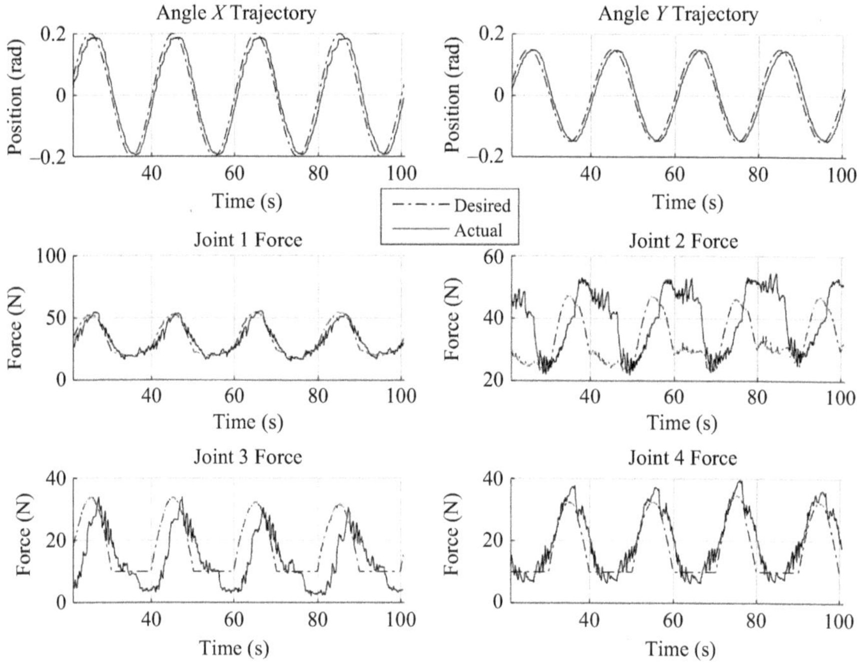

Figure 7.3 Trajectory and FFM force tracking responses of the mixed-axis training

model-free method may be better. Iterative feedback tuning (IFT) is a model-free learning control and it is very much suitable for repeated rehabilitation trajectories due to the requirement of the specially designed experiments. It appears that IFT method satisfies the requirements of such a PAMs-driven parallel rehabilitation robot control.

As the ankle rehabilitation robot has multiple actuators to be controlled, the implementation of multiple instances of the IFT technique is explored. The base control structure is presented in Figure 7.4, where inverse kinematics is used to obtain the joint space trajectories $l_i, i = 1, 2, 3, 4$ for each actuator. The reference and actual trajectory of each link are evaluated from the desired orientation $\theta_{d,XYZ}$ and the measured end-effector orientation θ_{XYZ} respectively by using inverse kinematics. These actuators are then controlled individually using a proportional-integral-derivative (PID) controller with the parameter vector being tuned by IFT technique. In the control structure, the same set of starting parameters of $\rho = \begin{bmatrix} K_P & K_I & K_D \end{bmatrix}^T$ was applied to all four controllers. The outer control loop regulates the angular position, and each of the inner control loops regulates air pressure in each PAM. The PAM model converts the control signal u_i into air pressure p_i for each proportional regulator.

For each PAM, a block diagram of the closed loop system is shown in Figure 7.5. We consider the PAM as an unknown system G, and r the reference

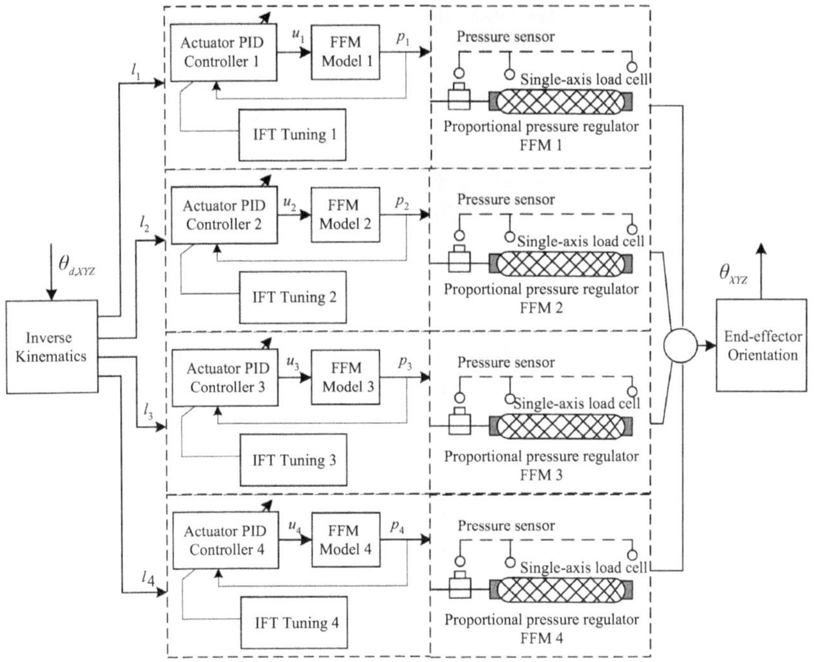

Figure 7.4 Control structure of multiple DOF IFT on the parallel robot

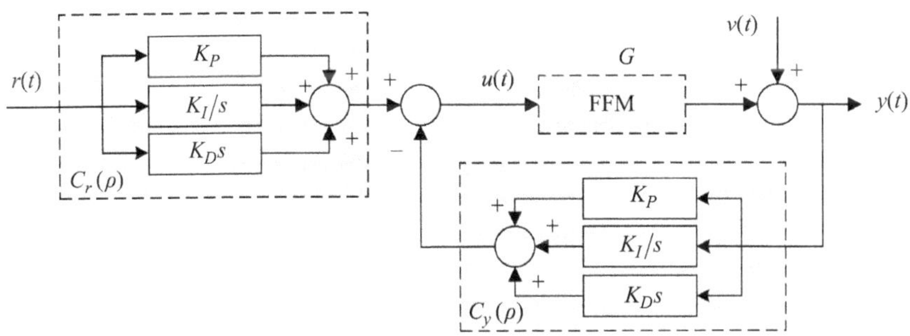

Figure 7.5 Block diagram of the controlled system for each FFM

input, u the output from the controller, and y the system output, v the unmeasurable disturbance. The controller designs a two DOF one in the form $C(\rho) = [C_r(\rho),\ C_y(\rho)]$, where $C_r(\rho)$ and $C_y(\rho)$ are PID controllers. The two controllers share the same parameters. The parameters for C_r and C_y are collected and optimised in a vector of controller parameters: $\rho = [K_P \quad K_I \quad K_D]^{\mathrm{T}}$.

The objective for an ILC is to generate a sequence of appropriate control inputs $u_t(i)$ to drive the system output $y_t(i)$ approaches a given reference trajectory y_d, for iteration i. Each iteration of control input generation should take the output $y_t(i)$ closer to the reference trajectory by the IFT algorithm learning about the properties of the system being controlled. Details of the general IFT algorithm can be found in [16]. In this subsection, only those expressions that are necessarily important for the controller development are given. The used design criterion or objective function $J(\rho)$ takes into account both the error response as well as the controller input magnitude. λ is a predetermined weighting factor.

$$J(\rho) = \frac{1}{2N}\left(\sum_{t=1}^{N} \tilde{y}_t(\rho)^2 + \lambda \sum_{t=1}^{N} u_t(\rho)^2\right) \tag{7.4}$$

Here ρ is a vector of process parameters to be optimised, $\tilde{y}_t(\rho)$ is the error between the actual output and the desired output signal, and N is the total number of samples collected. The optimised controller parameter vector ρ^* is defined as shown in (7.5). The design criterion is to be calculated after each optimisation iteration to quantify the performance of the system response.

$$\rho^* = [\arg \min_{\rho}](\rho) \tag{7.5}$$

The partial derivative of $\tilde{y}_t(\rho)$ and $u_t(\rho)$ with respect to the parameters ρ is:

$$\frac{\partial \tilde{y}_t}{\partial \rho}(\rho) = \frac{1}{C_r(\rho)}\left[\frac{\partial C_r}{\partial \rho}(\rho) T_0 r_t - \frac{\partial C_y}{\partial \rho}(\rho) T_0 y_t\right] \tag{7.6}$$

$$\frac{\partial u_t}{\partial \rho}(\rho) = S_0\left[\frac{\partial C_r}{\partial \rho}(\rho) r_t - \frac{\partial C_y}{\partial \rho}(\rho) y_t\right] \tag{7.7}$$

The partial derivatives $\frac{\partial y_t(\rho_i)}{\partial \rho}$ and $\frac{\partial u_t(\rho_i)}{\partial \rho}$ can be obtained by performing actual experiments on the system. Normally, three experiments are required to complete each iteration of the optimisation process. The estimated gradient of the design criterion $J(\rho)$ for the ith iteration based entirely on experimental data can be constructed from the estimated partial derivatives:

$$\text{est}\left[\frac{\partial J}{\partial \rho}(\rho_i)\right] = \frac{1}{N}\sum_{t=1}^{N}\left(\tilde{y}_t(\rho_i)\text{est}\left[\frac{\partial y_t}{\partial \rho}(\rho_i)\right] + \lambda u_t(\rho_i)\text{est}\left[\frac{\partial u_t}{\partial \rho}(\rho_i)\right]\right) \tag{7.8}$$

The next iterate $\rho_{i+1} = \left[K_P^{i+1} \quad K_I^{i+1} \quad K_D^{i+1}\right]^T$ is calculated by using the Gauss-Newton optimisation algorithm, based on the gradient of $J(\rho)$ and previous ρ_i.

$$\rho_{i+1} = \rho_i - \gamma_i R_i^{-1}\text{est}\left[\frac{\partial J}{\partial \rho}(\rho_i)\right] \tag{7.9}$$

where γ_i is a positive scalar step size, and R_i is some positive definite matrix:

$$R_i = \frac{1}{N}\sum_{t=1}^{N}\left(\text{est}\left[\frac{\partial y_t}{\partial \rho}(\rho_i)\right]\text{est}\left[\frac{\partial y_t}{\partial \rho}(\rho_i)\right]^T + \lambda\text{est}\left[\frac{\partial u_t}{\partial \rho}(\rho_i)\right]\text{est}\left[\frac{\partial u_t}{\partial \rho}(\rho_i)\right]^T\right) \tag{7.10}$$

As the ankle stiffness for a patient is high, the participant may not have adequate ROM. The trajectory used for testing the effectiveness of the proposed IFT method was a sinusoidal waveform about the X Euler axis with an amplitude of 0.2 rad and a period of 20 s. The rationale behind the use of rotation about a single axis only is that all four actuators will need to be utilised no matter what the trajectory is. Furthermore, this waveform ensures that all four actuators have a smooth and cyclical trajectory after the inverse kinematics, which improves the performance of the IFT algorithm when it is implemented on the control system [17].

In this experiment, IFT with normalised design criterion is used to tune the robot for position control performance in task space. A PID form of the IFT algorithm was directly applied to individual controllers in the control system. The starting value for the PID parameter vector was set to be $\rho = \begin{bmatrix} 15 & 9 \times 10^{-3} & 5 \times 10^{-4} \end{bmatrix}^T$, which gave an over-damped response. Usually, very few iterations are needed for the IFT method to achieve a good performance. More iterations seem to be needed for smaller sampling intervals, but the result will be about the same. Thus ten iterations of online optimisation were performed, with the results taken directly from the tuning process.

The IFT tuning result is shown in Figure 7.6, where a positive angle in the X Euler axis denotes the dorsiflexion direction and a negative angle denotes the

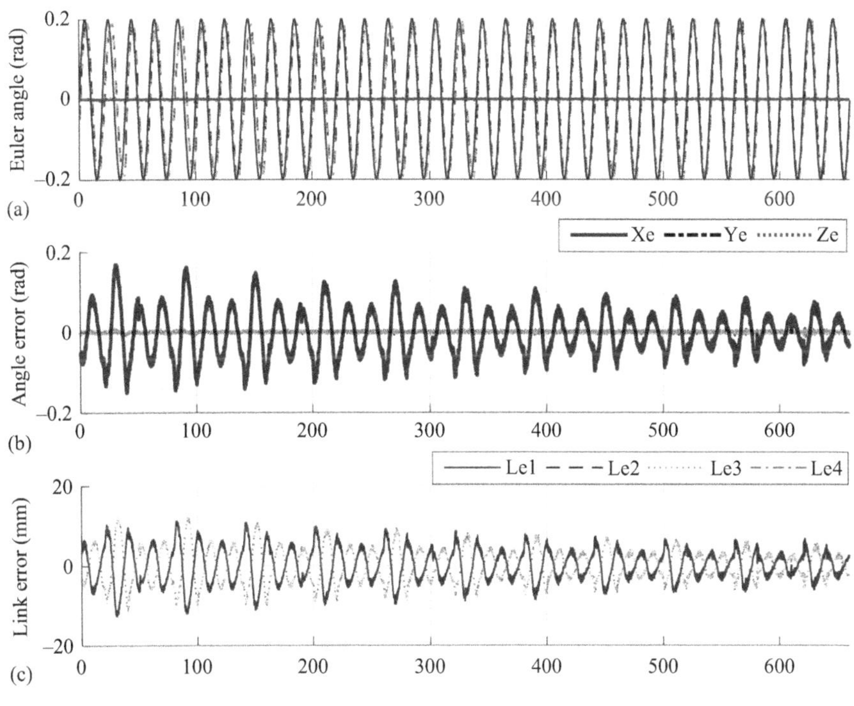

Figure 7.6 Repetitive control result using IFT tuning: (a) End-effector orientation tracking result. (b) End-effector tracking error. (c) Actuator tracking error in joint space

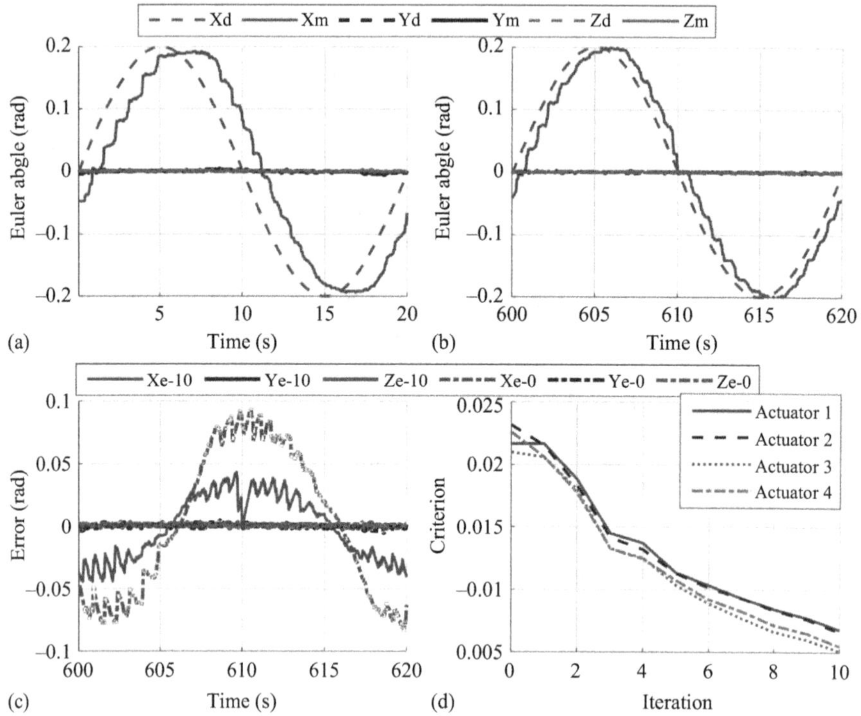

Figure 7.7 IFT tuning test. (a) End-effector orientation before tuning. (b) End-effector orientation after tuning. (c) End-effector error. (d) Design criterion profiles. IEEE. Adapted from [17] with permission

plantarflexion. For such a repetitive trajectory, the robot tracking control performance becomes better and better during the ten iterations, as shown by Figure 7.6(a). The end-effector orientation error in Figure 7.6(b) and the link tracking error of each actuator shown in Figure 7.6(c) also provide evidence that the IFT technique is able to tune the controller parameters towards a high-performance tracking results within several minutes. It can be seen that there is a significant improvement in the trajectory tracking response when comparing the before tuning and end of tuning results in Figure 7.7(a) and (b), respectively. The errors for all three Euler angle axes at iteration zero and at iteration 10 are shown in Figure 7.7(c) by the dotted and the solid line respectively. The profile of how the value of the design criterion decreases is shown in Figure 7.7(d), where there is a steady decrease in the value of $J(\rho)$ from over 0.02 to around 0.005.

7.3 Active training control

In the early to middle stage of rehabilitation, in order to realise the active and passive combination training of robot-assisted ankle rehabilitation, this section will propose an intelligent control method that can be switched between passive and active modes. The passive training of the robot is maintained when the patient does not produce the active intention, and the active trajectory of the robot is changed to realize the active training when the intention is generated by the patient. In the middle and late stages of rehabilitation, the patient has the ability to continuously change the movement of the robot. Here the robot impedance model is adjusted adaptively according to the patient's rehabilitation status, then two kinds of cooperative control methods are designed to integrate the patient's intention into the virtual game.

7.3.1 Trajectory adaptation-based intelligent control

In order to realize the above-mentioned intelligent training strategy integrating passive and active mode, the patient can switch the training mode according to the recovery level in the early and middle stage of rehabilitation. In this section, we propose a control method based on trajectory adjustment. The method is able to implement two types of robot training modes, which means the robot will remain in a passive periodicity when the patient did not intend to change the current movement. In contrast, if a motive force is applied to change the current motion of the robot, the robot will switch to the active training mode, by modifying the reference trajectory according to the interaction of the patient.

The periodic trajectory with sinusoidal function is adopted as the initial reference trajectory of the SARR, as its motion direction and velocity can be easily realised by adjusting its phase and frequency parameters. The initial reference trajectory of the robotic device is defined in (7.11), where A_x is the amplitude of trajectory along X, f the frequency, and t the time variable.

$$x_{init}(t) = A_x \sin(2\pi f t) \tag{7.11}$$

Suppose the patient attempts to change the robot movement at time t_1, by exerting an interaction force that exceeds the threshold F_0, the modified trajectory $x_{\mathrm{adap}}(t)$ is generated. In the proposed scheme, we distinguish between two cases. In Case 1, the interactive force is in the same axis as the current trajectory, for example, both along X. If the applied force is trying to resist the robot movement, the new adapted trajectory will reverse its direction to facilitate patient-in-charge control. Define x_1 the current displacement of trajectory, x_1' the velocity, t_1 the time of force event, the trajectory adaption law can be expressed by (7.12), in which the modified phase can be obtained from (7.13), where F_x is the X-axis component of interaction force.

$$x_{adap}(t) = x_{init}(t + \varphi_{xadap}) \tag{7.12}$$

$$\varphi_{xadap} = \begin{cases} \dfrac{1}{2f} - \sin^{-1}\dfrac{|x_1|}{\pi f}, & if\ x_1 \geq 0,\ x_1' \geq 0,\ F_x < -F_0 \\ \dfrac{-1}{2f} + \sin^{-1}\dfrac{|x_1|}{\pi f}, & if\ x_1 \geq 0,\ x_1' > 0,\ F_x \geq -F_0 \\ \dfrac{1}{2f} + \sin^{-1}\dfrac{|x_1|}{\pi f}, & if\ x_1 < 0,\ x_1' < 0,\ F_x \geq -F_0 \\ \dfrac{-1}{2f} + \sin^{-1}\dfrac{|x_1|}{\pi f}, & if\ x_1 < 0,\ x_1' \geq 0,\ F_x < -F_0 \end{cases} \tag{7.13}$$

In Case 2, the interactive force is in a different axis with the current trajectory, for example, the triggered force event along *Y* occurs during the robot's movement towards *X*, and the new adapted trajectory is expected to switch to another axis and be constructed as a new continuous function. Since trajectories along different axis are all centred at the zero-crossing point, the transition between these two trajectories is modulated here. Eventually, the new adapted trajectory is switched from *X* to *Y*, and then the new path adaptation control law is similar to that in *X*. The trajectory adaptation steps described above were integrated into the proposed intelligent training controller. Figure 7.8 explains the scheme of this trajectory adaption strategy.

Experiments were carried out on the actual SARR environment to verify the performance and effectiveness of the proposed trajectory regulation controller. The experiment setup and control structure is shown in Figure 7.9. The preliminary results of the intelligent training strategy implemented on the SARR in Cases 1 and 2 are presented in Figures 7.10 and 7.11, respectively. In both figures, the top and middle plots are the desired and measured trajectory of *X* and *Y*, respectively, and the bottom is the force trigger events. It is clear that the trajectory adaptation control law could guarantee the robot's movement keeping coincided with the patient's intended force. The robot was controlled in both passive and active modes by using the proposed method. With Case 1 in Figure 7.10, the robot exerts a reverse acting moment during the movement of the robot at 30, 70, 90 s, and the robot immediately changes its current direction of motion and continues its movement. With Case 2 in Figure 7.11, the robot was controlled to move along different axes. This strategy is able to encourage the participants' active efforts by changing the robot movement when the participant achieves a force threshold.

7.3.2 Game guided training control

Virtual-reality games have been developed recent years to be used combined with robot-assisted joint rehabilitation. This technique can improve the efficiency of ankle rehabilitation by making the repetitive and tedious training process more interesting to the patients and promoting their enthusiasm in participating the training [18].

The virtual reality game here for SARR-assisted training is developed in LABVIEW. It is a step-on-gopher game. The main purpose for the patient is to move their ankle to a desired angle to step on the gopher comes out of a hole. The patient interface is shown in Figure 7.12. The indicators on the top are round, timer and score.

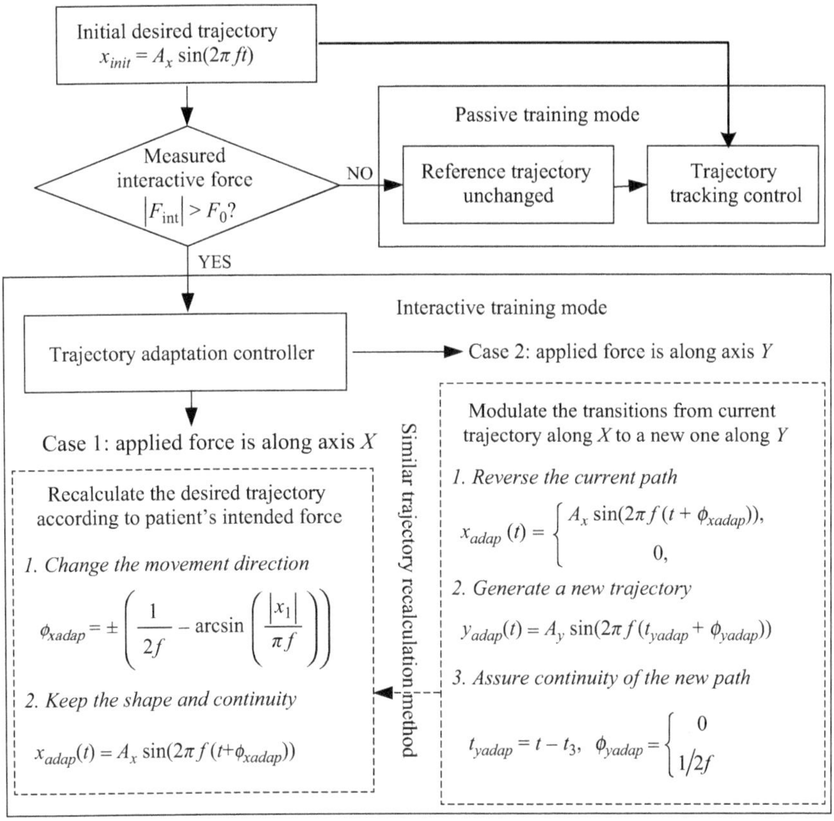

Figure 7.8 Scheme of the proposed intelligent training strategy

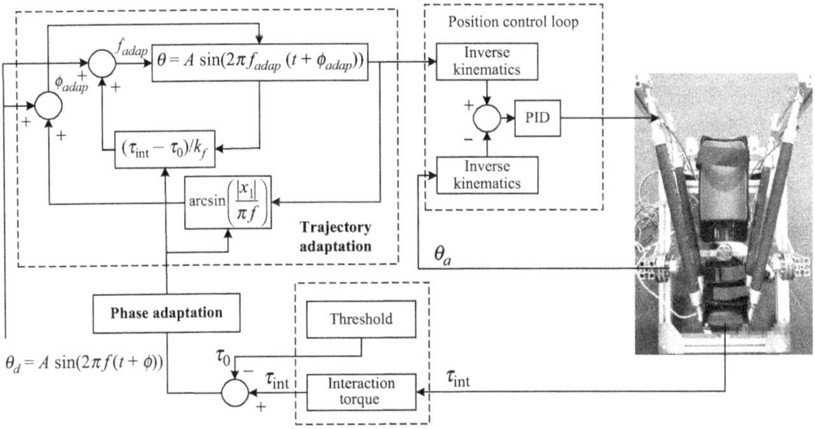

Figure 7.9 Experiment setup and control structure of the rehabilitation robot

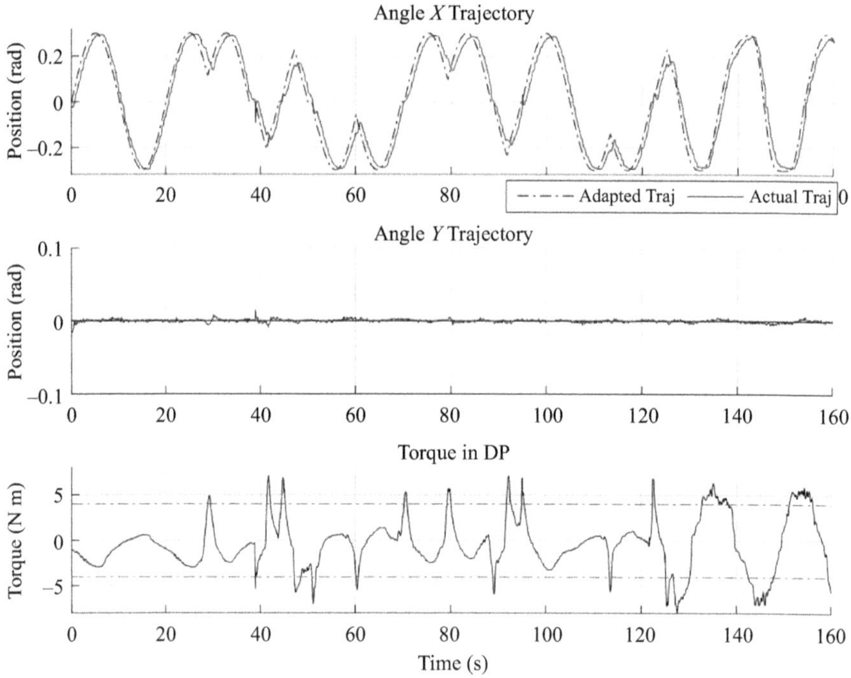

Figure 7.10 Trajectory tracking responses of the intelligent training along single-axis

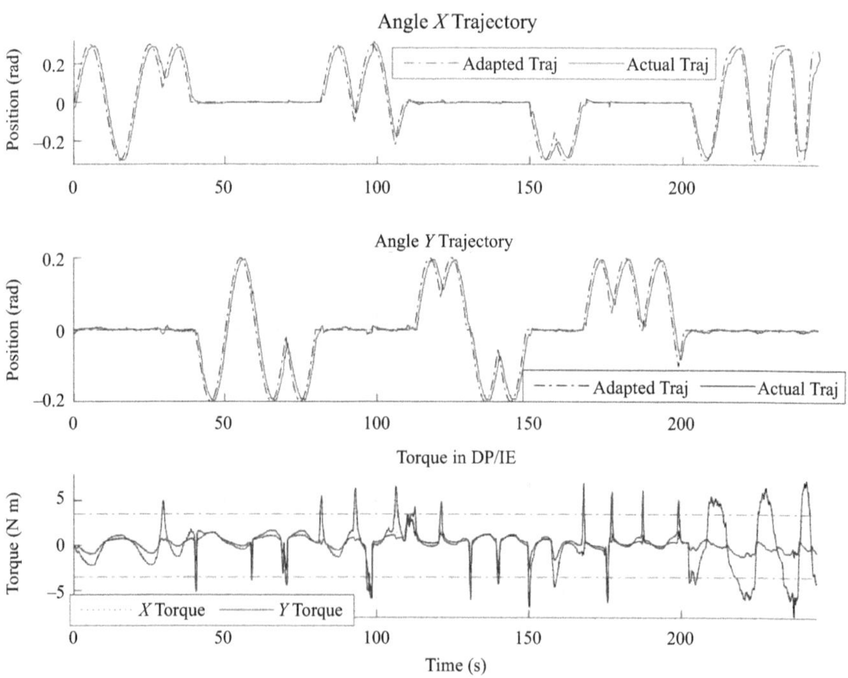

Figure 7.11 Trajectory tracking responses of the intelligent training along mixed-axes

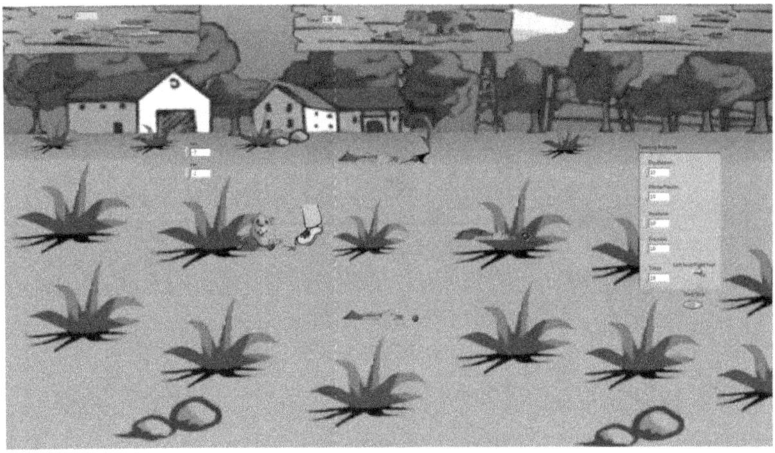

Figure 7.12 Patient interface for the game

Round indicator will give how many repetitions of movement the patient has performed. Timer indicator will tell the participant how many seconds remained for him or her to achieve the goal. Once the patient steps on a gopher within the time limit, he will get one score and the total score will be shown by the score indicator. The two numeric controls on the left give the current position of the platform: the control with the label 'hor' indicates dorsiflexion (positive value) and plantarflexion (negative value); the control with the label 'ver' indicates inversion and eversion. The four holes around the tent are targets that the patient needs to move their ankle to. The tent is the equilibrium position of the platform. On the right of the patient interface is the therapist interface which allows the therapist to put in training protocols.

An interactive training scheme is developed by combining the intelligent control methods into the visual game. The robot movement is embodied in the virtual reality game, which can greatly stimulate the interest of the patients to participate in rehabilitation training and make it easy to understand the control process of the robot. In intelligent control mode, when the patient applies the active torque, the trajectory of the robot can be corrected to move more quickly or directly to the target point. When the robot reaches the target, the game scores, and then randomly generates another target position. In the case of passive training, patients can see the process of the game and a steady score. In the case of active training, the patient can, by his or her own efforts, speed up the movement of the robot towards the target point.

The game guided training programme will be implemented based on intelligent control scheme. Then the training phase consists of four subsystems: (1) dorsiflexion, (2) plantarflexion, (3) inversion and (4) eversion. The main structure and principle for the four subsystems is similar. Take dorsiflexion subsystem for example. When the programme gets a zero in the start phase, it will go to dorsiflexion state. The gopher-hole control will be given a true value and the gopher on the top will appear. The timer indicator starts counting down. The patient needs to perform a dorsiflexion to a desired angle to step on the gopher. When the patient

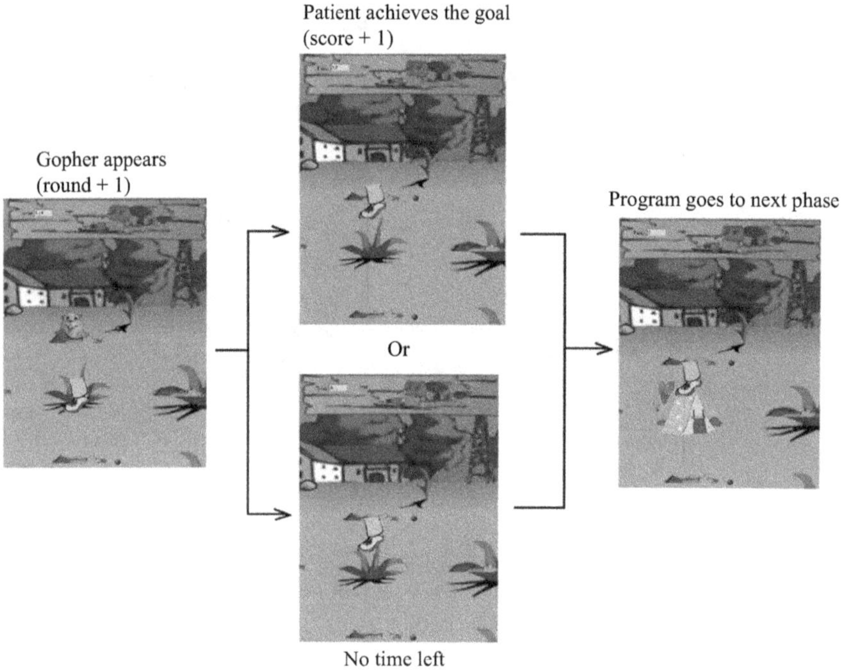

Figure 7.13 The process of game-guided training phase

Table 7.1 Experimental statistics of the game-guided training

	Trial 1	Trial 2	Trial 3	Trial 4
Game scores	10	13	17	23
Intended attempts	16	16	19	23
Success rate (%)	62.5	81.25	89.47	100
Average time cost (s)	30	23.08	17.65	13.04

achieves the goal or there is no time left, the gopher-hole control will be given a false value and the gopher turns to a hole. After that, the programme goes to back home phase. The process is illustrated in Figure 7.13.

Experiments were conducted on a healthy male subject with 170 mm height and 62 kg weight to verify the above-mentioned virtual game-guided robot training control. This trial has been approved by the University of Auckland Human Participants Ethics Committee (reference 011904). Set the vertical range of the game 0.3 rad, the horizontal movement range of 0.2 rad with a period of 20 s. If the subject cannot reach the gopher within 20 s, the attempt will not score and need to return to the home position for the next attempt. The total game time is set to 5 min. For the participant, each game trial lasts 5 min, and the output data of the game is shown in Table 7.1. Experimental results are presented in Figure 7.14, in which Figure 7.14(a) is the

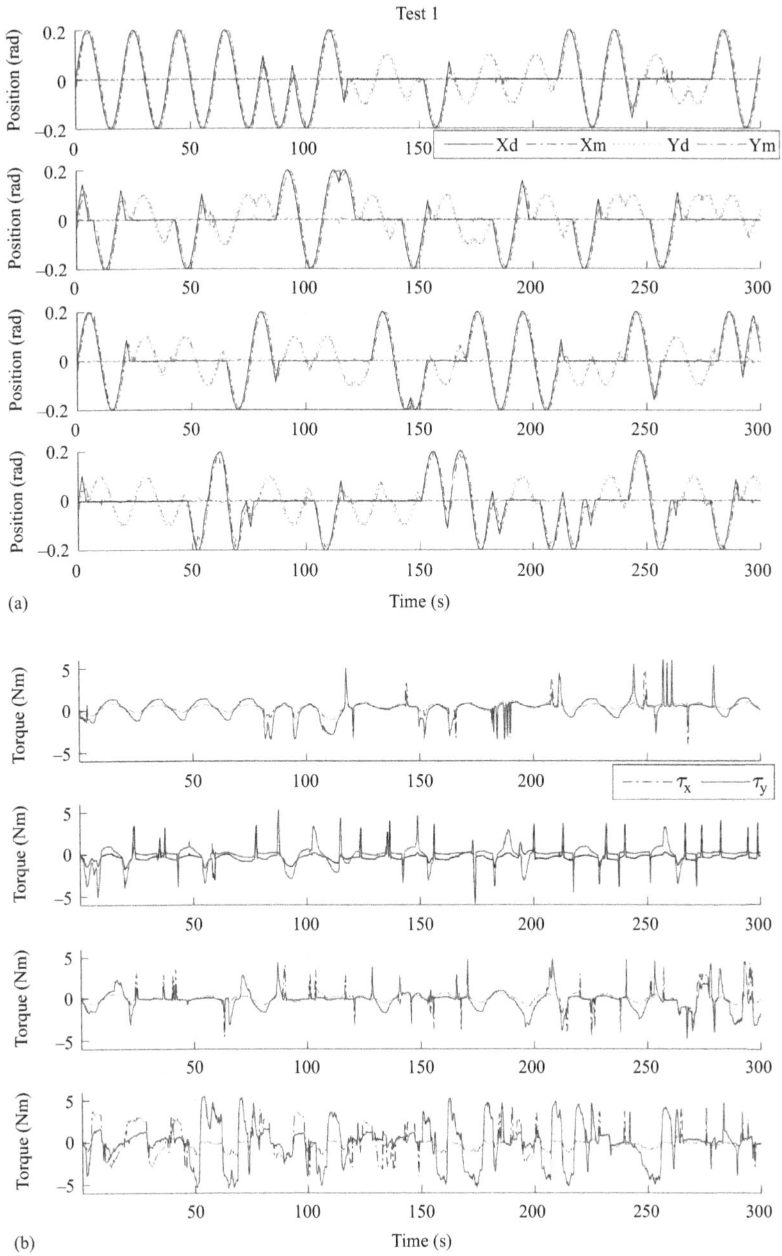

Figure 7.14 Experimental results of the game-guided training. (a) Trajectory tracking responses of the game-guided training: trial 1–4. (b) Torque records of the game-guided training: trial 1–4

trajectory tracking responses of the game-guided training of four trials from top to bottom, and Figure 7.14(b) is the torque records during the four game trials.

From the results of the above-mentioned game experiments, it can be seen that with the increase of the number of games, the subject learned how to effectively control the robot to track the target position better. It means that the patient can gradually get higher game scores and success rates. And the average time spent on each score was reduced, in this way the participants are more willing to participate in the game. As the subject is more and more familiar with the rules of the game, it can generate more trajectory changes by active action and increased active torque to complete the game task. Therefore, such a step-on-gopher game used with an ankle rehabilitation robot can make the training process more attractive to the patients. The programme allows the therapist to put in different training protocols. It can be well connected to the robot and can be used in voluntary ankle rehabilitation exercise. This scheme of patient-cooperative control can effectively promote the patients' active participation, so as to improve the motivation and effectiveness of robot training.

7.4 Summary

This chapter proposes and discusses the implementation of control strategies on the SARR for the treatment of a variety of ankle injuries. The cascade position control shows good trajectory tacking performance, and guarantees FFMs in tension during the robotic operation. The intelligent algorithm aims to adapt the predefined trajectory based on the movement intention of the patient. If no movement intention is detected, the SARR operates in a passive mode along the pre-defined trajectory. If movement intention is detected, the SARR runs in an active interaction model based on the adapted trajectory, wherein the movement ROM, direction, and velocity are adaptively adjusted. By the proposed virtual game-guided training together with the impedance controller, the SARR can deliver virtual reality training based on the patient-robot interaction. The active training strategy is also expected to make the robotic training more interesting and effective and promote the outcomes. One of the limitations in this chapter is that only one patient was recruited in the present experiments to simulate clinical human-robot interaction. Future work will further optimise the proposed control methods through clinical trials involving a large sample of participants with injured ankles when evaluating its therapeutic effects.

References

[1] Zhang M, Davies TC, Xie S. Effectiveness of robot-assisted therapy on ankle rehabilitation–a systematic review. J Neuroeng Rehabil. 2013;10(30):1–16.

[2] Zhang LQ, Chung SG, Bai Z, *et al*. Intelligent stretching of ankle joints with contracture spasticity. IEEE Trans Neural Syst Rehabil Eng. 2002; 10(3):149–57.

[3] Wu YN, Hwang M, Ren YP, *et al.* Combined passive stretching and active movement rehabilitation of lower-limb impairments in children with cerebral palsy using a portable robot. Neurorehabil Neural Repair. 2011; 25(4):378–85.
[4] Waldman G, Yang CY, Ren Y. Effects of robot-guided passive stretching and active movement training of ankle and mobility impairments in stroke. NeuroRehabil. 2013;32(5):625–34.
[5] Tsoi YH, Xie SQ, Graham AE. Design, modeling and control of an ankle rehabilitation robot. Stud Comput Intell. 2009;177:377–99.
[6] Jamwal PK, Xie SQ, Hussain S, *et al.* An adaptive wearable parallel robot for ankle injury treatments. IEEE Trans Mechatronics. 2014;19(1):64–75.
[7] Riener R, Lunenburger L, Jezernik S, *et al.* Patient-cooperative strategies for robot-aided treadmill training: first experimental results. IEEE Trans Neural Syst Rehabil Eng. 2005;13(3):380–94.
[8] Blaya JA, Herr H. Adaptive control of a variable-impedance ankle-foot orthosis to assist drop-foot gait. IEEE Trans Neural Syst Rehabil Eng. 2004;12(1):24–31.
[9] Duschau-Wicke A, Caprez A, Riener R. Patient-cooperative control increases active participation of individuals with SCI during robot-aided gait training. J Neuroeng Rehabil. 2010;7:43.
[10] Hassan M, Khajepour A. Analysis of bounded cable tensions in cable-actuated parallel manipulators. IEEE Trans Robot. 2011;27(5):891–900.
[11] Pott A, Bruckmann T, Mikelsons L. Closed-form force distribution for parallel wire robots. Comput Kinematics. 2009;26(1):25–34.
[12] Taghirad HD, Bedoustani YB. An analytic-iterative redundancy resolution scheme for cable-driven redundant parallel manipulators. IEEE Trans Robot. 2011;27(6):1137–43.
[13] Van Peppen RP, Kwakkel G, Wood-Dauphinee S, *et al.* The impact of physical therapy on functional outcomes after stroke: what's the evidence? Clin Rehabil. 2004;18(8):833–62.
[14] Balasubramanian S, Wei R, Perez M, *et al.* RUPERT: an exoskeleton robot for assisting rehabilitation of arm functions. Virt Rehabil. 2008:163–7. IEEE: Vancouver, BC, Canada. DOI: 10.1109/ICVR.2008.4625154.
[15] Lu CZ. Advanced iterative learning algorithm for control of rehabilitation robots. Auckland: The University of Auckland; 2015.
[16] Hjalmarsson H, Gevers M, Gunnarsson S, *et al.* Iterative feedback tuning: theory and applications. IEEE Control Syst. 1998;18(4):26–41.
[17] Meng W, Xie SQ, Liu Q, *et al.* Robust iterative feedback tuning control of a compliant rehabilitation robot for repetitive ankle training. IEEE/ASME Trans Mechatronics. 2017;22(1):173–84.
[18] Zhang M, Zhu G, Nandakumar A, *et al.* A virtual-reality tracking game for use in robot-assisted ankle rehabilitation. IEEE/ASME 10th international conference on mechatronic and embedded systems and applications. ASME: Seattle, WA; 2014. p. 1–4.

Chapter 8
Design of a GAit Rehabilitation EXoskeleton

Pneumatic artificial muscle (PAM) actuated rehabilitation robots have been widely researched, because of PAM's intrinsic compliance and high power-to-weight ratio. Task-specific gait rehabilitation training imposes strict torque, range of motion (ROM) and bandwidth requirements to the robotic exoskeleton design. However, the PAM's nonlinear and hysteresis behaviour, slow pressure dynamics and negative correlation between its force output and contracting length make the development even more challenging. To address such challenges, a new robotic GAit Rehabilitation EXoskeleton (GAREX) has been developed in order to facilitate task-specific gait rehabilitation with controlled intrinsic compliance. GAREX was designed for the experiments with human subjects. Several implementations ensure the safety of the subject, which is of paramount importance. GAREX has modular design to accommodate anthropometrics of most of the population.

8.1 Introduction

The PAM provides a good option to reduce exoskeleton inertia as well as achieve variable actuation stiffness, due to the actuators' high power-to-weight ratio [1] and intrinsic compliance [2]. With such properties, PAMs have been employed in various rehabilitation robotic applications [3–5].

To achieve effective robotic gait rehabilitation, the training is required to be as task-specific as possible [6]. Hence, the robots need to assist or guide the subjects to walk in or similar to normal gait speed and pattern. Transferring this to the robot development, the following specifications are to be satisfied: (1) multiple actuated degrees of freedom (DOF) to reproduce desired gait patterns; (2) sufficient ROM for the powered joints; (3) sufficient joint actuation torque to guide severely impaired subjects during training and (4) adequate controlled bandwidth. Moreover, the intrinsic compliance property is one of the main motivations of adapting PAMs in rehabilitation robotics. It is equally important to investigate how the intrinsic compliance can be controlled or adjusted to facilitate the training.

In the past, GAREXs actuated by PAMs have been developed. Beyl *et al.* [4,7] developed a lower limb exoskeleton (LLE), named KNEXO, actuated by pleated PAM. Both torque and trajectory control approaches were investigated. However, with the only actuated DOF at the knee joint, the device's potential use in clinical trials is limited.

Hussain *et al.* [5] developed a treadmill-based robotic GAREX with both the hip and knee joints actuated in the sagittal plane. Only the peak torque was reported which may not be sufficient to justify the torque requirement of task-specific gait rehabilitation had been met.

There are needs to develop a new PAM actuated robotic GAREX with the requirements of task-specific training in mind. This chapter will firstly briefly describe the support structure and trunk mechanism of the GAREX system. This will be followed by actuation system and mechanism design of the unilateral LLE. Pneumatic system and instrumentations will be presented next. Lastly the safety features of the GAREX system will be covered.

8.2 Support structure and trunk mechanism

To meet the specifications stated in the last section as well as advance the robotic gait rehabilitation research towards clinical trials. GAREX has been developed. The robot system consists of three mechanical modules: (1) the support structure, (2) the trunk mechanism and (3) most importantly the unilateral LLE which are illustrated in Figure 8.1.

The support structure is constructed with MiniTec frames. All the mechanical, pneumatic and electronic components are mounted to the structure. The structure is usually rigidly connected to the rehabilitation treadmill for treadmill-based gait

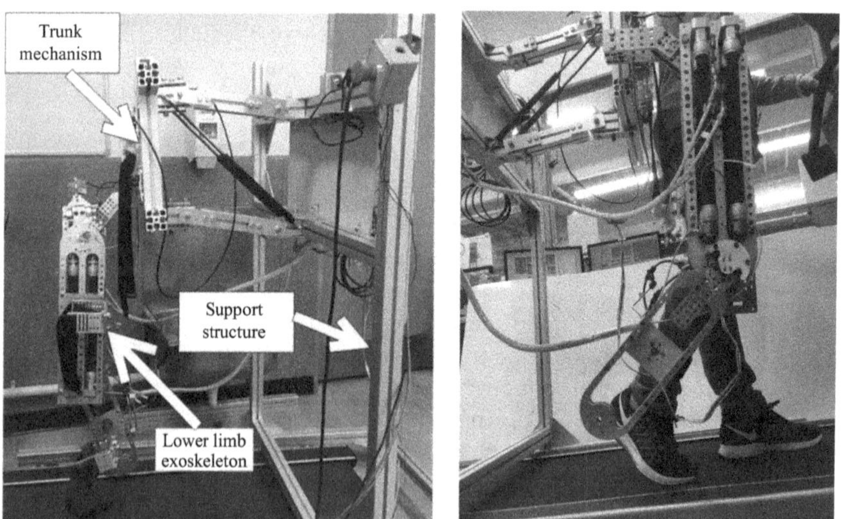

Figure 8.1 Left: the photo of GAREX with all the mechanical modules illustrated. Right: a healthy subject walking with GAREX

rehabilitation experiments. It also has four wheels, so over-ground training with GAREX is also made possible. Because of the modular mechanical design, the trunk mechanism's vertical and horizontal position relative to the support structure can be easily adjusted to suit various patients or switch between treadmill-based or over-ground gait training.

During gait rehabilitation experiments, subject's upper body was attached to the trunk mechanism by means of straps. One of the main functions of the trunk mechanism is to have three unactuated or passive DOFs, which are vertical and lateral translations as well as the rotation around the vertical axis. During normal walking, the trunk a healthy subject usually has ROMs of less than 10 cm in both translational DOFs and a ROM of 20° in the rotational DOF. Hence, the trunk mechanism was design with 15-cm ROMs for both translating DOFs and a 30° ROM for the rotational DOFs.

Another main function of the trunk mechanism is to suspend the LLE, so the patient does not have to bear any weight of the mechanism during training. The suspension is achieved by a pair of two air springs whose stiffness was adjusted to an appropriate level. The connection between the trunk mechanism and the LLE allows two unactuated DOFs of the hip joint which are the abduction and the rotation in the transverse plane. These two DOFs are loaded torsional springs. When both springs are in neutral position the LLE will be aligned with the sagittal plane. Such design can accommodate the natural movements in these dimensions and meanwhile constraining excessive or unnecessary ad-/abduction of hemiplegic gait [8]. Moreover, all the unactuated DOFs of the trunk and connection mechanisms can be blocked to suit the requirements of different gait rehabilitation tasks.

8.3 Lower limb exoskeleton

The main module of the robotic platform is the LLE which has a unilateral design. In order to help patients reproduce gait patterns, the sagittal plane rotations of the exoskeleton's hip and knee joints are actuated by the soft PAMs, taking the advantaged offered by such actuators discussed in Section 8.1. The major challenge of exoskeleton design also comes from the PAM actuation system.

There are three main design criteria of the LLE. Firstly, it should be able to provide sufficient assisting torque and ROM to facilitate robotic gait rehabilitation. Secondly, it should have compact and lightweight design that fit the anthropometric data of a large range of population. Finally, it needs to be designed and built efficiently; and meanwhile be robust enough for further experiments with human subjects.

8.3.1 Actuation of the lower limb exoskeleton

Before getting into the design process, it is worthwhile to briefly mention the operation principles of the PAM actuators. PAMs tend to contract and apply unidirectional pulling actuation to the attached objects, when inflated. Hence, it is common practice to adopt antagonistic configurations of PAMs to actuate rotational joints for bi-directional actuation [9–11]. The antagonistic PAMs of the exoskeleton are comparable to the extensor and flexor muscle groups of the human hip and knee joints. Therefore, regarding to the torque requirement of a joint, the extension and flexion PAMs were analysed separately. The force generated by a PAM actuator is positively correlated to its diameter and inflating pressure and negatively correlated to the contracting percentage with respect to its original length. In other words, there is a trade-off between the ROM and peak torque a certain PAM system can provide.

To meet the first design criterion, PAMs need to be longer and thicker in order to provide more torque and greater ROM. However, such design could potentially violate the second criterion. Hence, the design problem was simplified into determining the quantity, type, diameter and length of PAMs actuators for the actuated joints, as well as the radii of the pulleys, so both criteria mentioned previously could satisfied.

The PAMs manufactured by FESTO were selected. Compared to in-house manufactured PAMs, commercially available PAMs would provide better reliability, reduce the inter-PAM variance and hence reduce the uncertainty in modelling. The FESTO PAMs can be made in three diameters 10, 20 and 40 mm and their length can be customised, which provides good design flexibility. In the same situation (pressure, original PAM length and contraction percentage), the 40-mm diameter PAMs would provide sufficient pulling force and hence joint torque. However, due to their bulky end fittings, mounting them to the exoskeleton would result much lengthier and bulkier exoskeleton segment than actual human lower limb segments. One solution to this problem is to have Bowden cables as transmission and mount the PAMs at a remote location [12]. Bowden cable power transmission however conflicts with one of the initial motivations for employing PAMs, which is being light for direct mounting. Nonetheless, the Bowden cable would add modelling uncertainties and reliability issues.

Simple pulley and cable based antagonistic PAM designs were adopted to actuate the joints of the exoskeleton. The moment arms are the radii of the pulleys. The PAM's distal ends to the pulleys have fixed connections. The design is easy to implement and reliable in testing and also simplifies the modelling and controller development processes later on. In the finalised design, the hip and knee joints of GAREX each has two pairs of 20 mm diameter PAMs for sufficient torque output. In order to maximise the joint ROM without resulting over-lengthy exoskeleton segments, 300 mm (excluding end fittings) PAMs (FESTO: DMSP-20-300N-RM-CM) were selected. The pulley radii are 30 mm for both the hip and knee joints. The designed actuation system of GAREX is illustrated in Figure 8.2. The reasoning of choosing such a design will be detailed in the following paragraphs.

Based on the gait data published by Perry and Burnfield [13], the actuated ROM of both the hip and knee joints was determined and listed in Table 8.1. Such ROM ensures that the exoskeleton can help reproduce a large variety of gait patterns as well as limit the maximum PAM contraction in order to meet the torque requirement. It is designed that the extensor PAMs are at their original length (no contraction or stretch) when the joint reaches maximum flexion, and vice versa.

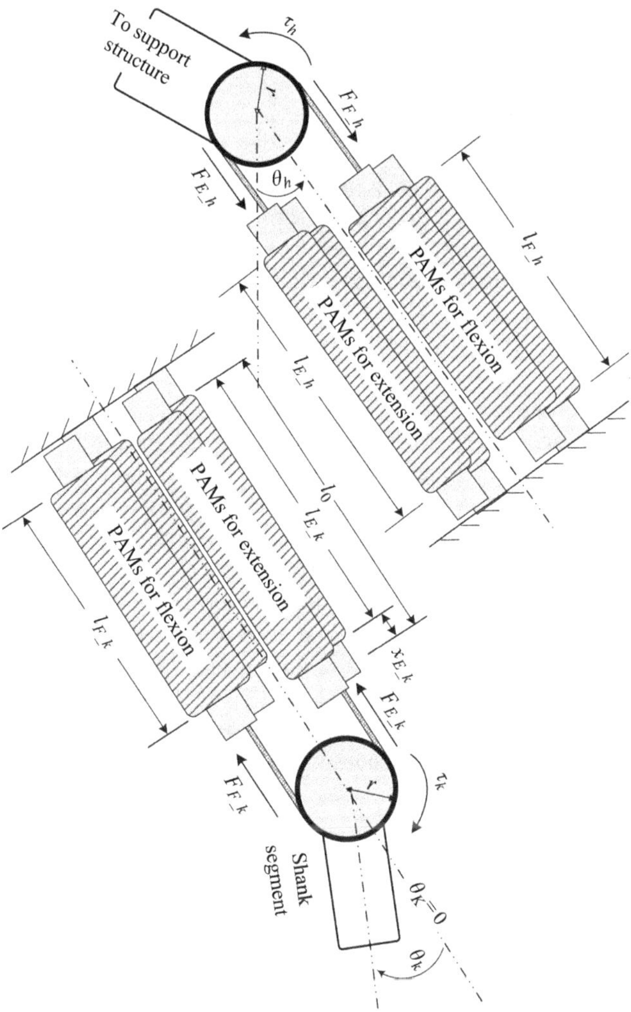

Figure 8.2 Illustrations of the joint actuation systems for the hip (top) and knee (bottom) joints. Useful variable definitions are illustrated arrows showing their positive directions

Table 8.1 Torque and range of motion design parameters of GAREX

	Hip	Knee
ROM (θ_{F0} to θ_{E0})	−20–40°	−3–69°
Linear ROM PAM (mm)	31.4 (10.5%)	37.7 (12.6%)
Equilibrium position ($x_E = x_F$)	10°	33°
Minimum peak torque PAM	47 Nm	40 Nm
Peak torque at equilibrium position	62 Nm	60 Nm

Hence the contraction of the extension and flexion PAM can be expressed as a function of joint angular position as:

$$\begin{cases} x_{Fi} = r_i(\theta_i - \theta_{F0i}) \\ x_{Ei} = r_i(\theta_{E0i} - \theta_i) \end{cases} \quad \text{with} \quad (i = h, k) \tag{8.1}$$

where r_i is the joint radius; θ_i is the joint angular position; θ_{E0i} and θ_{F0i} are the joint angular positions when the extensor and flexor PAMs are at their original length; x_{Ei} and x_{Fi} and are the length of the extensor and flexor PAMs. In this manuscript, the subscripts h and k denote attributes of hip and knee joints, respectively. In this chapter, the subscripts E and F denote attributes of extensor and flexor PAMs, respectively. The subscripts h and k denote attributes of the hip and knee joint, respectively.

In terms of torque requirement, the exoskeleton is designed to provide enough guidance for hip and knee joint torque to help a subject reproduce desired gait pattern. The problem can hence be articulated as comparing the torque generation capacity of the actuation system and the maximum possible required torque for both joints throughout a gait cycle (GC). A healthy subject's joint space gait pattern and joint torque published in [14] is used as reference. It has also been reported in [13] that the joint torque during walking can be normalised by body weight. With this normalisation technique, the walking joint torque requirement for healthy subjects of various body weight can be approximated and plotted in Figure 8.3.

The maximum contractile force ($F_{\max}$) one PAM when inflated to maximum pressure (six bar) can be approximated as a function of its contracting percentage to its original length ($l_0 = 0.3$ m), according to the datasheet of the FESTO PAM. Thus, the maximum joint actuation torque ($\tau_{\max}$) can also be calculated:

$$F_{\max\_ij} = 16{,}236\frac{x_{ij}^2}{l_0^2} - 9{,}405\frac{x_{ij}}{l_0} + 1{,}578 \tag{8.2}$$

$$\tau_{\max\_ij} = 2r_j F_{\max\_ij} \quad \text{with} \quad (i = F, E) \quad \text{and} \quad (j = h, k) \tag{8.3}$$

By combining the joint trajectory data through a GC with (8.1) and (8.2), the actuators capability of providing extension and flexion torque through the GC can be calculated in (8.3) and illustrated with the shaded areas in Figure 8.3. It can be viewed from the figure that the actuation system is able to cover hip and knee joint torque requirement of a 71-kg healthy subject during level walking. For the simulated subject with 100 kg body weight, the designed actuation system is still capable of providing sufficient torque for most of the GC except the peak extension torque requirement for the knee joints and the peak flexion and extension torque for the hip joint. By analysing the plots shown in Figure 8.3, it is observed that the peak torques all occur within the first 60% of the GC which is the stance phase, when there are needs to support the body weight. Body weight support systems are commonly used in conjunction with robotics exoskeleton and treadmill to provide gait rehabilitation training. The body weight unloading is up to 60–80% for patients with severe paralysis [15]. This implies that the exoskeleton only needs to bear a

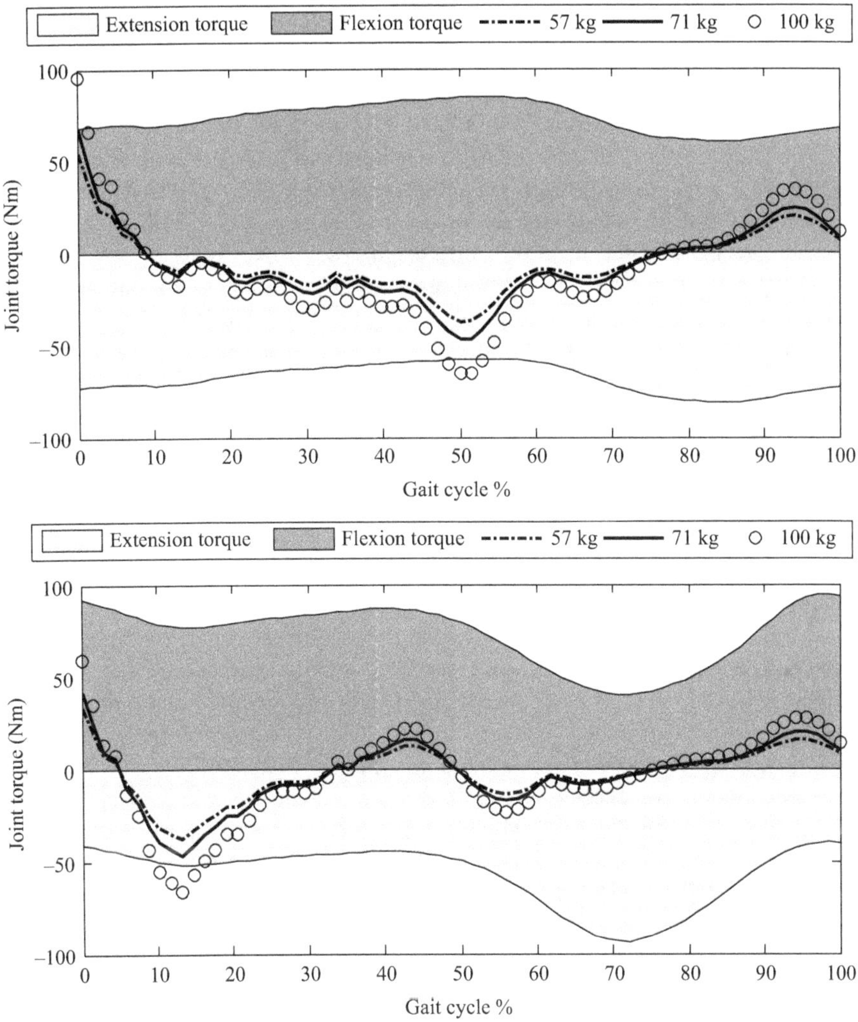

Figure 8.3 Joint torque versus gait cycle (GC) plots for the hip (top) and knee (bottom) joints. The joint torque requirement data of the 57 kg healthy subject during normal walking are adopted from [14] The data of the 71 kg and 100 kg are calculated from the 57 kg subject with normalisation of body weight. The shaded areas in the plots are indicating the joint torque output capability of both the extension and flexion PAMs throughout the GC

fraction of the torque requirement of supporting body weight. Hence, it can be confidently concluded that the designed actuation system is capable of providing sufficient torque to facilitate robotic gait training for patients of up to 100 kg body weight.

8.3.2 Mechanical and pneumatic system design of the lower limb mechanism

After selecting the pneumatic actuators, the following step was to design and construct the LLE that integrates with the antagonistic PAM actuators.

The LLE also has a modular design as shown in Figure 8.4. The knee and hip modules each contains it corresponding joint actuation system. The two modules are connected to form the thigh segment of the LLE. The relative position of the two modules can be adjusted to ensure that the hip and knee joints of the LLE are aligned with the subject's joints during an experiment. Each of the module has a rigid leg brace attached. During training, one of the subject's legs is attached to the braces via straps. The sizes and positions of the braces are adjustable according to the subject's anthropometric measurements. The braces were designed to be rigid to prevent any relative movement between the exoskeleton and the leg attached to it.

The designs by Hussain *et al.* [5] and Choi *et al.* [16] have PAMs located at both the thigh and shank segments of the exoskeleton for actuation of the hip and knee joints, respectively. On GAREX, all eight PAM actuators were located to the thigh segments of LLE. Such design transfers the actuators' inertia from the shank to the thigh segment, thus reducing the torque requirements of both the hip and knee joints for producing the same movement.

In order to accomplish a robust working prototype in a short timeframe, most of the parts of the LLE were made of laser cut aluminium parts. Some key structure parts were machined steel parts such as the shafts and bearing houses of the actuated joints.

The key part of the pneumatic system is the valves controlling the air flow to the PAMs. Mainly two types of valves have been used on this role. One is pressure-controlled proportional valves, which have embedded software to regulate their output pressures to the desired levels. The other type is analogue proportional valve, which effectively changes their orifice areas by changing the spool positions. When used in controlling PAM-driven mechanism, the pressure regulator type of valves appears to be black boxes in control loops, which leads to simpler the system models by ignoring the details of PAM's pressure characteristics. However, there could be unpredictable transient behaviour of the controlled PAM pressure.

To overcome this, four 3/5 analogue valves (FESTO: MPYE-5-1/8-LF-010-B) were adopted in this research, two for each actuated joint, as shown in Figure 8.5. The pneumatic flow through the valve can be controlled by changing the valve orifice area which depends on its input voltage. Compared to Shen [17] which used a single 3/5 analogue valve for an antagonistic pair of PAMs, the design in this research is a redundant actuation system if only implementing trajectory control. However, it leaves the possibilities open for more sophisticated controller development to cater various robotic gait rehabilitation modes.

Similar to the analogue valves, pressure sensors were installed, one for each side of the antagonistic PAMs of an actuated joint. The pressure sensors are used for both feedback control and status monitoring. It can also be viewed from

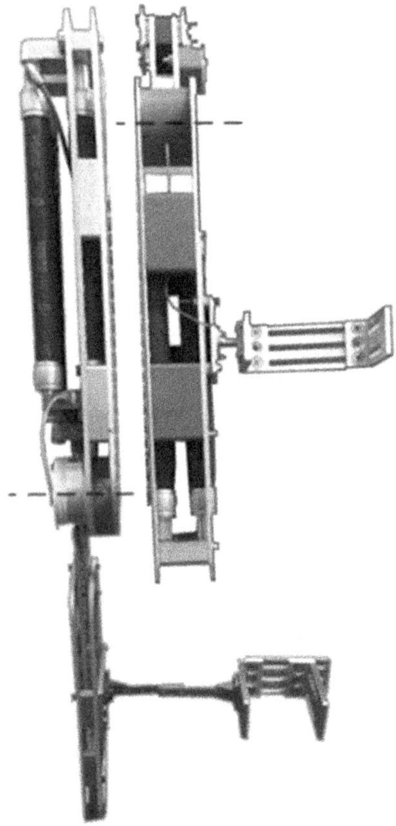

Figure 8.4 The front view of the lower limb exoskeleton (LLE) with the thigh (right) and shank (left) modules separated. The relative position of the two modules can be adjusted in order to align the rotational axes (marked with dashed lines) of the knee and hip with the subject's ones

Figure 8.5 that a main solenoid valve in between the pneumatic source and the analogue valves is for the PAMs. The solenoid valve is used to switch the pneumatic flow to the actuation system based a digital signal sent from the control software.

8.4 Instrumentation

All major components including the pneumatic components described in the previous paragraphs are included in the block diagram in Figure 8.6, which shows the hardware architecture for the entire GAREX system, myRIO from National Instrument is used as the main control platform. Inside the myRIO, there is an FPGA module and a micro-processor. The FPGA has been programmed to conduct

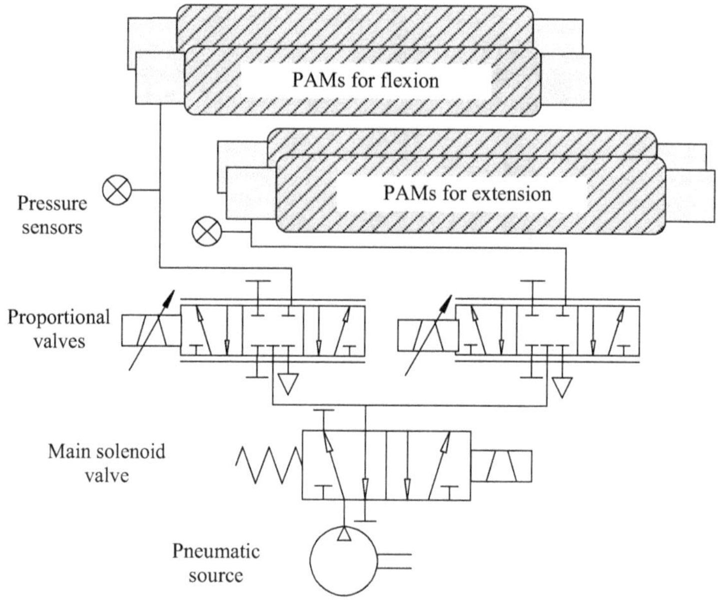

Figure 8.5 The pneumatic flow diagram for one of the actuated exoskeleton joint. The other joint has an identical configuration. The two actuated joints share the same pneumatic source and main solenoid valve

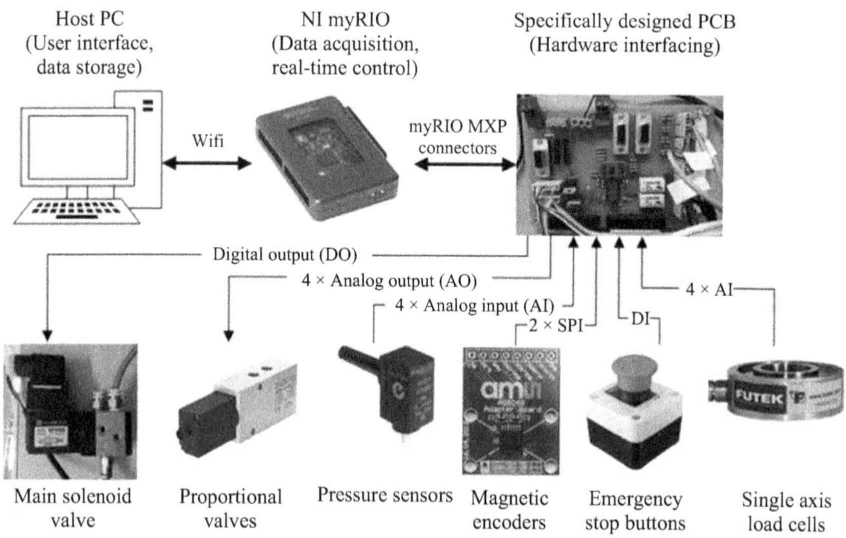

Figure 8.6 Hardware configuration block diagram. Major components of the instrumentation hardware system are listed with connectors indicating the types of interfaces and directions of data flows

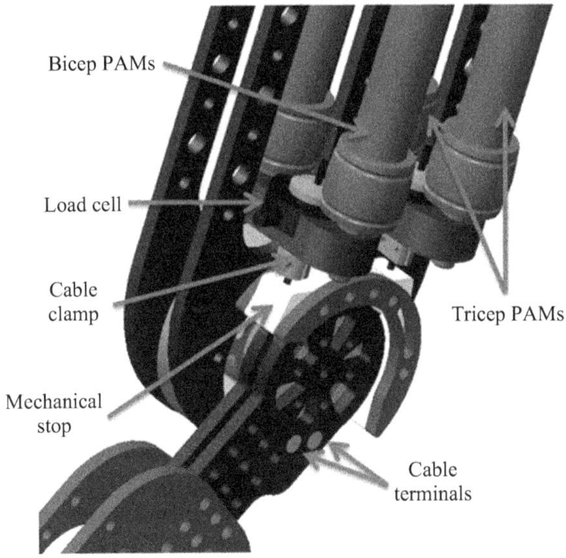

Figure 8.7 Detailed computer-aided-design of the knee joint mechanism. All the major components of the mechanism are illustrated

hardware interfacing and sensor signal processing at a rate of 1 kHz. The processor could then be used to focus on model-based controller processing at a rate of 100 Hz. For physical hardware interface, a custom-printed circuit board (PCB) was designed. The PCB contains connectors for various components which are illustrated in Figure 8.6, together with their types of interface. The PCB was also designed with circuits to handle the emergency stop situation which will be discussed later.

For the joint space position feedback, magnetic encoders were mounted to be co-axial with the two actuated joints. The filtered derivatives of the angular positions are computed through the FPGA module for the potential use in controller development. Single axis load cells are mounted as shown in Figure 8.7 to monitor the pulling forces of the antagonistic PAMs at the knee joint and thus the joint's actuation torque.

8.5 Safety of GAREX

The safety is of paramount importance. A variety of features have been designed and implemented to ensure the safety of the patients if any unexpected incident happens.

Mechanical ROM-limiting stops shown in Figure 8.7 were designed for both the actuated hip and knee joints of the exoskeleton to ensure that the exoskeleton cannot move beyond the allowed ROM of corresponding human joints.

Emergency stop buttons are made accessible to both the training subject and the supervising therapists or engineers. Once any of the stop buttons is pressed, 2-fold safety actions will take place. At hardware level, relay circuits have been designed on the custom PCB. The press of a stop button grounds the voltage input to the main solenoid valve, so the pneumatic flow to the actuation system can be cut off. Meanwhile, the analogue signal input to all the proportional valves would be suppressed with a 0 V signal which essentially deflates all the PAMs at the valves' full capacity. At the software level, the controller recognises the stop button press, idles all the control process, sends signals to the hardware to cut-down pneumatic follow and deflates the PAMs, as well as displays warning message on the graphical user interface.

8.6 Summary

A unilateral robotic gait rehabilitation system actuated by PAMs has been designed and built. Only a few PAM-driven gait rehabilitation robots have been reported. To the author's knowledge, none of them have conducted detailed torque analysis to verify the system's ability to provide task-specific gait training. GAREX was designed with future clinical application in mind. The system is capable of providing sufficient torque for the knee and hip joint rotations in the sagittal planes to facilitate gait rehabilitation for a patient weighing up to 100 kg.

Four analogue valves were selected to allow detailed modelling of the entire controlled plant in the following research. Position, pressure and force sensors were installed for both control feedback and system monitoring. Safe training was achieved through system monitoring as well as dedicated features such as mechanical limit stops and emergency stop buttons.

To ensure that GAREX can provide training to a wide population range, the system was designed to be modular and telescopic. The knee and hip actuation modules' relative position can be adjusted to accommodate variable lengths of patients' lower limb segments. To fit subjects with different builds, the horizontal and vertical position of the exoskeleton module to the trunk manipulation module was made adjustable, together with the vertical position of the trunk manipulation module relative to the supporting frame.

References

[1] Chou CP, Hannaford B. Measurement and modeling of McKibben pneumatic artificial muscles. IEEE Trans Robot Autom. 1996;12(1):90–102.

[2] Choi TY, Choi BS, Seo KH. Position and compliance control of a pneumatic muscle actuated manipulator for enhanced safety. IEEE Trans Control System Technol. 2011;19(4):832–42.

[3] Sugar TG, He J, Koeneman EJ, Koeneman JB, *et al.* Design and control of RUPERT: a device for robotic upper extremity repetitive therapy. IEEE Trans Neural Syst Rehabil Eng. 2007;15(3):336–46.

[4] Beyl P, Damme MV, Ham RV, Vanderborght B, Lefeber D. Pleated pneumatic artificial muscle-based actuator system as a torque source for compliant lower limb exoskeletons. IEEE/ASME Trans Mechatronics 2014;19(3):1046–56.
[5] Hussain S, Xie SQ, Jamwal PK, Parsons J. An intrinsically compliant robotic orthosis for treadmill training. Med Eng Phys. 2012;34(10):1448–53.
[6] Cao J, Xie SQ, Das R, Zhu GL. Control Strategies for effective robot assisted gait rehabilitation: the state of art and future prospects. Med Eng Phys. 2014;36(12):1555–66.
[7] Beyl P, Van Damme M, Cherelle P, Lefeber D. Safe and compliant guidance in robot-assisted gait rehabilitation using proxy-based sliding mode control. ICORR-IEEE International conference on rehabilitation robotics; 2009.
[8] Kuan TS, Tsou JY, Su FC. Hemiplegic gait of stroke patients: the effect of using a cane. Arch Phys Med Rehabil. 1999;80(7):777–84.
[9] Chang MK. An adaptive self-organizing fuzzy sliding mode controller for a 2-DOF rehabilitation robot actuated by pneumatic muscle actuators. Control Eng Pract. 2010;18(1):13–22.
[10] Andrikopoulos G, Nikolakopoulos G, Manesis S. Advanced nonlinear PID-based antagonistic control for pneumatic muscle actuators. IEEE Trans Ind Electron. 2014;61(12):6926–37.
[11] Lilly JH, Yang L. Sliding mode tracking for pneumatic muscle actuators in opposing pair configuration. IEEE Trans Control Syst Technol. 2005;13 (4):550–8.
[12] Kora K, McDaid A, Xie S. Non-linear model-based control for the human-inspired robotic exoskeleton (HuREx) gait trainer.World congress of the international federation of automatic control. HuREx:Cape Town, South Africa; 2014.
[13] Perry J, Burnfield JM. Gait analysis: normal and pathological function. Thorofare, NJ: SLACK, c2010; 1992.
[14] Winter DA. Biomechanics and motor control of human movement. Philadelphia, PA: John Wiley & Sons; 2009.
[15] Frey M, Colombo G, Vaglio M, Bucher R, Jorg M, Riener R. A novel mechatronic body weight support system. IEEE Trans Neural Syst Rehabil Eng. 2006;14(3):311–21.
[16] Choi T-Y, Lee J-J. Control of manipulator using pneumatic muscles for enhanced safety. IEEE Trans Ind Electron. 2010;57(8):2815–25.
[17] Shen X. Nonlinear model-based control of pneumatic artificial muscle servo systems. Control Eng Pract. 2010;18(3):311–7.

Chapter 9

Modelling and control strategies development of GAREX

This chapter focuses on a multi-input-multi-output (MIMO) sliding mode (SM) controller which is aimed to simultaneously control the angular trajectory and compliance of the GAit Rehabilitation Exoskeleton (GAREX). The MIMO controller is developed based on the complete model of GAREX system which consists of four sub-system models. They are flow dynamics of the valves, pressure and force dynamics of the antagonistic pneumatic artificial muscles, as well as the load dynamics of the exoskeleton. Experiments with and without healthy subjects are conducted a GAREX to validate the developed SM controllers. The experimental results indicate good multivariable tracking performance of this controller.

9.1 Introduction

Pneumatic artificial muscle (PAM) actuators are intrinsically compliant and with high force/power to weight ratio. These advantages make PAMs suitable for rehabilitation robots, especially exoskeleton type of robotic devices. Ferris *et al.* [1] developed an ankle-foot orthosis actuated by PAM to assist the ankle planar flexion during walking. This orthosis was further developed into a knee-ankle-foot orthosis with the knee flexion/extension and ankle dorsi-/planar-flexion all actuated [2]. A PAM actuated upper limb rehabilitation robot, named RUPERT, was developed by a research group from Arizona State University. The robot had four degrees of freedom (DOF) each actuated by a PAM actuator [3]. In the authors' research group, a robotic exoskeleton for gait rehabilitation has also been developed, with both the hip and knee joints of the exoskeleton powered by antagonistic PAM actuators [4]. Despite their advantages, dynamics of PAMs is highly non-linear and also subject to hysteresis; therefore, it becomes a challenging task to model them precisely.

In order to develop more effective controllers, a number of researchers have investigated different modelling method of PAMs. Chou and Hannaford [5] developed the simple but widely used geometrical model on McKibben PAM. Tondu and Lopez [6] further improved the model in [5] by compensating the end deformation (PAM is not a cylindrical shape when inflated) and attempting to offset the hysteretic behaviour between inflation and deflation of a PAM. Another commonly adopted model of PAM is the phenomenological model developed by Reynolds *et al.* [7]. The PAM model is similar to the Hill's muscle model in biomechanics. It contains parallel force generation, spring and damping elements.

Although modelling of PAM has been extensively investigated, researchers [8,9] still claimed that models tend to be highly nonlinear and subject to uncertainties, mainly due to friction, temperature and change of properties overtime. To cope with these problems, a variety of controllers have been implemented on PAM-driven mechanisms, which include adaptive pole-placement controller by Caldwell *et al.* [10], robust and adaptive back-stepping controller by Carbonell *et al.* [11], fuzzy PD + I controller by Chan *et al.* [12], neural network-based PID controller by Thanh and Ahn [13] and more recently echo state network-based predictive controller with particle swarm optimisation by Huang *et al.* [14].

Sliding mode control and its variations have also been implemented in several applications to control mechanism-driven PAM actuators, because SM controllers are robust to modelling uncertainties and disturbances. Van Damme *et al.* [15] applied proxy-based SM control on a two-DOF serial robotic manipulator actuated by antagonistic pleated PAMs. Lilly and Yang [9] applied SM approach to control the trajectory of a single DOF rotational mechanism driven by McKibben PAM actuators. Their dynamic model was based on the work reported in [7]. Xing *et al.* [16] developed SM trajectory control with nonlinear disturbance observer to a PAM-driven mechanism. Chang [17] reported an adaptive self-organising fuzzy SM controller for a two-DOF serial robot manipulator. In [9,15,17], the rotational joints were all actuated by antagonistic PAMs. Single-input-single-output (SISO) SM approaches were dedicated for trajectory control. It is common that the desired pressures of individual PAMs can be calculated by the controllers' output Δp and a fixed desired average pressure (P_{0d}) of the antagonistic PAMs as:

$$\begin{cases} P_{Fd} = P_{0d} + \Delta P \\ P_{Ed} = P_{0d} - \Delta P \end{cases} \tag{9.1}$$

where P_{Fd} and P_{Ed} are the reference pressures of the muscles for joint flexion and extension, respectively. These were fed into the pressure regulators which adjusted the PAM pressures to their desired values. Choi *et al.* [18] implemented both position and compliance control on a PAM actuated manipulator. The position control implementation was similar to the work reported by Lilly and Yang [9]. Instead of having fixed average pressure of the antagonistic PAMs, an open loop compliance controller was developed. Based on a dynamic model [7] of PAMs, the magnitude of joint space compliance can be derived from the desired compliance value. It is also noteworthy that the compliance control is independent from the SM trajectory controller.

In [9,15–18], the use of pressure regulators, which appears to be black boxes in control loops, simplified the system models by ignoring the details of the pressure characteristics of the PAM actuator. Hence, unpredictable errors or time delays could be introduced. Shen [19] eliminated these black boxes by modelling the whole system with four major processes, which were flow dynamics of the valve, pressure and force dynamics of the PAM actuators and the load dynamics of a linear antagonistic mechanism. With a single 3/5 analogue valve, the SISO control was made possible by merging the models of four processes and, letting the valve voltage as input and the trajectory as output. This control approach was verified with a linear mechanism actuated by antagonistic PAMs. Aschemann and Schindele [20] developed a cascade SM control algorithm to control a linear mechanism. The four major processes similar to [19] were also utilised to model the system. In the outer trajectory control loop, an SM controller was implemented with the force dynamics of the PAM actuators and the load dynamics of the mechanism. Equation (9.1) was then used to calculate the reference pressures for the PAM actuators from the controller output of the outer loop (ΔP) and the desired average pressure (P_0). For each individual PAM, a SM controller was implemented based on the flow dynamics of the valve and the pressure dynamics of the PAM actuator. Compared to [18], Aschemann and Schindele's approach [20] was able to vary the average pressure, in other words stiffness of the mechanism, while tracking the desired trajectory. However, substantial difference in time constant between the pressure SM controller and trajectory SM controller was needed to decouple the cascaded controller into two SISO controllers [21]. Hence, the bandwidth of the trajectory control was limited.

Goals of research are to make the robot assisted gait training more task specific or close to real walking and to have robot only assist patients as much as they need. In terms of control strategies, the intrinsic compliance property of PAMs can be utilised to adjust the level of assistance provided by the exoskeleton. Hence, controller of the exoskeleton should be able to control the joint space trajectory and the compliance of the exoskeleton simultaneously. Similar ideas has been implemented in [18,20]; however, these two approaches are both subject to certain limitations, which have been discussed in the previous paragraph.

The main contribution of this chapter is the novel application of a centralised MIMO SM controller to an antagonistic PAM actuated joint mechanism for robotic gait rehabilitation. Firstly, the complete model of GAREX's lower limb mechanism is introduced. This is followed by the development of the MIMO joint trajectory and compliance controller. Extensive experiments of the MIMO controller were conducted on the knee joint mechanism only, as well as on the entire GAREX system.

9.2 System modelling

A block diagram of the PAM-driven antagonistic robotic system has been presented in Figure 9.1. It is noteworthy that the subscripts '*h*' and '*k*' are for variables of hip and knee joint; '*F*' and '*E*' are for properties of the flexor and extensor PAMs. In this section the entire plant is divided into four sequential sub-systems which are each modelled individually.

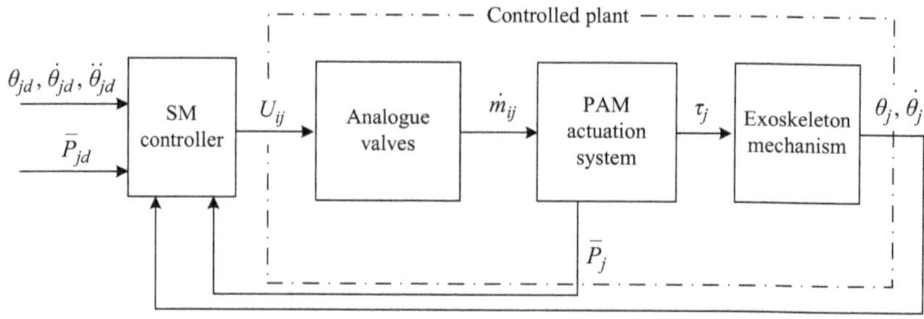

Figure 9.1 The control system block diagram of GAREX. In this Figure $i = F, E$ and $j = h, k$; U_{ij} is the voltage fed into the corresponding analogue valve; $\dot{m}_{ij}$ is the pneumatic mass flow rate to the corresponding PAMs; $\bar{P}_{jd}$ is the average pressure of the antagonistic PAMs of the corresponding joint. The subscript d indicates desired value of a property

9.2.1 Valve flow dynamics

Pneumatic mass flow through the 3/5 analogue valve is modelled as dimensional compressible flow through an orifice. The effective area of the orifice is controlled by the voltage signals applied to the valves. The mass flow rate through a valve is described as a function of the valve's opening area:

$$\dot{m}_{(E,F)}(P_u, P_d) = A_{(E,F)} \cdot \Lambda_{(E,F)}(P_u, P_d) \tag{9.2}$$

where:

$$\Lambda(P_u, P_d) = \begin{cases} \sqrt{\dfrac{\gamma}{RT}\left(\dfrac{2}{\gamma+1}\right)^{(\gamma+1)/(\gamma-1)}} C_f P_u & if \dfrac{P_d}{P_u} \le C_r \text{ (chocked)} \\ \sqrt{\dfrac{2\gamma}{RT(\gamma-1)}}\sqrt{1-\left(\dfrac{P_d}{P_u}\right)^{(\gamma-1)/\gamma}}\left(\dfrac{P_d}{P_u}\right)^{1/\gamma} C_f P_u & \text{otherwise (unchocked)} \end{cases} \tag{9.3}$$

In the two equations above, $A_{(E,F)}$ are the equivalent valve area for the PAMs on the extension and flexion sides; P_u and P_d are the upstream and downstream pressures, respectively; C_f is the discharge constant and C_r is the pressure ratio that divides the flow into choked and un-choked flow through the orifice.

During the inflating process of the PAM actuator, the pneumatic supply pressure (P_s) is regarded as the upstream pressure and the downstream pressure is equal to the pressure inside the PAM actuator, expressed in (9.4):

$$\begin{cases} P_u = P_s \\ P_d = P_{(E,F)} \end{cases} \tag{9.4}$$

During the deflating process, the pressure of inside the PAM is regarded as the upstream pressure and the atmospheric pressure (P_{atm}) is regarded as the downstream pressure:

$$\begin{cases} P_u = P_{(E,F)} \\ P_d = P_{atm} \end{cases} \tag{9.5}$$

It is noteworthy that the equivalent area of a valve is constrained by the maximum opening area. The applied voltage to the valve, U_i, which is the actual input to the physical system, is calculated using a linear piecewise function of the controller output A_i as:

$$U_i = \begin{cases} 178{,}592A_i + 5.255 \ (0.02A_{\max} \le A_i \le A_{\max}) \\ 10^6 A_i + 5 \ (-0.02A_{\max} \le A_i \le 0.02A_{\max}) \\ 178{,}592A_i + 4.745 \ (-A_{\max} \le A_i \le -0.02A_{\max}) \end{cases} \quad (i = E, F) \tag{9.6}$$

Ideally, a 5 V input to the valve would idle the pneumatic flow through the valve and the equivalent valve opening area would be proportional to $(U_i - 5)$. However, in actual operation, the proportional relationship is only valid if the input voltage is approximately more than 0.3 V away from the ideal idle voltage. Through trial and error, (9.6) was constructed to present the valve input voltage to equivalent opening areas conversion.

9.2.2 Pneumatic muscle pressure dynamics

The PAM actuation system block in Figure 9.1 can be further divided into models of the pressure dynamics and force dynamics. The pressure dynamics models the relation between the mass flow rate and the rate of pressure change of the PAMs. The force dynamics models the PAM's contracting force versus PAM pressure and kinematics relationship.

For the pressure dynamics model, It is assumed that pneumatic flow into and out of the PAM is an adiabatic process [19]. Thus, the rate of change of pressure in PAM can be described by the physics-based model as:

$$\dot{P}_{(E,F)} = \frac{(\gamma RT\dot{m}_{(E,F)} - \gamma P\dot{V}_{(E,F)})}{V_{(E,F)}} \tag{9.7}$$

$$V_{(E,F)} = 2\left(a_1 x_{(E,F)^2} + a_2 x_{(E,F)} + a_3\right) \tag{9.8}$$

$$\dot{V}_{(E,F)} = 4a_1 x_{(E,F)}\dot{x}_{(E,F)} + 2a_2\dot{x}_{(E,F)} \tag{9.9}$$

where γ and R are the ratio of specific heats and universal gas constant of air; T is the gas temperature; m_is the pneumatic mass flow rate of the PAMs which is positive for flow into the PAMs; and V is the volume of air inside the two PAMs of each side of the antagonistic pair. V is modelled as a function of muscle contraction length (x) in (9.8) and its time derivative is expressed in (9.9).

9.2.3 Pneumatic muscle force dynamics model

The task-specific robotic gait rehabilitation imposes bandwidth requirement to the actuation system. An appropriate dynamic model is essential for further controller development of the robotic GAREX. To the authors' best knowledge, there were no dynamic force models for the FESTO pneumatic muscle available for direct implementation [22,23]. To make better use of the FESTO PAMs in dynamic applications such as robotic gait rehabilitation, a more specific dynamic model for FESTO PAM still needs to be developed based on the original model by Reynolds *et al.* [7].

The dynamic PAM model developed by Reynolds *et al.* [7] is in a similar format to the well-known Hill's muscle model in biomechanics. It contains parallel force generation, spring and damping elements as shown in Figure 9.2. The dynamic force behaviour is represented by the following equation:

$$F(P) + B(P)\dot{x} + K(P)x = L + m\ddot{x} \tag{9.10}$$

where P is the inflating pressure of the PAM actuator; $F(P)$, $B(P)$, $K(P)$ are force, damping and spring elements which are all linearly dependent on pressure (as indicated in (9.11)) and determined experimentally; m is the mass of the load; x, and $\ddot{x}$ are the contracting length, velocity and acceleration of PAM, respectively; and L is the force exerted on the load.

$$\begin{cases} F(P) = F_0 + F_1 P \\ K(P) = K_0 + K_1 P \\ B(P) = B_{I0} + B_{I1} P \ \text{(Inflation)} \\ B(P) = B_{D0} + B_{I1} P \ \text{(Deflation)} \end{cases} \tag{9.11}$$

The parameters F_i, K_i, B_{Ii} and B_{Di} $(i = 0, 1)$ in (9.11) can be determined experimentally. The damping element of the inflation and deflation processes was modelled separately to address the hysteresis behaviour of the PAM.

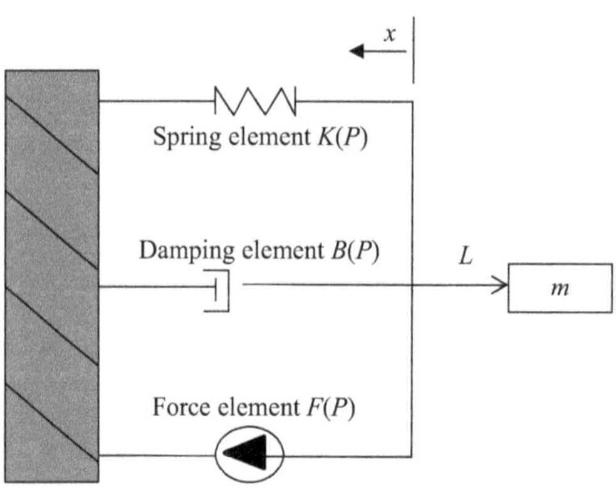

Figure 9.2 The Hill's type of dynamic PAM model adapted by Reynolds et al. [7]

The model published in [7] is a good benchmark of the development of a dynamic force model for the specific type of PAMs used in this research. Hence an experimental rig was constructed to investigate between the force generated by a PAM and its inflating pressure and kinematics. Based on the experimental rig, the research designed an automated experimental process to have the tested PAM operate in a wide range of dynamic scenarios and record data. In the data analysis, the research firstly investigated if the model in [7] is able to well present the gathered experimental data. If the fit was not ideal, the researcher would attempt to look for a new or improved dynamic model for the PAMs actuating GAREX.

A rig had been built to conduct automated experiments. The parameters of the model can be calculated in order to best present the experimental data. The experimental setup is shown in Figure 9.3. The PAM_1 at the bottom was the

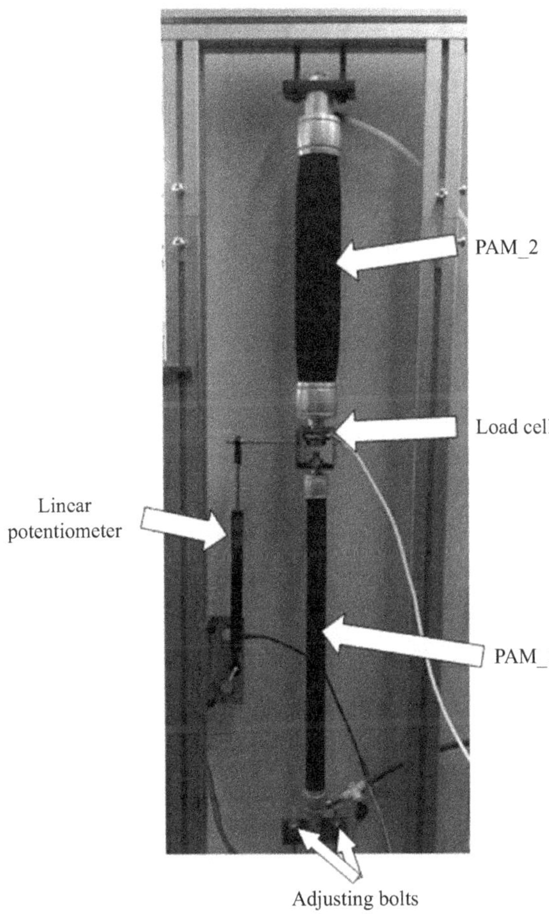

Figure 9.3 The experimental setup to find the dynamic model parameters of a PAM actuator

muscle to be modelled. A PAM (FESTO DMSP-20-300N-RM-CM) integrated in GAREX design was adopted as PAM_1. PAM_2 (FESTO DMSP-40-300N-RM-CM) was 40 mm in diameter, 300 mm length, which provides motions as required during the experiments. The pressure of PAM_1 was controlled by a pressure regulator (FESTO VPPAM-6L-L-1-G18-0L6H-A4N). The pneumatic flow rate of PAM_2 was changed via an analogue valve (MPYE-5-1/8-LF-010-B). A pressure sensor (SPTE-P10R-S6-V2.5K) was also placed next to the pneumatic connection to PAM_1 for more accurate pressure measurement. The linear potentiometer (Variohm VLP100) and the load cell (FUTEK LTH350) were used to measure contracting length of PAM_1 and interaction force between the two PAMs, respectively. The assumption of this testing setup was that masses of all moving components are negligible. This is because, in the worst scenario, the product of the entire moving mass (0.3 kg) of the rig and the maximum acceleration (3 m/s) is less than the noise of the load cell reading.

During one set of experiments, the pressure of PAM_1 was regulated to the fixed value P_1, while the PAM_2 was inflated and deflated at various rates in order to exert different load to PAM_1. Initially, PAM_2 was fully deflated. After the measurement of x_0 was completed, the step inflating voltage was applied to the analogue valve of PAM_2. The orifice size of the analogue valve is proportional to the applied. As a response, PAM_2 contracts to stretch PAM_1. After the movement was settled and a wait of 3 s, another step voltage was applied the analogue valve to deflate PAM_2, so PAM_1 contracted again back to x_0. It is worth to note that the inflating and deflating orifice areas were of same magnitude. During this process, kinematics, load cell reading and the pressure of PAM_1 were monitored and logged to a data file at a rate of 100 Hz.

The inflation-settling-deflation process repeated. The inflating (deflating) orifice areas were increased from 10% to 100% of the maximum opening of the valve in the step size of 10%. Up to this point, the experiment for the selected pressure of PAM_1 was completed. Figure 9.4 is showing the gathered data for the set of experimental data when PAM_1 is regulated to 3.2 bar. Only dynamic data (velocity magnitude greater than 0.005 m/s) are gathered. The contracting and stretching data points are separated, so hysteresis can be considered in the proposed model. The same experimental procedure was repeatedly conducted to various pressures of PAM_1 ranging from 0.8 bar to 5 bar, with three experiments for each pressure. A total of 51 valid experiments have been conducted.

For each of the 51 experiments conducted, the data for the contracting and stretching processes of PAM_1 were separated. Curve fitting was the conducted for both sets of data in the same method of producing Figure 9.4. As a result, 102 combinations of $K(P)$, $B(P)$ and $F(P)$ could be calculated. These parameter combinations were all plotted against their corresponding PAM_1 pressures in order to investigate the parameters are dependent on PAM pressure. The plots are shown in Figure 9.5.

The initial investigation was on the first-order linear relationships between PAM pressure and the parameters as described in (9.11). The first-order linear model is represented using grey lines in Figure 9.5. Its modelling coefficients are

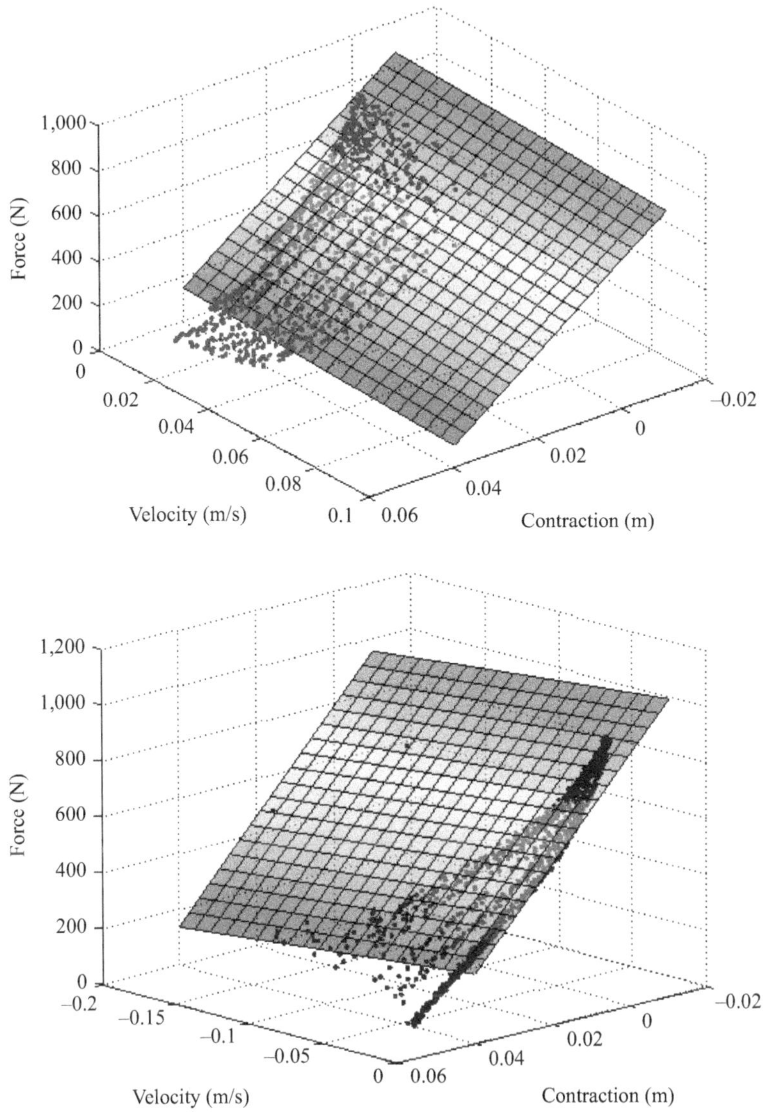

Figure 9.4 The first-order polynomial representation curve fitting result of PAM force versus its contracting length and velocity when its pressure was regulated to 3.2 bar. The upper plot is for the contracting process of PAM_1 and the lower plot is for the stretching process

shown in the third column of Table 9.1. As it can be seen from Figure 9.5, the grey lines are well-correlated to the experimental data except the one for the spring element. To further quantify the how well the dynamic model by Reynolds *et al.* [7] fits the experimental data. Regression analysis was performed to calculate the R^2

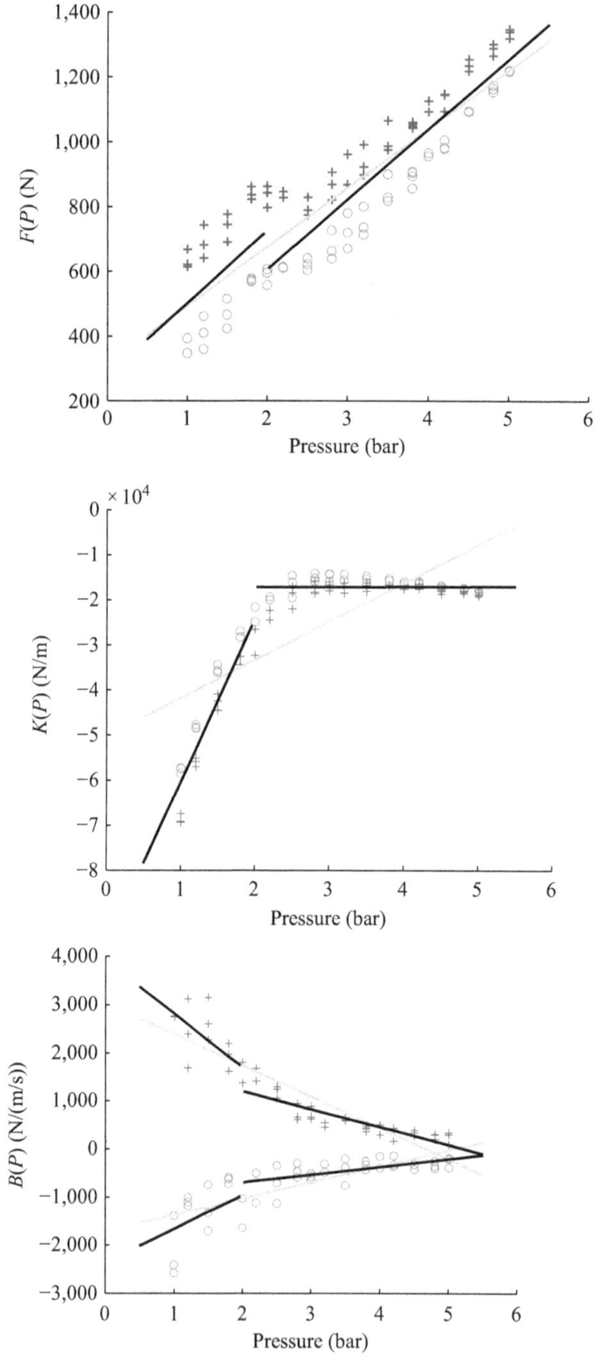

Figure 9.5 F(P) (top), K(P) (middle) and B(P) (bottom) versus PAM_1 pressure plots, respectively. The scatters represent the parameters gathered from the 51 experiments. The 'o' scatters are for the contracting processes of PAM_1 and '+' scatters for the stretching processes

Table 9.1 Parameters of different dynamic models and regression analysing results of the models, for the 300 mm PAM used in GAREX

Factor		Coefficient	First-order linear model	Piecewise model	
				Below 2 bar	Above 2 bar
Force element		(N)	311.8	276.8	173.6
		F_1 (N/bar)	181.9	224.7	216.2
Spring element		K_0 (N/m)	−39,085	−96,524	−17,253
		K_1 (N/m/bar)	24,634	36,121	47.1
Damping element	Contraction	B_0 (N s/m)	−1,704	−2,363	−1,022
		B_1 (N s/m/bar)	336.5	702.2	163.2
	Stretch F_0	B_0 (N s/m)	3,041	3,930	1,931
		B_1 (N s/m/bar)	−649.8	−1,117	−368.7
Regression analysis	Contraction	R^2	0.5719	0.9430 (0.9130)	
	Stretch		0.5106	0.9507 (0.9227)	

values (shown in the bottom row of Table 9.1) of the entire population of experimental data. For every valid data point, the force calculated via (9.10) and (9.11) was compared with the measured force. A total of 38,745 and 38,217 data points are included in the analysis for stretch and contraction of PAM_1, respectively. The result of regression analysis indicates that the model could be improved to better represent the dynamic behaviour of the PAM.

Firstly, by analysing the plots in Figure 9.5, it was realised that the spring parameter versus pressure relationships have different trends when the pressure is below or above 2 bar. The linear representations of $K(P)$, $B(P)$ and $F(P)$ were modified into two-stage piecewise linear functions, which are shown as the black lines in Figure 9.5. The constants of the piecewise model as well as the R^2 values of the regression analysis are listed in the columns titled 'Piecewise Model' of Table 9.1. The R^2 values are calculated in the same way as the ones for the original model. The R^2 values outsides the brackets are computed with all three elements from the proposed piecewise model; meanwhile, the ones inside the brackets are computed through a hybrid model with only the spring element from the piecewise model and the other elements from the original model. The regression analysis indicated that the modified piecewise model and the hybrid model fitted better to the experimental data compared to the original dynamic model. The difference between the pure piecewise model and the hybrid model was less obvious.

9.2.4 Load dynamics of the mechanism

The low limb exoskeleton can be treated as be treated as a serial robot and the well-established Lagrangian Formulation was adopted to calculate the actuated joint torque requirement from the kinematics of the exoskeleton as:

$$\mathbf{M}\underline{\ddot{\theta}} + \underline{V} + \underline{G} = \underline{\tau} \tag{9.12}$$

$$\text{or}\quad \begin{bmatrix} M_{11} & M_{12} \\ M_{21} & M_{22} \end{bmatrix} \begin{bmatrix} \ddot{\theta}_1 \\ \ddot{\theta}_2 \end{bmatrix} + \begin{bmatrix} V_1 \\ V_2 \end{bmatrix} + \begin{bmatrix} G_1 \\ G_2 \end{bmatrix} = \begin{bmatrix} \tau_1 \\ \tau_2 \end{bmatrix} \tag{9.13}$$

The first term in (9.13) is the inertial component of the joint torques. The second term $\underline{V}$ represents the Coriolis and centrifugal forces, which is followed by the gravitational component. The Lagrangian Formulation was adopted to calculate the symbolic representations of **M**, $\underline{V}$ and $\underline{G}$ at any given instant of the exoskeleton operation.

Figure 9.6 was created to visualise the modelling representation. Two coordinate systems have been created. One is a base coordinate system, whose

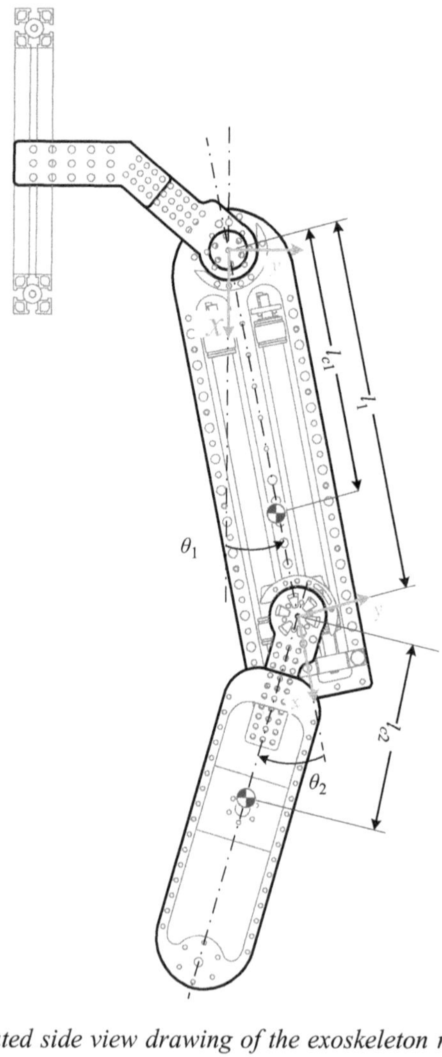

Figure 9.6 Illustrated side view drawing of the exoskeleton module for dynamics analysis of the mechanism. The z-axes of the two coordinate systems are both pointing out of the page

z-axis is co-axial with the hip joint of the exoskeleton, with its x-axis pointing down vertically and y-axis pointing right horizontally. The other coordinate system's z-axis is co-axial with the knee joint with x-axis long the thigh segment. The centre of mass (COM) of the thigh and shank segments are also illustrated in the figure using the “” symbol. Detailed calculating process of the dynamics of the mechanism can be found in Appendix A. The following processed parameters are:

$$M_{11} = \mathrm{m}_2 l_1^2 + 2\mathrm{m}_2 \cos\theta_2 l_1 l_{c2} + \mathrm{m}_1 l_{c1}^2 + \mathrm{m}_2 l_{c2}^2 + I_{1z} + I_{2z} \tag{9.14}$$

$$M_{12} = I_{2z} + l_{c2}\mathrm{m}_2 \left(l_{c2} + l_1 \cos\theta_2\right) \tag{9.15}$$

$$M_{21} = I_{2z} + l_{c2}\mathrm{m}_2 \left(l_{c2} + l_1 \cos(\theta_2)\right) \tag{9.16}$$

$$M_{22} = \mathrm{m}_2 l_{c2}^2 + I2_z \tag{9.17}$$

$$V_1 = -l_1 l_{c2}\mathrm{m}_2 \dot{\theta}_2^2 \sin\theta_2 - 2l_1 l_{c2}\mathrm{m}_2\, \dot{\theta}_1\dot{\theta}_2 \sin\theta_2 \tag{9.18}$$

$$V_2 = l_1\, l_{c2}\mathrm{m}_2\, \dot{\theta}_1^2 \sin\theta_2 \tag{9.19}$$

$$G_1 = \left(g_c \mathrm{m}_2 (l_{c2} \cos(\theta_1 + \theta_2) + l_1 \cos\theta_1) + g_c l_{c1}\mathrm{m}_1 \cos\theta_1\right) \tag{9.20}$$

$$G_2 = \left(g_c l_{c2}\mathrm{m}_2 \cos(\theta_1 + \theta_2)\right) \tag{9.21}$$

It is also worthy to note that the variable definitions used for the exoskeleton design and control development are different for the ones used in the dynamics modelling. The following conversions are adopted for ease of further controller implementation:

$$\begin{cases} \theta_1 = \theta_h - 90^\circ \\ \theta_2 = -\theta \end{cases} \begin{cases} \dot{\theta}_1 = \dot{\theta}_h \\ \dot{\theta}_2 = -\dot{\theta}_k \end{cases} \begin{cases} \ddot{\theta}_1 = \ddot{\theta}_h \\ \ddot{\theta}_2 = -\ddot{\theta}_k \end{cases} \begin{cases} \tau_1 = \tau_h \\ \tau_2 = -\tau_k \end{cases} \tag{9.22}$$

Upon substituting (9.22) into (9.13), the model can then be expressed in (9.23).

$$\begin{bmatrix} M_{11} & -M_{12} \\ -M_{21} & M_{22} \end{bmatrix} \begin{bmatrix} \ddot{\theta}_h \\ \ddot{\theta}_k \end{bmatrix} + \begin{bmatrix} V_1 \\ -V_2 \end{bmatrix} + \begin{bmatrix} G_1 \\ -G_2 \end{bmatrix} = \begin{bmatrix} \tau_h \\ \tau_k \end{bmatrix} \tag{9.23}$$

9.3 Multi-input-multi-output sliding mode control for GAREX

For the MIMO SM control system, the two model outputs are the position and the average pressure of the antagonistic PAMs of exoskeleton's knee joint. The two inputs are the equivalent areas of the two valves. A state–space model representation of the system was also constructed for the ease of MIMO SM control implementation. The SS variable ($\underline{x}$), system input ($\underline{u}$) and output ($\underline{y}$), vectors are given in the following three equations:

$$\underline{x} = \begin{bmatrix} \theta_k & \dot{\theta}_k & P_F & P_E \end{bmatrix}^T = [x_1 \quad x_2 \quad x_3 \quad x_4]^T \tag{9.24}$$

$$\underline{u} = [A_F \quad A_E]^T \tag{9.25}$$

$$\underline{y} = \begin{bmatrix} y_1(\underline{x}) \\ y_2(\underline{x}) \end{bmatrix} = \begin{bmatrix} x_1 & \dfrac{x_3 + x_4}{2} \end{bmatrix}^T \tag{9.26}$$

By combining the sub-models developed previously, the nonlinear state–space model can be written in the form of:

$$\dot{\underline{x}} = f(\underline{x}) + g(\underline{x})\underline{u} \tag{9.27}$$

or
$$\dot{\underline{x}} = f(\underline{x}) + \sum_{k=1}^{2} g_k(\underline{x})u_k \tag{9.28}$$

where,

$$f(\underline{x}) = \begin{bmatrix} \dot{\theta}_k \\ \begin{pmatrix} 2r\big(F(P_F) + r(\theta_{F0} - \theta_k)K(P_F) - r\dot{\theta}_k B(P_F)\big)/J \\ -2r\big(F(P_E) - r(\theta_{E0} - \theta_k)K(P_E) + r\dot{\theta}_k B(P_E)\big)/J \end{pmatrix} \\ \dfrac{0.5KP_F\big(4ar^2\dot{\theta}_k(\theta_{F0} - \theta_k) - 2a_2 r\dot{\theta}_k\big)}{V_F} \\ \dfrac{0.5KP_E\big(4ar^2\dot{\theta}_k(\theta_{E0} - \theta_k) + a_2 r\dot{\theta}_k\big)}{V_E} \end{bmatrix} \tag{9.29}$$

$$g(\underline{x}) = \begin{bmatrix} 0 & 0 \\ 0 & 0 \\ \dfrac{KRT\Lambda_F}{V_F} & 0 \\ 0 & \dfrac{KRT\Lambda_E}{V_E} \end{bmatrix} \tag{9.30}$$

$$V_F = 2a_3 + 2a_1 r^2(\theta_{F0} - \theta_k)^2 - 2a_2 r(\theta_{F0} - \theta_k) \tag{9.31}$$

$$V_F = 2a_3 + 2a_1 r^2(\theta_{F0} - \theta_k)^2 - 2a_2 r(\theta_{F0} - \theta_k) \tag{9.32}$$

A coordinate transformation [24] is performed with the following equation to make the system outputs and their derivatives as new state variable vector ($\underline{z}$).

$$\underline{z} = \mu(\underline{x}) = \begin{bmatrix} y_1(\underline{x}) \\ L_f y_1(\underline{x}) \\ L_f^2 y_1(\underline{x}) \\ y_2(\underline{x}) \end{bmatrix} = \begin{bmatrix} x_1 \\ x_2 \\ \dot{x}_2 \\ \dfrac{x_3 + x_4}{2} \end{bmatrix} \tag{9.33}$$

where the expression of $L_f(y_i)$ stands for the directional derivative of scalar y_i with respect to vector $f(\underline{x})$, which has the following properties:

$$L_f(y_i) = \frac{\partial y_i}{\partial x_1} f_1(\underline{x}) + \cdots + \frac{\partial y_i}{\partial x_n} f_n(\underline{x}) \quad \text{with } (i = 1, 2) \tag{9.34}$$

$$L_f^k(y_i) = L_f\left(L_f^{k-1}(y_i)\right) \quad \text{with } (i = 1, 2) \tag{9.35}$$

Based on (9.28), the time derivative of output y_i is calculated in (9.36) and the time derivative of the new state space variable vector is calculated in (9.37) to (9.42).

$$\begin{aligned} \frac{dy_i}{dt} &= \frac{\partial y_i}{\partial \underline{x}} \frac{\partial \underline{x}}{\partial t} = \frac{\partial y_i}{\partial \underline{x}} [f(\underline{x}) + g_1(\underline{x}) u_1 + g_2(\underline{x}) u_2] \\ &= L_f(y_i) + L_{g_1}(y_i) u_1 + L_{g_2}(y_i) u_2 \end{aligned} \quad \text{with } (i = 1, 2) \tag{9.36}$$

$$\dot{\underline{z}} = \begin{bmatrix} \dot{\theta}_k \\ \ddot{\theta}_k \\ L_f^3(y_1(\underline{x})) + L_{g_1} L_f^2(y_1(\underline{x})) u_1 + L_{g_2} L_f^2(y_1(\underline{x})) u_2 \\ L_f(y_2(\underline{x})) + L_{g_1}(y_2(\underline{x})) u_1 + L_{g_2}(y_2(\underline{x})) u_2 \end{bmatrix} \tag{9.37}$$

$$L_f^3(y_1(\underline{x})) = \frac{\partial \ddot{\theta}_k}{\partial \theta_k} f_1(\underline{x}) + \frac{\partial \ddot{\theta}_k}{\partial \dot{\theta}_k} f_2(\underline{x}) + \frac{\partial \ddot{\theta}_k}{\partial P_F} f_3(\underline{x}) + \frac{\partial \ddot{\theta}_k}{\partial P_E} f_4(\underline{x}) \tag{9.38}$$

where,

$$\frac{\partial \ddot{\theta}_k}{\partial \theta_k} = -\frac{2r^2(K_F(P_F) + K_F(P_F))}{J}$$

$$\frac{\partial \ddot{\theta}_k}{\partial \dot{\theta}_k} = -\frac{2r^2(B_F(P_F) + B_E(P_E))}{J}$$

$$\frac{\partial \ddot{\theta}_k}{\partial P_F} = \frac{2r\left(F_{F1} - B_{F1}\dot{\theta}_k r + K_{F1}(\theta_{F0} - \theta_k) r\right)}{J}$$

$$\frac{\partial \ddot{\theta}_k}{\partial P_E} = -\frac{2r\left(F_{E1} + B_{E1}\dot{\theta}_k r - K_{E1}(\theta_{E0} - \theta_k) r\right)}{J}$$

$$L_{g_1}L_f^2(y_1(\underline{x})) = \frac{\partial \ddot{\theta}_k}{\partial P_F} \cdot g_{31}(\underline{x}) > 0 \tag{9.39}$$

$$L_{g_2}L_f^2(y_1(\underline{x})) = \frac{\partial \ddot{\theta}_k}{\partial P_E} \cdot g_{42}(\underline{x}) < 0 \tag{9.40}$$

$$L_f(y_2(\underline{x})) = \frac{(f_3(\underline{x}) + f_4(\underline{x}))}{2} \tag{9.41}$$

$$L_{g_1}(y_2(\underline{x})) = \frac{g_{31}(\underline{x})}{2} > 0; \quad L_{g_2}(y_2(\underline{x})) = \frac{g_{42}(\underline{x})}{2} > 0 \tag{9.42}$$

To apply the SM control to the modelled system, two sliding surface variables (σ_1, σ_2) are firstly defined:

$$\sigma_1 = \lambda^2(\theta_k - \theta_{kd}) + 2\lambda(\dot{\theta}_k - \dot{\theta}_{kd}) + (\ddot{\theta}_k - \ddot{\theta}_{kd}) \tag{9.43}$$

$$\sigma_2 = \frac{P_F}{2} + \frac{P_E}{2} - P_{0d} \tag{9.44}$$

where σ_1 represents the sliding surface for the joint space trajectory; σ_2 is for the average pressure; λ is a tuning parameter of the sliding surface; θ_k, $\dot{\theta}_{kd}$, $\ddot{\theta}_{kd}$ are desired knee joint angular position, velocity and acceleration, respectively; P_{0d} is the desired average pressure of the antagonistic PAM actuators.

With the selected sliding surfaces, the control law can be designed in order to drive the state–space trajectories to the sliding surface. Once reached, the trajectories are forced to stay on the sliding surfaces by the controller. A classic controller design [25] is described as:

$$\frac{1}{2}\frac{d}{dt}\sigma_i^2 = \sigma_i\dot{\sigma}_i \le -\eta_i|\sigma_i| \tag{9.45}$$

in which η_i is strictly positive. The time derivatives of (9.43) and (9.44) can be expressed in the vector form of:

$$\begin{aligned}\begin{bmatrix}\dot{\sigma}_1 \\ \dot{\sigma}_2\end{bmatrix} &= \left[\lambda^2(\dot{\theta}_k - \dot{\theta}_{kd}) + \lambda(\ddot{\theta}_k - \ddot{\theta}_{kd}) - \dddot{\theta}_{kd} + L_f^3(y_1(\underline{x}))L_f(y_2(\underline{x})) - \dot{P}_{0d}\right] \\ &\quad + \begin{bmatrix} L_{g_1}L_f^2(y_1(\underline{x})) & L_{g_2}L_f^2(y_1(\underline{x})) \\ L_{g_1}(y_2(\underline{x})) & L_{g_2}(y_2(\underline{x}))\end{bmatrix}\begin{bmatrix}u_1 \\ u_2\end{bmatrix} \\ &= \mathbf{H} + \mathbf{S} + \mathbf{Q}\underline{u}\end{aligned} \tag{9.46}$$

with $$\mathbf{H} = \begin{bmatrix}h_1 \\ h_2\end{bmatrix} = \begin{bmatrix}L_f^3(y_1(\underline{x})) \\ L_f(y_2(\underline{x}))\end{bmatrix} \tag{9.47}$$

$$\mathbf{Q} = \begin{bmatrix} q_1 & q_2 \\ q_3 & q_4 \end{bmatrix} = \begin{bmatrix} L_{g_1}L_f^2(y_1(\underline{x})) & L_{g_2}L_f^2(y_1(\underline{x})) \\ L_{g_1}(y_2(\underline{x})) & L_{g_2}(y_2(\underline{x})) \end{bmatrix} \tag{9.48}$$

$$\mathbf{S} = \begin{bmatrix} \lambda^2(\dot{\theta}_k - \dot{\theta}_{kd}) + \lambda(\ddot{\theta}_k - \ddot{\theta}_{kd}) & -\dot{P}_{0d} \\ -\dddot{\theta}_{kd} & \end{bmatrix} \tag{9.49}$$

Hence, the SM control law can be applied. The control action vector ($\underline{u}$) contains two components:

$$\underline{u} = \mathbf{Q}^{-1}(\underline{u}_{eq} + \underline{u}_{rob}) \tag{9.50}$$

where is a continuous equivalent control element, which helps reaching of the sliding surfaces for desired motions; is the discontinuous robust element, which makes sure that the desired motions are sustained by sticking to the sliding surface. By zeroing $\dot{\underline{\sigma}}$, the expression of can be derived as:

$$\underline{u}_{eq} = -\mathbf{H} - \mathbf{S} \tag{9.51}$$

$$\underline{u}_{rob} = -\begin{bmatrix} k_1\,\mathrm{sgn}(\sigma_1) \\ k_2\,\mathrm{sgn}(\sigma_2) \end{bmatrix} \tag{9.52}$$

Based on (9.39), (9.40) and (9.42), matrix $\mathbf{Q}$ is non-singular. Here, it is necessary to remind that all the modelling parameter mentioned previous are based on the ideal situations. All the uncertainties of the model are contained by ideal matrices $\mathbf{H}$ and $\mathbf{Q}$.

Hence, for any instant, the actual representation derivatives of the sliding surfaces are given as:

$$\begin{bmatrix} \dot{\sigma}_1 \\ \dot{\sigma}_2 \end{bmatrix} = \hat{\mathbf{H}} + \mathbf{S} + \hat{\mathbf{Q}}\underline{u} \tag{9.53}$$

$$\hat{\mathbf{H}} = \begin{bmatrix} \hat{h}_1 \\ \hat{h}_2 \end{bmatrix}; \quad \hat{\mathbf{Q}} = \begin{bmatrix} \hat{q}_1 & \hat{q}_2 \\ \hat{q}_3 & \hat{q}_4 \end{bmatrix} \tag{9.54}$$

where $\hat{\mathbf{H}}$ and $\hat{\mathbf{Q}}$ are the instantaneous actual values of the model estimated $\mathbf{H}$ and $\mathbf{Q}$. The estimation errors of these matrices are bounded by the known function in the following ways:

$$|h_i - \hat{h}_i| \leq H_i \quad \text{with } (i = 1, 2) \tag{9.55}$$

$$\forall i = 1, 2, 3, 4 \qquad \beta^{-1} \leq \frac{\hat{q}_i}{q_i} \leq \beta \tag{9.56}$$

$$\beta = \left(\frac{q_{i\_\max}}{q_{i\_\min}}\right)^{1/2}_{\max} \tag{9.57}$$

To ensure the control law (9.50), satisfy the design criteria stated by (9.45). Equation (9.50) is substituted into (9.53), for $i = 1,\ 2$:

$$\dot{\sigma}_i = (1 - \zeta_i)s_i + \left(h_i - \zeta_i\hat{h}_i\right) - \zeta_i k_i \operatorname{sgn}(\sigma_i) \tag{9.58}$$

$$\zeta_1 = \frac{\hat{q}_1 q_4 - \hat{q}_2 q_3}{q_1 q_4 - q_2 q_3} > 0 \tag{9.59}$$

$$\zeta_2 = \frac{q_1 \hat{q}_4 - q_2 \hat{q}_3}{q_1 q_4 - q_2 q_3} > 0 \tag{9.60}$$

Hence, (9.58) is substituted into (9.45) and the following relationship can be generated:

$$\zeta_i k_i \geq \operatorname{sgn}(\sigma_i)\left((1 - \zeta_i)s_i + \left(h_i - \zeta_i\hat{h}_i\right)\right) + \eta_i \tag{9.61}$$

In order to ensure (9.61) is valid, k_i needs to be selected to satisfy the following condition:

$$k_i \geq \left|(\zeta_i^{-1} - 1)s_i + (\zeta_i^{-1} - 1)h_i + \zeta_i^{-1}\left(\hat{h}_i - h_i\right)\right| + \zeta_i^{-1}\eta_i \tag{9.62}$$

Due to the use of switch functions $\operatorname{sgn}(\sigma_i)$ in (9.52), the system is prone to high frequency chattering along the sliding surfaces. The solution to this problem is replacing the switching element along the sliding surface with piece-wise saturation function with a boundary layer [25,26]. Hence, the robust control element can now be expressed as:

$$\underline{u}_{rob} = -\begin{bmatrix} k_1\, sat\left(\dfrac{\sigma_1}{\phi_1}\right) \\ k_2\, sat\left(\dfrac{\sigma_2}{\phi_2}\right) \end{bmatrix} \tag{9.63}$$

where ϕ_i, $(i = 1, 2)$ are the boundary layer thicknesses for their corresponding sliding surfaces.

9.4 Experimental validation

The experiments were conducted with two different experimental setups. The first setup is focused on the knee joint of the exoskeleton only. It was aimed to investigate the controller's capability to track both desired objective trajectories simultaneously. The second experiment setup was for the pilot experiments of GAREX for treadmill-based gait rehabilitation.

9.4.1 Experiments with the knee joint mechanism

To conduct experiments with the controller, the knee joint mechanism of GAREX was mounted to an aluminium stand with its thigh segment in horizontal position Figure 9.7(a) and (b). The trajectory experiments were performed with and without human limb attached to the mechanism. Both squared and sinusoidal trajectories at various frequencies are used to characterise the performance of the controller implemented. For experiments without human leg attached, the mechanism only actuates the shank segment of the exoskeleton. The other experiments were

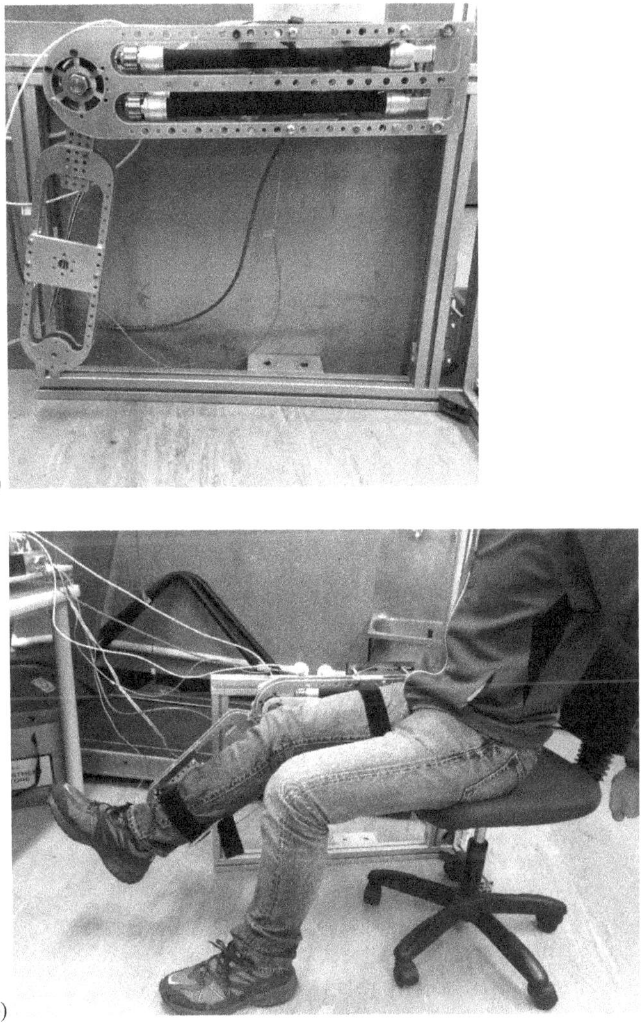

(a)

(b)

Figure 9.7 (a) Structure of the knee joint mechanism; (b) a healthy subject participating validation experiment with the mechanism conducted with human leg attached, in which the mechanism needs to drive the human shank and the shank segment of the exoskeleton as a rigid body. It is also assumed that the subject's knee joint is aligned with the knee joint of the mechanism. All the experiments with leg attached were conducted with the help of one healthy subject (male, height: 1.85 m, weight: 100 kg). A written consent has been obtained from the subject. The ethics approval for experiments with health subjects has been granted University of Auckland Human Participants Ethics Committee (Ref. 014970). The experimental setup was shown in Figure 9.7(b). The one of the subject's lower limbs was securely strapped to the leg holders of the knee joint mechanism. The knee joint rotational axes of the human limb and the mechanism were aligned. During the experiments, the subject was asked to relax the leg and let the mechanism to guide its motions.

The first experiment was conducted without leg attached experiment was designed to have the knee joint mechanism follow a reference sinusoid trajectory while maintaining its average pressure of the PAM actuators. Step changes of the desired average pressure were also adapted to study the system's behaviour. Result of the experiment is displayed in Figure 9.8. The figure indicates both the trajectory and pressure tracking are effective. The step changes of the desired average pressure

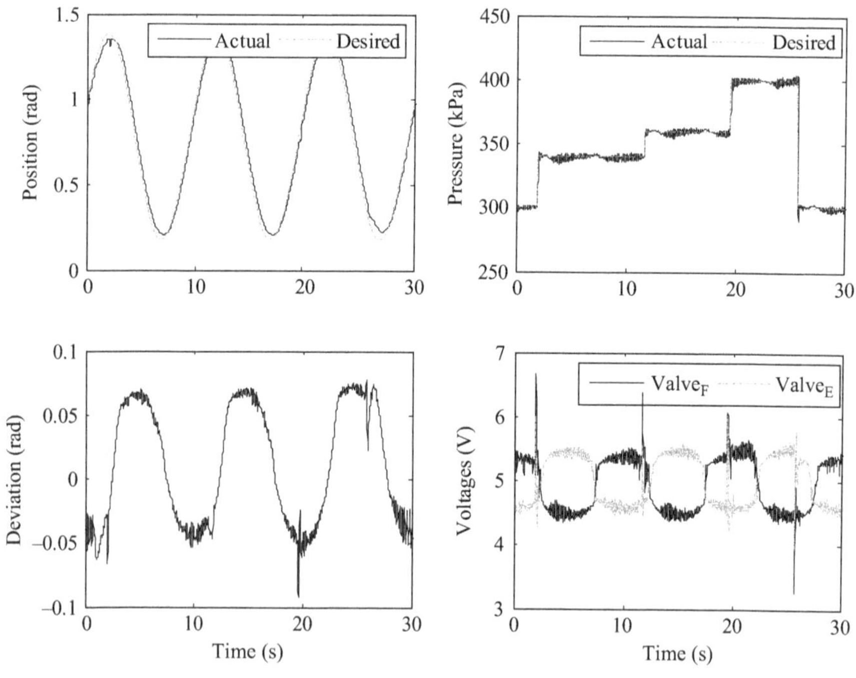

Figure 9.8 SM controller tracking performance. Top-left: knee joint trajectory tracking of a 0.1 Hz sinusoid wave. Top-right: step responses of the average pressure. Bottom-left: difference between the actual and desired joint angular trajectory. Bottom-right: the controlled valve voltages during the experiment

were quickly reacted by the controller's actions shown in the bottom-right plot of the figure. This resulted in good step response behaviour of the pressure tracking together with some oscillations in the joint trajectory. It is observed that the oscillation amplitude is positively correlated to step size of the reference pressure. Therefore, such oscillation can be significantly reduced by specifying the maximum change rate of the reference pressure. It is notable that the peak-to-peak amplitude of the reference sinusoid trajectory is ranging from 0.2 to 1.4 radians for all the experiments described in this manuscript. This is specially selected to simulate the actual knee joint range of motion during gait [27]. Meanwhile, the frequency of the reference sinusoid wave is varied in different experiments to examine the performance of the system.

The multivariable tracking performances are also compared between with and without leg situations. For the experiment with human leg attached, the subject was fitted to the exoskeleton as in the right-hand side of Figure 9.7. He was asked to relax the leg strapped to the exoskeleton and just let the exoskeleton guide his shank movement. Both sets of experiments were conducted with the identical 0.2 Hz reference joint trajectory and 400 kPa average pressure and the experimental results are illustrated. The plots of Figure 9.9 are for the experiment without leg

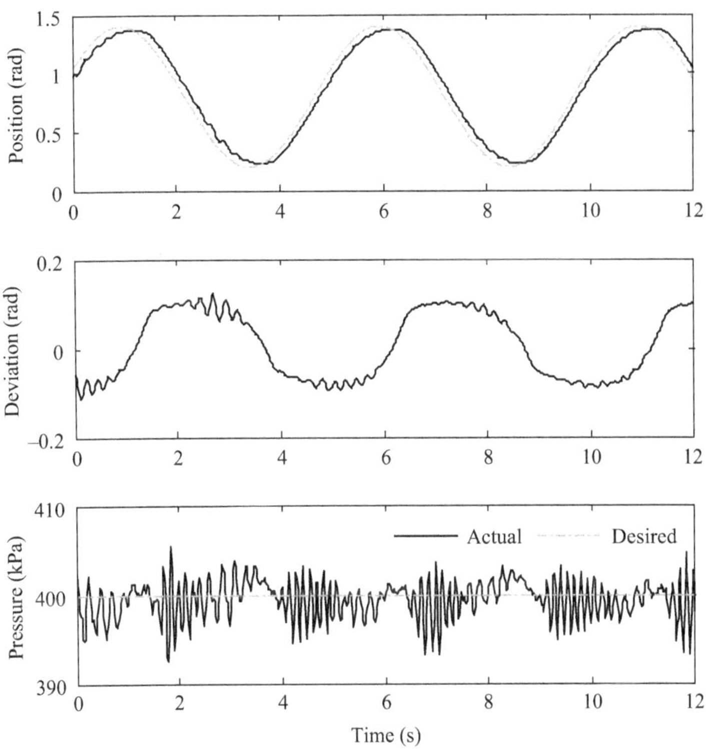

Figure 9.9 Joint trajectory and pressure tracking performances without leg attached. Top: desired (dashed line) versus actual (solid line) joint trajectory; middle: the trajectory deviation; bottom: desired versus actual average pressure (= 0.0751)

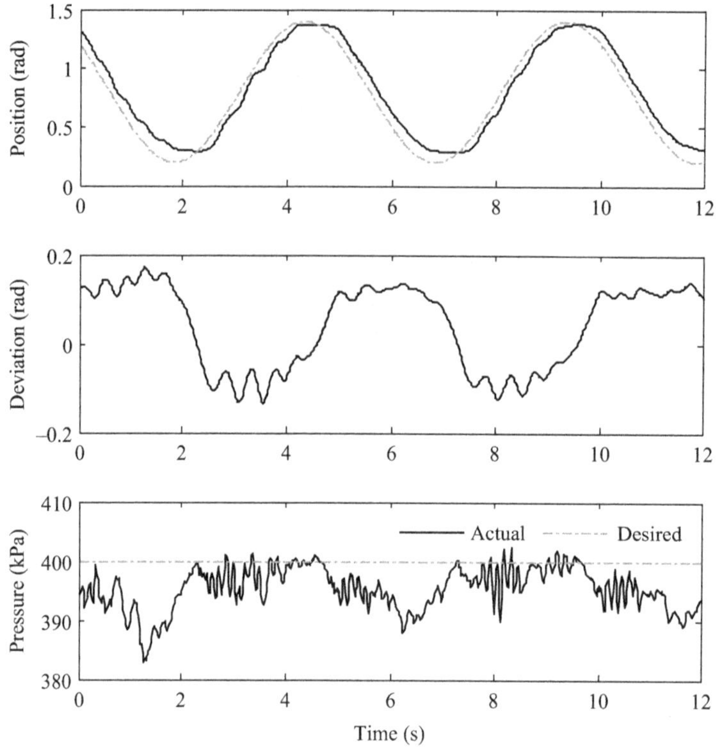

Figure 9.10 Joint trajectory and pressure tracking performances with leg attached. Top: desired (dashed line) versus actual (solid line) joint trajectory; middle: the trajectory deviation; bottom: desired versus actual average pressure (= 0.1022)

attached and the plots of Figure 9.10 are for the other experiment. A few comments can be made on the results. Firstly, the added human leg can be treated as disturbance the system (especially in terms of the un-modelled inertia of the moving part). With the presence of such disturbance, the controller was still able to provide good tracking performance. Compared to the without leg experiment, the increase in errors for the joint trajectory and pressure tracking was not significant. The change of compliance due to the change of the average pressure was investigated in the next set of experiments, whose results are shown in Figures 9.11 and 9.12.

The experiments shown in Figures 9.11 and 9.12 are conducted with the subject under the same conditions to the experiment shown in the right column of Figure 9.10. The experiment of Figure 9.10 had the reference average pressure of 400 kPa and the ones of Figures 9.11 and 9.12 were 300 and 200 kPa, respectively. By analysing the three sets of plots, larger joint deviations, which is expressed in terms of root-mean-square trajectory error (e_{RMS}), were observed as decrease in the

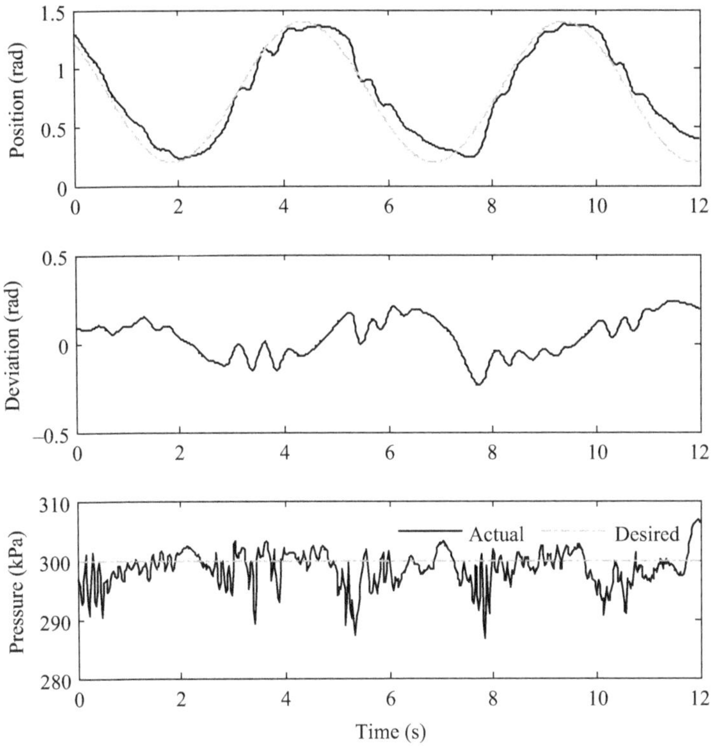

Figure 9.11 Joint trajectory and pressure tracking performances without leg attached ($e_{RMS} = 0.1174$)

average pressure and increase in actuator compliance. This further means the control of the actuation system's intrinsic compliance can be achieved. The behaviours are comparable to controller simulated variable impedance or virtual tunnels reported on motor-driven gait rehabilitation robots [28,29].

9.5 Pilot study of gait training with GAREX

9.5.1 Generating reference gait trajectory

The experiment-based reference gait trajectory generation method will be presented first, as it is important to have suitable desired trajectories for the upcoming pilots of the control system with healthy subjects.

Experiments were conducted to record healthy subjects' hip and knee joint trajectories as potential reference trajectories for upcoming controller system development. To conduct such experiments, a subject was strapped to GAREX,

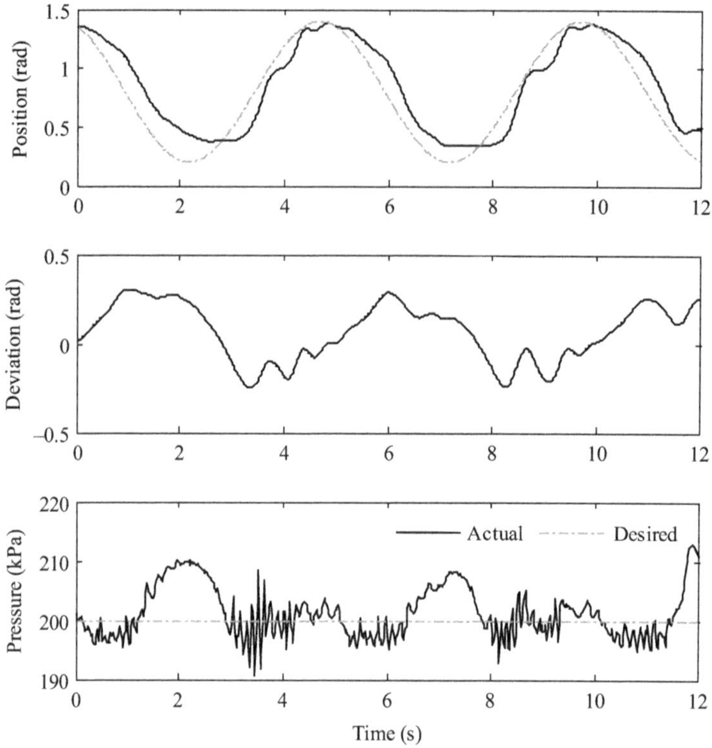

Figure 9.12 Joint trajectory and pressure tracking performances without leg attached right ($e_{RMS} = 0.1726$)

which had been adjusted according to the subject's anthropometric data. It was ensured the hip and knee joints of the subject and the exoskeleton were coaxial and their thigh and shank segments were also aligned, so the angular positions of the exoskeleton were assumed to be equal to the ones of the attached limb.

During the experiments, the subject was asked to walk on the treadmill with the un-actuated lower limb exoskeleton attached. When the exoskeleton was un-actuated, the cables of both sides of the antagonistic PAM actuation system were never in tension; hence, no torque was exerted on the hip or knee joints by the PAM actuation systems. The gravity of the lower limb exoskeleton module was compensated by the air spring suspension system of the trunk mechanism. It was aimed to minimise the disturbance of the subject, so he/she could feel like free walking on the treadmill.

The goal of the experiment was to record periodical joint space trajectories by the subject during free walking. In terms of instrumentation, the hip and knee joint encoders were utilised to record the angular positions throughout the experiments. In order to extract the periodic trajectories over gait cycles, it was necessary to identify the starting instant of every gait cycle. In biomechanics, the heel strike or initial contact between the foot and the walking surface is usually regarded as the starting point of a gait cycle of the respective lower limb [27]. Hence it is a common practice to utilise ground reaction force or pressure sensors to the identification. However, due to the time constraint of the research, such sensors were not implemented to the system. Instead, the researcher monitoring the experiment visually identified the instant of heel strikes and toggled a hand-held switch at the starting point of every gait cycle. The system recorded the digital input from the switch as well as the encoder readings for post-experiment analysis.

The post-experiment analysis was conducted through MATLAB. Based on the toggle switch input, the average gait cycle length in seconds could first be calculated. Then, the effective recorded joint space trajectories could be sliced to fit into the gait cycle length. The sliced data are presented as blue scatters in Figures 9.13–9.22.

A sum of four sinusoidal functions in the format of (9.64) was decided to represent experimental data:

$$\theta_d(t) = \sum_{i=1}^{4} a_i \sin(b_i t + c_i) \tag{9.64}$$

where t is the time elapsed since the start of the gait cycle; a_i, b_i and c_i ($i = 1, 2, 3, 4$) are the curve fitting parameters calculated from the experimental data; is the function describing the fitted desired joint space trajectory.

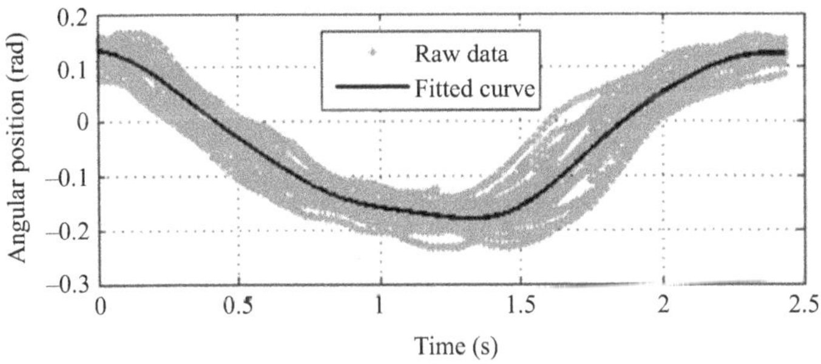

Figure 9.13 The record trajectory data and generated desired trajectory curve of Subject_A's hip joint when walking at 1.2 km/h. The period of the average gait cycle (T_{GC}) is 2.43 s. The coefficient of determination (R^2) of the regression curve is 0.92

Table 9.2 Parameters of the fitted curve in Figure 9.13

0.155	2.45	1.82	0.0382	0.264	5.06
0.0146	6.43	–5.09	0.00439	10.6	–4.58

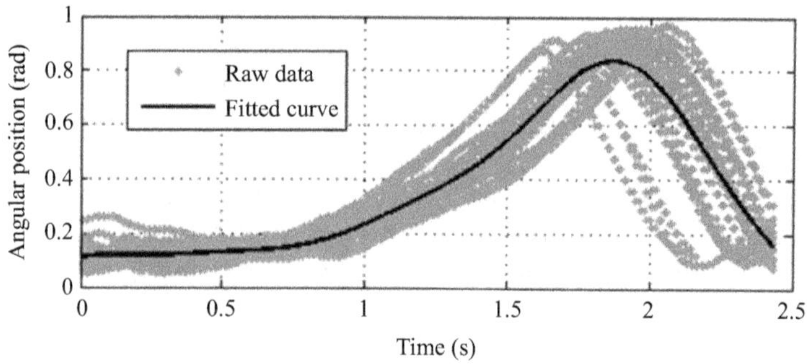

Figure 9.14 The record trajectory data and generated desired trajectory curve of Subject_A's knee joint when walking at 1.2 km/h. $T_{GC} = 2.43$ s. $R^2 = 0.87$

Table 9.3 Parameters of the fitted curve in Figure 9.14

0.744	1.58	−0.473	0.455	2.69	1.99
0.124	7.35	−4.81	0.104	7.91	−2.09

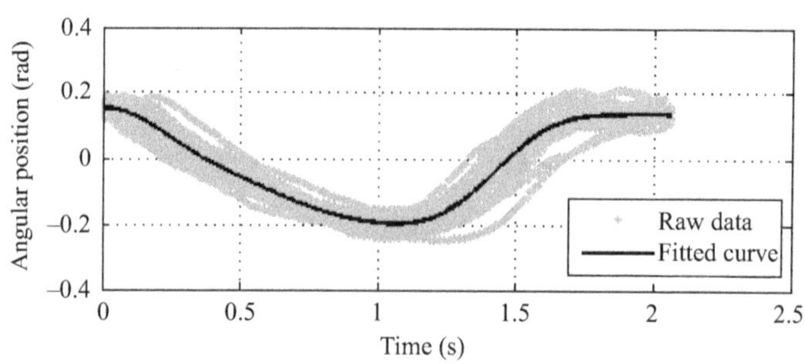

Figure 9.15 The record trajectory data and generated desired trajectory curve of Subject_A's hip joint when walking at 1.5 km/h. $T_{GC} = 2.06$ s. $R^2 = 0.92$

Table 9.4 Parameters of the fitted curve in Figure 9.15

0.0163	3.29	1.50	0.446	0.995	4.28
0.0237	7.89	−4.77	0.00579	12.0	−4.69

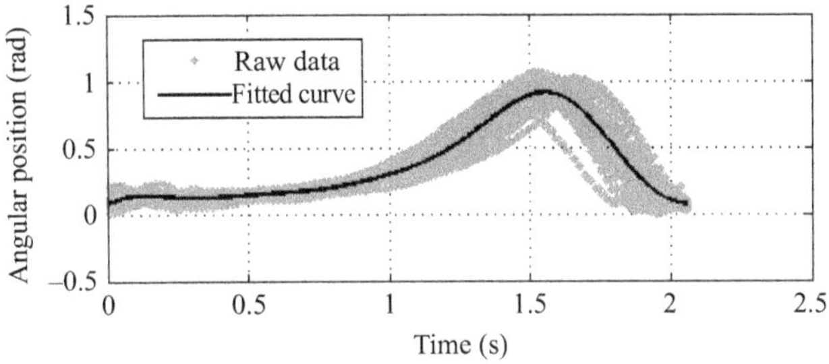

Figure 9.16 The record trajectory data and generated desired trajectory curve of Subject_A's knee joint when walking at 1.5 km/h. $T_{GC} = 2.06$ s. $R^2 = 0.90$

Table 9.5 Parameters of the fitted curve in Figure 9.16

0.57	1.52	−0.448	0.256	4.38	0.995
0.514	9.18	−5.48	0.461	9.45	−2.54

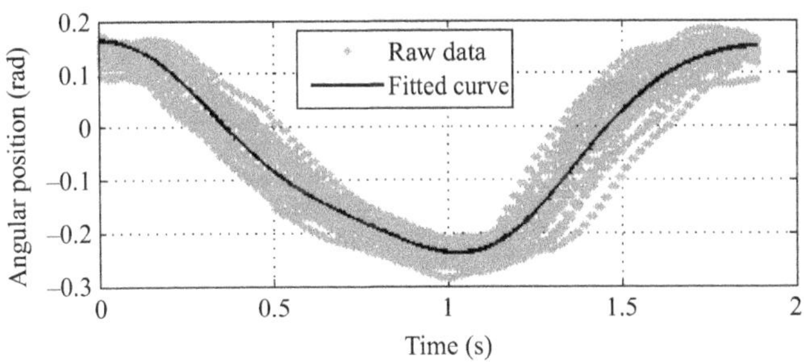

Figure 9.17 The record trajectory data and generated desired trajectory curve of Subject_A's hip joint when walking at 1.8 km/h. $T_{GC} = 1.90$ s. $R^2 = 0.93$

Table 9.6 Parameters of the fitted curve in Figure 9.17

0.57	1.52	−0.448	0.256	4.38	0.995
0.514	9.18	−5.48	0.461	9.45	−2.54

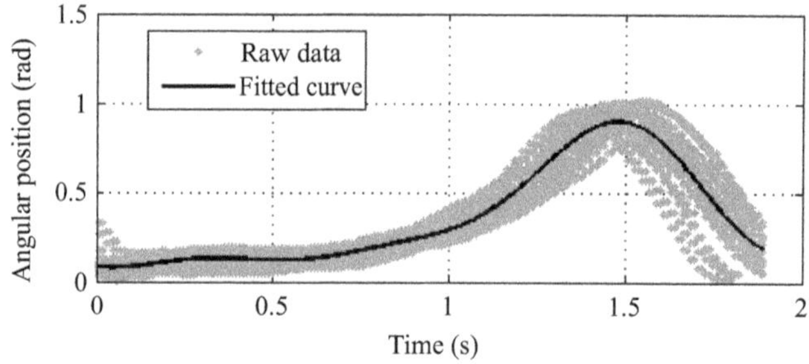

Figure 9.18 The record trajectory data and generated desired trajectory curve of Subject_A's hip joint when walking at 1.8 km/h. $T_{GC} = 1.90$ s. $R^2 = 0.91$

Table 9.7 Parameters of the fitted curve in Figure 9.18

0.655	1.77	−0.193	0.451	3.15	2.42
1.04	8.44	−3.20	0.995	8.60	−0.153

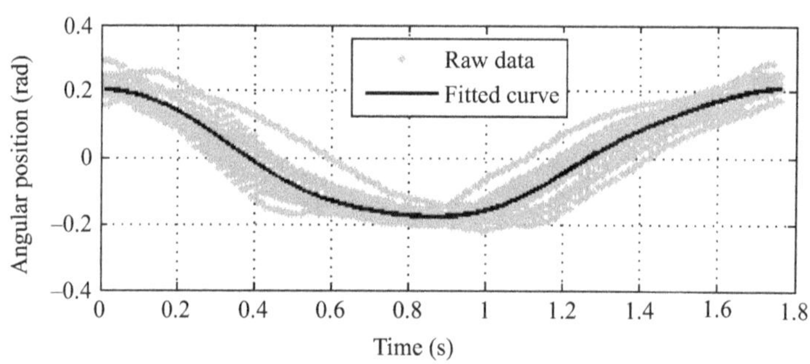

Figure 9.19 The record trajectory data and generated desired trajectory curve of Subject_B's hip joint when walking at 1.5 km/h. $T_{GC} = 1.76$ s. $R^2 = 0.91$

Table 9.8 Parameters of the fitted curve in Figure 9.19

8.19	3.54	1.40	0.0282	5.40	2.82
7.99	3.53	−1.74	0.00933	11.0	−0.392

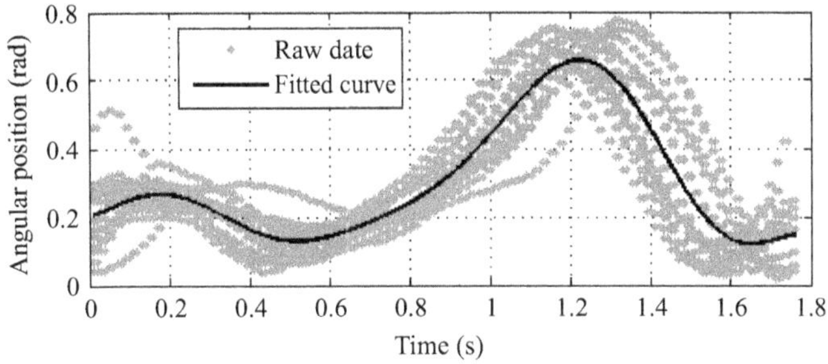

Figure 9.20 The record trajectory data and generated desired trajectory curve of Subject_B's knee joint when walking at 1.5 km/h. $T_{GC} = 1.76$ s. $R^2 = 0.80$

Table 9.9 Parameters of the fitted curve in Figure 9.20

27.7	2.11	0.809	18.28	9.29	−1.99
27.57	2.13	3.94	18.23	9.3	1.15

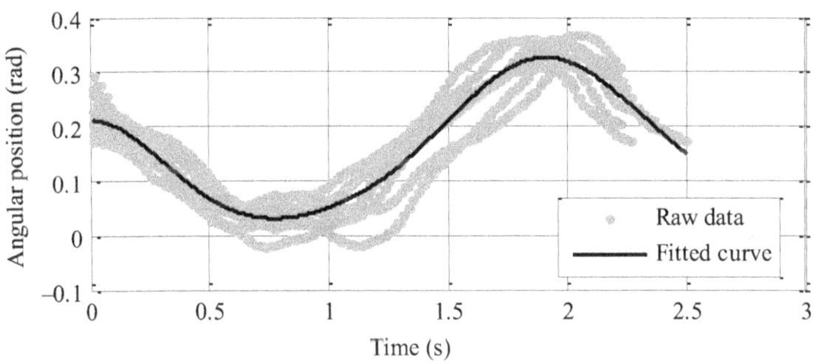

Figure 9.21 The record trajectory data and generated desired trajectory curve of Subject_C's hip joint when walking at 1.5 km/h. $T_{GC} = 2.5$ s. $R^2 = 0.89$

Table 9.10 Parameters of the fitted curve in Figure 9.21

0.223	0.947	0.0605	0.422	2.80	0.3539
0.457	2.91	3.05	0.0126	6.58	1.71

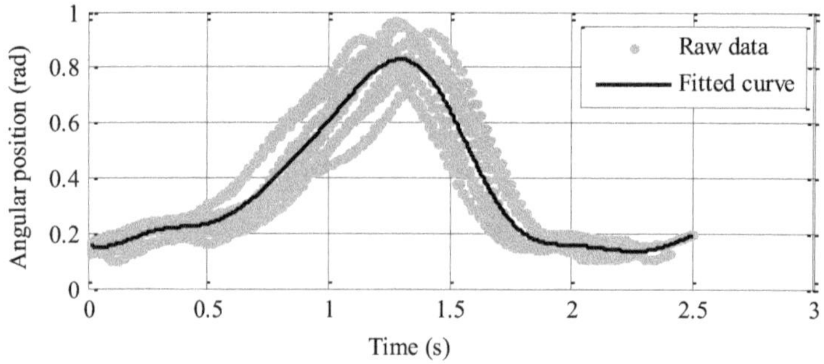

Figure 9.22 The record trajectory data and generated desired trajectory curve of Subject_C's knee joint when walking at 1.5 km/h. $T_{GC} = 2.5$ s. $R^2 = 0.90$

Table 9.11 Parameters of the fitted curve in Figure 9.22

0.457	0.584	0.971	0.0846	6.90	−1.15
0.291	3.48	−2.72	0.0245	10.7	−0.896

The selected format not only can well fit to the raw data, but also in simple form for real-time implementation. The derivatives of the function are smooth and can be calculated analytically. Curve fitting parameters of (9.64) were computed from the sliced experimental data using the curve fitting toolbox of MATLAB.

Experiments were conducted to acquire the gait trajectories of three male subjects (Subject_A: 188 cm, 80 kg; Subject_B: 172 cm, 68 kg and Subject_C: male, 185 cm, 100 kg) when walking at various walking speeds. The sliced raw data of the experiments and the best fitted gait trajectory of a gait cycle are plotted in the following ten figures. The curve fitting parameters used to describe the generated reference trajectory are listed below each figure (Tables 9.2–9.11). Regression analysis results expressed using coefficient of determination, are also listed in the figure captions. Figures 9.13–9.18 are for the experimental results of Subject_A. Three experiments were conducted at different walking speed (1.2, 1.5 and 1.8 km/h) and the results are plotted for both the hip and knee joints. For comparison reasons, the experimental results of Subject_B and Subject_C walking at 1.5 km/h are also shown in Figures 9.19–9.22.

It can be seen from the figures that regression analysis indicates that the developed method was able to generate a reference trajectory to well present the recorded gait patterns. All the generated reference trajectories were stored for future application. In the upcoming experiments of the GAREX system, an appropriate reference trajectory can be selected based on the training subject's build.

Because the starting moments of the gait cycles were identified by the researcher, more uncertainties were introduced than using ground reaction force sensors. Due to such uncertainties, the raw data show some obvious phase differences in difference gait cycles in all the plots. Such phase differences are regarded as the main affecting factor for the curve fitting quality. For 1.5 km/h walking speed, less phase differences are observed in the knee joint result of Subject_A (Figure 9.16) than Subject_B (Figure 9.20). Hence, the better regression result was obtained from Subject's result.

9.5.2 Treadmill-based gait experiment with healthy subject

One healthy subject (male, 172 cm, 68 kg) participated in the validation experiment. During the preparation phase of the experiment, the subject was instructed to stand on the treadmill and a researcher measured the dimension of his lower limb and adjusted the exoskeleton according to the subject's anthropometric data. The researcher then securely strapped the subject's trunk and right leg to the back support and exoskeleton respectively. It was made sure that the subject's hip and knee joints are coaxial with the respective joints of the exoskeleton.

During the experiment, programmed with the MIMO SM controller, GAREX guided the subject to walk in a predefined gait trajectory on the treadmill with a speed of 1.5 km/h. To conduct the experiment, the subject was asked to relax the leg strapped to the exoskeleton and let GAREX guide its movement. The subject also adapted un-actuated leg's movements to achieve stable walking on the treadmill.

The subject was able to walk on the treadmill comfortably with the guidance from GAREX in all four experimental conditions. The subject's gait trajectories of the two actuated joints are presented in Figures 9.23–9.26. It can be observed from the figure that the controller was capable of tracking the desired gait trajectory in order to facilitate gait rehabilitation in all the experimental conditions. The trajectory tracking performance was evaluated with the root-mean-square (RMS) error between the desired and actual trajectory and the results are listed in Table 9.12. It is obvious from the table that the RMS errors had a trend of decrease as the controlled average PAM pressure increased. This is an indication that the exoskeleton became less compliant and gave the subject less freedom around the desired trajectory.

The average antagonistic PAM pressure tracking results of the hip and knee joints are also shown in Figures 9.23 and 9.25. It can be seen from the figures that the MIMO SM controller was able to regulate the desired average PAM pressures during task-specific gait training experiment with the healthy subject. It is also observed that the better pressure control was achieved by the hip joint in the same experiment. This is likely caused by tuning of the MIMO SM control system. Considering the safety and nature of robotic gait rehabilitation, angular trajectory tracking needs to be prioritised among the two control objectives. This was realised by the tuning parameters that let angular trajectory tracking take the dominate role in the overall control actions. Compared to the hip joint, the desired trajectory of

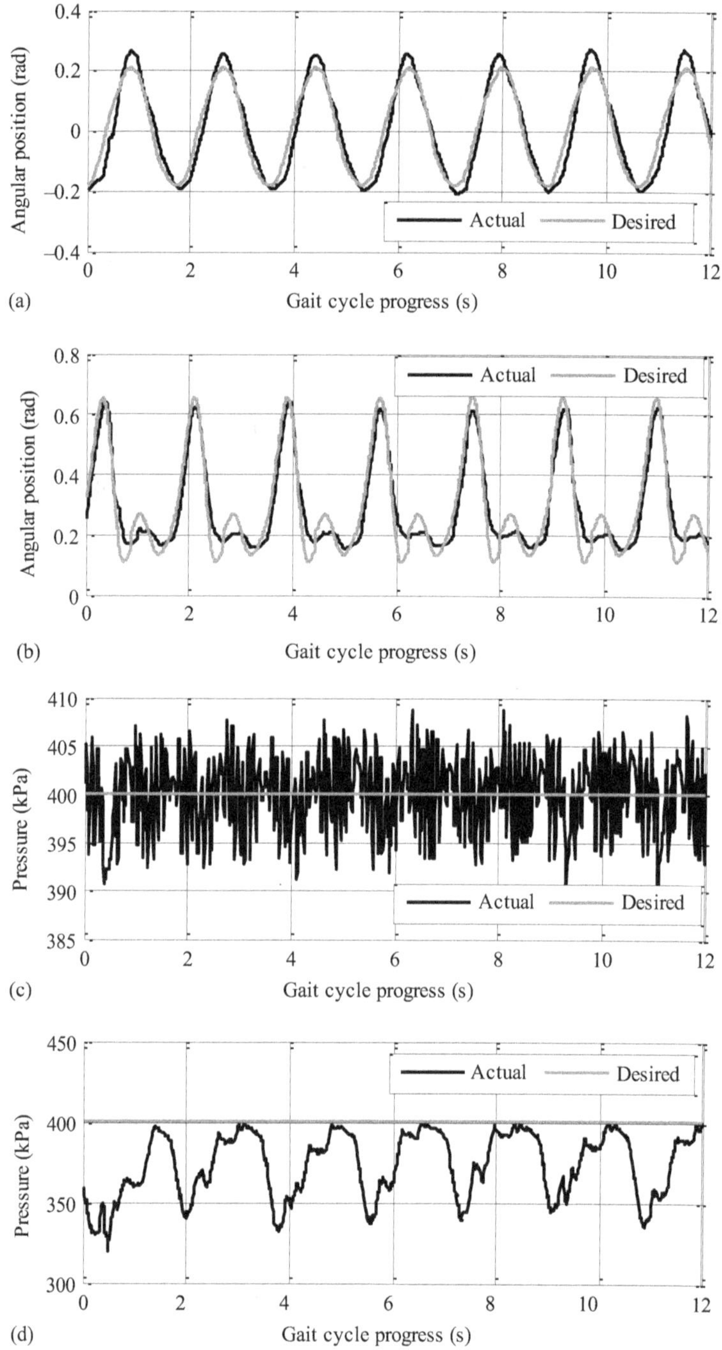

Figure 9.23 Results of gait training experiment with healthy subject when the average antagonistic PAM pressure of the hip and knee joints were both regulated to 400 kPa. (a) and (c) the trajectory tracking results for the hip and knee joints, respectively. (b) and (d) the average PAM pressure control results for the hip and knee joints

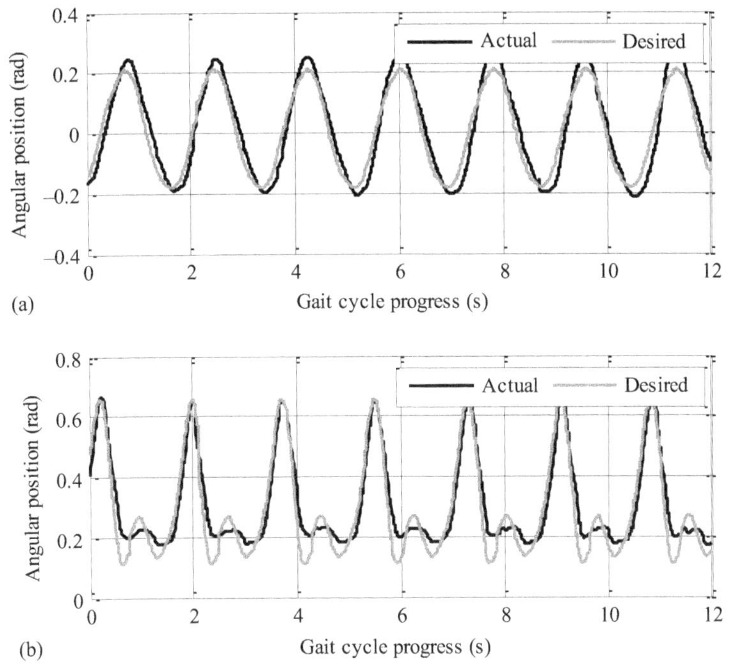

Figure 9.24 Results of gait training experiment with healthy subject when the average antagonistic PAM pressure of the hip and knee joints were both regulated to 320 kPa. (a) and (b) are the trajectory tracking results for the hip and knee joints, respectively

the knee joint is more difficult to track for the system. More control action is needed to tracking the knee joint trajectory. Hence, the control action to maintain the average pressure thus became less effective.

9.6 Summary

The MIMO SM controller was developed based on the model of the complete system of the exoskeleton. It was hypothesised that lower average PAM pressure leads to less compliant the joint. The MIMO SM controller was initially implemented to the knee joint mechanism and extensive experiments were conducted either without subject or with healthy subject to investigate its performance. Apart from investigating the ability of simultaneous angular trajectory and average pressure tracking, novel experiments were performed by five healthy subject to demonstrate that the MIMO SM controller was able to adjust the joint compliance by controlling the average PAM pressure.

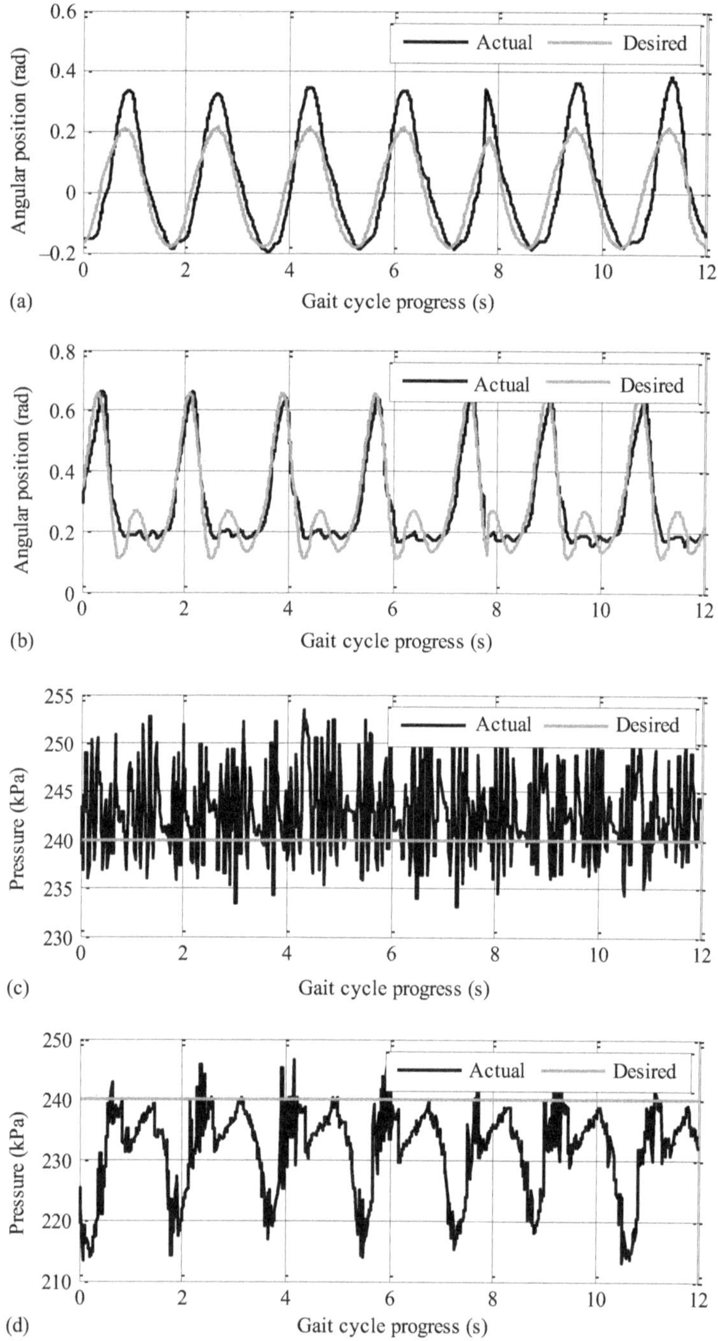

Figure 9.25 Results of gait training experiment with healthy subject when the average antagonistic PAM pressure of the hip and knee joints were both regulated to 240 kPa. (a) the trajectory tracking results for the hip joint (b) trajectory tracking results for the knee joint (c) and (d)

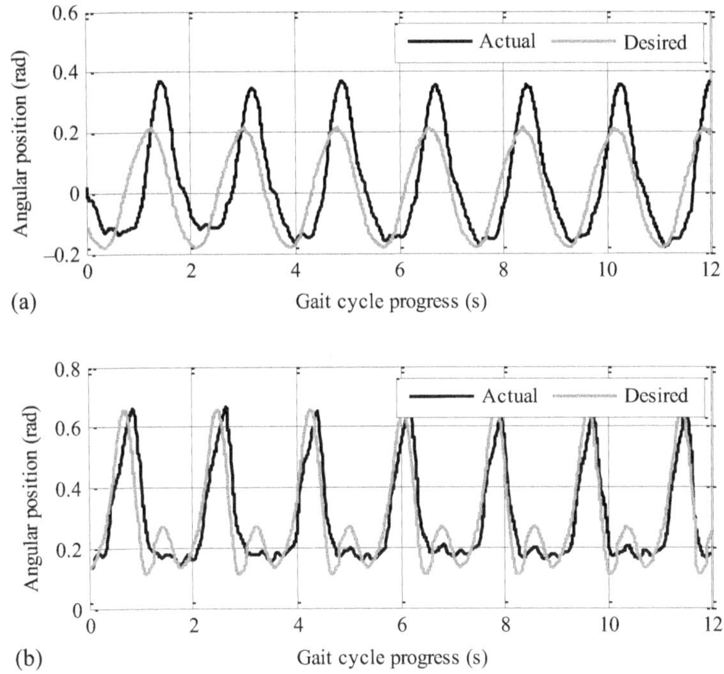

Figure 9.26 Results of gait training experiment with healthy subject when the average antagonistic PAM pressure of the hip and knee joints were both regulated to 160 kPa. (a) the trajectory tracking results for the hip joint and (b) trajectory tracking results for the knee joint

Table 9.12 The RMS errors (rad) of both actuated joints under all four experimental conditions

	160 kPa	240 kPa	320 kPa	400 kPa
Knee	0.127	0.110	0.097	0.092
Hip	0.136	0.111	0.0718	0.066

After initial validation with the knee joint mechanism, the MIMO SM controller were then implemented to both the hip and knee joints of GAREX to facilitate task specific gait rehabilitation. The pilot experiments showed that the exoskeleton could comfortably guide healthy subjects to complete treadmill based gait experiments in a speed adopted for clinical trials on a motor driven gait rehabilitation robot. Such result revealed the potential of taking GAREX to the clinical trial stage in the near future.

Appendix A The mechanism dynamics calculation

The low limb exoskeleton can be treated as be treated as a serial robot and the well-established Lagrangian Formulation was adopted to calculate the actuated joint torque requirement from the kinematics of the exoskeleton as:

$$\mathbf{M}\ddot{\underline{\theta}} + \underline{V} + \underline{G} = \underline{\tau} \tag{A.1}$$

or
$$\begin{bmatrix} M_{11} & M_{12} \\ M_{21} & M_{22} \end{bmatrix} \begin{bmatrix} \ddot{\theta}_1 \\ \ddot{\theta}_2 \end{bmatrix} + \begin{bmatrix} V_1 \\ V_2 \end{bmatrix} + \begin{bmatrix} G_1 \\ G_2 \end{bmatrix} = \begin{bmatrix} \tau_1 \\ \tau_2 \end{bmatrix} \tag{A.2}$$

Figure 1.3 was constructed to help the description of the dynamics model. Equation (A.3) is the inertia matrix of segment i ($i = 1$ for thigh segment; $i = 2$ for shank segment) about its COM. ${}^{i}I_i$ can be expressed with respect to the base coordinate system by the transformation in (A.4).

$${}^{i}\mathbf{I}_i = \begin{bmatrix} I_{ix} & 0 & 0 \\ 0 & I_{iy} & 0 \\ 0 & 0 & I_{iz} \end{bmatrix} \tag{A.3}$$

$$\mathbf{I_i} = {}^{0}R_i{}^{i}R_i\left({}^{0}R_i\right)^T \tag{A.4}$$

where ${}^{0}R_i$ is the rotation matrix from COM of segment I to the base frame, which can be expressed as:

$${}^{0}R_1 = \begin{bmatrix} \cos\theta_1 & -\sin\theta_1 & 0 \\ \sin\theta_1 & \cos\theta_1 & 0 \\ 0 & 0 & 1 \end{bmatrix} \tag{A.5}$$

$${}^{0}R_2 = \begin{bmatrix} \cos(\theta_1+\theta_2) & -\sin(\theta_1+\theta_2) & 0 \\ \sin(\theta_1+\theta_2) & \cos(\theta_1+\theta_2) & 0 \\ 0 & 0 & 1 \end{bmatrix} \tag{A.6}$$

The kinetic energy of the entire exoskeleton system can thus be expressed as:

$$K_e = \frac{1}{2}\dot{\underline{\theta}}^T\mathbf{M}\dot{\underline{\theta}} \tag{A.7}$$

where $\mathbf{M}$ is aninertia matrix defined as:

$$\mathbf{M} = \sum_{i=1}^{2}\left(\mathbf{J_{vi}^T}m_i\mathbf{J_{vi}} + \mathbf{J_{\omega i}^T}\mathbf{I_i}\mathbf{J_{\omega i}}\right) \tag{A.8}$$

where m_i is the mass of segment i; J_{vi} and $J_{\omega i}$ are the Jacobian sub-matrices of segments i which can be calculated as:

$$\underline{J_{v1}^1} = \underline{z} \times \underline{{}^1P_{c1}}; \underline{J_{v1}^2} = [0 \quad 0 \quad 0]^T \tag{A.9}$$

$$\underline{J_{v2}^1} = \underline{z} \times \underline{{}^1P_{c2}}; \underline{J_{v2}^2} = \underline{z} \times \underline{{}^2P_{c2}} \tag{A.10}$$

$$\mathbf{J_{vi}} = \begin{bmatrix} \underline{J_{vi}^1} & \underline{J_{vi}^2} \end{bmatrix} \text{ with} \tag{A.11}$$

$$\mathbf{J}_{\omega 1} = \begin{bmatrix} 0 & 0 \\ 0 & 0 \\ 1 & 0 \end{bmatrix}; \mathbf{J}_{\omega 2} = \begin{bmatrix} 0 & 0 \\ 0 & 0 \\ 1 & 1 \end{bmatrix} \tag{A.12}$$

In (A.9) and (A.10), $\underline{{}^jP_{ci}}$ is a position vector of the COM of segment relative to the coordinate system (for the base coordinate system and for the other).

$$\underline{{}^1P_{c1}} = [l_{c1}\cos\theta_1 \quad l_{c1}\sin\theta_1 \quad 0]^T \tag{A.13}$$

$$\underline{{}^1P_{c2}} = [l_{c2}\cos(\theta_1+\theta_2) + l_1\cos\theta_1 \quad l_{c2}\sin(\theta_1+\theta_2) + l_1\sin\theta_1 \quad 0]^T \tag{A.14}$$

$$\underline{{}^2P_{c2}} = [l_{c2}\cos(\theta_1+\theta_2) \quad l_{c2}\sin(\theta_1+\theta_2) \quad 0]^T \tag{A.15}$$

The potential energy stored in the exoskeleton with respect to the base coordinate system can be expressed as in (A.16) with the vector of gravity coefficient $\underline{g} = [0 \quad g_c \quad 0]$.

$$U = -\sum_{i=1}^{2} m_i \underline{g}^{T} \underline{{}^1P_{ci}} \tag{A.16}$$

The Lagrangian function of the mechanism is then defined in (A.17) and the actuation torques of the hip and knee joint can be calculation in (A.18), which can be re-arranged into matrix representation expressed in (A.2).

$$L = K_e - U \tag{A.17}$$

$$\frac{d}{dt}\left(\frac{\partial L}{\partial \dot{\theta}_i}\right) - \frac{\partial L}{\partial \theta_i} = \tau_i \qquad \text{for} \tag{A.18}$$

The V and G terms of (A.2) can further be calculated as:

$$V_i = \sum_{j=1}^{2}\sum_{k=1}^{2}\left(\frac{\partial M_{ij}}{\partial \theta_k} - \frac{1}{2}\frac{\partial M_{jk}}{\partial \theta_i}\right)\dot{\theta}_j\dot{\theta}_k \qquad \text{for} \tag{A.19}$$

$$G_i = -\sum_{j=1}^{2} m_j \underline{g}^T \underline{J_{vj}^i} \qquad \text{for} \tag{A.20}$$

The symbolic representations of the parameters in (A.2) are listed as below:

$$M_{11} = \mathrm{m}_2 l_1{}^2 + 2\mathrm{m}_2 \cos\theta_2 l_1 l_{c2} + \mathrm{m}_1 l_{c1}{}^2 + \mathrm{m}_2 l_{c2}{}^2 + I_1 z + I_2 z \tag{A.21}$$

$$M_{12} = I_2 z + l_{c2}\mathrm{m}_2(l_{c2} + l_1 \cos\theta_2) \tag{A.22}$$

$$M_{21} = I_2 z + l_c 2\mathrm{m}_2(l_c 2 + l_1 \cos(\theta_2)) \tag{A.23}$$

$$M_{22} = \mathrm{m}_2 l_{c2}{}^2 + I_2 z \tag{A.24}$$

$$V_1 = -l_1 l_{c2}\mathrm{m}_2\dot{\theta}_2{}^2 \sin\theta_2 - 2l_1 l_{c2}\mathrm{m}_2\dot{\theta}_1\dot{\theta}_2 \sin\theta_2 \tag{A.25}$$

$$V_2 = l_1 l_{c2}\mathrm{m}_2\dot{\theta}_1{}^2 \sin\theta_2 \tag{A.26}$$

$$G_1 = (g_c\mathrm{m}_2(l_{c2}\cos(\theta_1 + \theta_2) + l_1 \cos\theta_1) + g_c l_{c1}\mathrm{m}_1 \cos\theta_1) \tag{A.27}$$

$$G_2 = (g_c l_{c2}\mathrm{m}_2 \cos(\theta_1 + \theta_2)) \tag{A.28}$$

References

[1] Ferris DP, Czerniecki JM, Hannaford B, System VPSH of Washington U. An ankle-foot orthosis powered by artificial pneumatic muscles. J Appl Biomech. 2005;21(2):189.

[2] Sawicki GS, Ferris DP. A pneumatically powered knee-ankle-foot orthosis (KAFO) with myoelectric activation and inhibition. J Neuroeng Rehabil. 2009;6(1):23.

[3] Sugar TG, He J, Koeneman EJ, *et al.* Design and control of RUPERT: a device for robotic upper extremity repetitive therapy. IEEE Trans Neural Syst Rehabil Eng. 2007;15(3):336–46.

[4] Hussain S, Xie SQ, Jamwal PK, Parsons J. An intrinsically compliant robotic orthosis for treadmill training. Med Eng Phys. 2012;34(10):1448–53.

[5] Chou CP, Hannaford B. Measurement and modeling of McKibben pneumatic artificial muscles. IEEE Transac Robot Autom. 1996;12(1):90–102.

[6] Tondu B, Lopez P. Modeling and control of McKibben artificial muscle robot actuators. IEEE Control Syst. 2000;20(2):15–38.

[7] Reynolds D, Repperger D, Phillips C, Bandry G. Modeling the dynamic characteristics of pneumatic muscle. Ann Biomed Eng. 2003;31(3):310–17.

[8] Choi TY, Lee JJ. Control of manipulator using pneumatic muscles for enhanced safety. IIEEE Trans Ind Electron. 2010;57(8):2815–25.

[9] Lilly JH, Yang L. Sliding mode tracking for pneumatic muscle actuators in opposing pair configuration. IEEE Trans Control Syst Technol. 2005; 13(4):550–58.

[10] Caldwell DG, Medrano-Cerda GA, Goodwin M. Control of pneumatic muscle actuators. IEEE Control Syst. 1995;15(1):40–48.

[11] Carbonell P, Jiang Z, Repperger D, editors. Nonlinear control of a pneumatic muscle actuator: backstepping vs. sliding-mode. Control Applications, 2001 (CCA'01) Proceedings of the 2001 IEEE international conference. IEEE: Mexico City, Mexico; 2001.
[12] Chan SW, Lilly JH, Repperger DW, Berlin JE, editors. Fuzzy PD+I learning control for a pneumatic muscle. Fuzzy Systems, 2003 FUZZ '03 the 12th IEEE international conference. IEEE: St Louis, MO; 2003.
[13] Thanh TDC, Ahn KK. Nonlinear PID control to improve the control performance of 2 axes pneumatic artificial muscle manipulator using neural network. Mechatronics. 2006;16(9):577–87.
[14] Huang J, Qian J, Liu L, Wang Y, Xiong C, Ri S. Echo state network based predictive control with particle swarm optimization for pneumatic muscle actuator. J Franklin Inst. 2016;353(12):2761–82.
[15] Van Damme M, Vanderborght B, Van Ham R, Verrelst B, Daerden F, Lefeber D. Proxy-based sliding mode control of a manipulator actuated by pleated pneumatic artificial muscles. IEEE Int Conf Robot Autom. 2007.
[16] Xing K, Huang J, Wang Y, Wu J, Xu Q, He J. Tracking control of pneumatic artificial muscle actuators based on sliding mode and non-linear disturbance observer. IET Control Theory & Appl. 2010;4(10):2058–70.
[17] Chang MK. An adaptive self-organizing fuzzy sliding mode controller for a 2-DOF rehabilitation robot actuated by pneumatic muscle actuators. Control Eng Pract. 2010;18(1):13–22.
[18] Choi TY, Choi BS, Seo KH. Position and compliance control of a pneumatic muscle actuated manipulator for enhanced safety. IEEE Tras Control Syst Technol. 2011;19(4):832–42.
[19] Shen X. Nonlinear model-based control of pneumatic artificial muscle servo systems. Control Eng Pract. 2010;18(3):311–17.
[20] Aschemann H, Schindele D. Sliding-mode control of a high-speed linear axis driven by pneumatic muscle actuators. IEEE Trans Ind Electron. 2008;55(11):3855–64.
[21] Sala A. Multivariable control systems an engineering approach. London: Springer; 2004.
[22] Sarosi J. New approximation algorithm for the force of Fluidic Muscles. 7th IEEE International Symposium on Applied Computational Intelligence and Informatics (SACI). IEEE; Politehnica University of Timisoara, Timisoara, Romania; 2012.
[23] McDaid A, Kora K, Xie S, Lutz J, Battley M, editors. Human-inspired robotic exoskeleton (HuREx) for lower limb rehabilitation. IEEE international conference Mechatronics and Automation (ICMA). IEEE; Takamatsu, Japan; 2013.
[24] Smaoui M, Brun X, Thomasset D. Systematic control of an electropneumatic system: integrator backstepping and sliding mode control. IEEE Trans Control Syst Technol. 2006;14(5):905–13.

[25] Slotine JJE, Li W. Applied nonlinear control. Englewood Cliffs, NJ: Prentice-Hall; 1991.

[26] Young KD, Utkin VI, Ozguner U. A control engineer's guide to sliding mode control. IEEE Trans Control Syst Technol. 1999;7(3):328–42.

[27] Perry J. Gait analysis: normal and pathological function. Burnfield JM, editor. Thorofare, NJ: SLACK; 2010.

[28] Banala SK, Agrawal SK, Kim SH, Scholz JP. Novel gait adaptation and neuromotor training results using an active leg exoskeleton. IEEE/ASME Trans Mechatronics 2010;15(2):216–25.

[29] Duschau-Wicke A, von Zitzewitz J, Caprez A, Lunenburger L, Riener R. Path control: a method for patient-cooperative robot-aided gait rehabilitation. IEEE Trans Neural Syst Rehabil Eng. 2010;18(1):38–48.

Chapter 10
Conclusion and future work

This chapter seeks to summarise the main outcomes and conclusion of the research presented within this book. Various aspects including the design, modelling and control of some soft and compliant rehabilitation robots have been presented and discussed in previous chapters, as well as the modelling and development of the Peano muscle. This chapter also provides a discussion of future work that can be further explored to extend and advance the research presented in this book.

10.1 Book contributions

10.1.1 Physical modelling and embedded sensing for the Peano muscle

The large, heavy and rigid form of traditional electric, hydraulic and pneumatic actuators are ill-suited to actuating rehabilitation devices worn on the body. Many alternative actuators have a more promising form, but do not share the reliability and availability of their counterparts. Recently, there has been an initiative of developing soft, biologically capable, sheet-like, reactive actuators that enable valuable new robotic technologies for healthcare applications. Before contributing knowledge towards an actuator with the four desired properties, an actuator with those properties had to be found or invented. Mettam's Peano muscle was found as a solution in Chapters 2 and 3. This kind of actuator is a sheet-like fluid powered actuator that shares the form, fabrication and materials of everyday clothing. Hence, it can give clothing the ability to move the body, whether for assistance or rehabilitation.

Relatively little research has been done on the Peano muscle and there are several key areas where contributions can be made. These include the absence of modelling tools that use the Peano muscle's material properties to predict its static behaviour and the inability of the Peano muscle to sense its strain, pressure and force.

Chapter 3 proposes the MECHanical Approximation Lumped Parameter (MECHALP) static model, which captures the relationship between the Peano muscle's behaviour and several key material and geometry properties not found in existing Peano muscle models. Including these properties in the muscle model enables them to be optimised for maximum force or stroke in a given application. As literature shows these additional properties significantly influence the muscle's performance, their inclusion in the MECHALP static model can not only improve its usefulness and accuracy for design of the Peano muscle, but also for its control.

Current rehabilitation devices require many sensors to assess their users' physical ability and ensure they move precisely and safely. Unfortunately, these sensors add to the devices' cost, complexity and bulk. In Chapter 4, the design of the reactive Peano muscle is presented. Inspired by biological muscles' embedded sensors, the reactive Peano muscle measures its strain, pressure and force with novel dielectric elastomer (DE) sensors. We describe how to fabricate these sensors and embed them into a Peano muscle. We then characterise the resulting Peano muscle's actuation and sensing performance and demonstrate that embedded DE sensors do not compromise its form or function. Thus, the reactive Peano muscle concept has the potential to replace passive clothing with clothing that not only actuates, but also provides feedback on the physical ability and state of its wearer. The proposed actuator can monitor and control its interaction with uncertain environments. These abilities are essential to robots working in the real world, for example, wearable exoskeletons and autonomous search and rescue vehicles. Core to this technique is that, unlike previous fluidic muscles with embedded sensors, it enables the Peano muscle to attain reactivity without compromising its softness, biological capability and sheet-like form.

10.1.2 Design and control of a soft wrist rehabilitation robot

Affected wrist joints often show an increased spasticity and stiffness, caused by impairments of the surrounding muscles and tendons. The goal of Chapter 5 is to develop and control a robotic orthosis to assist the patient's wrist to perform rehabilitation exercise in a compliant way. A one-degree of freedom (DOF) robotic device using a parallel mechanism was designed for the human wrist by utilising soft pneumatic artificial muscles (PAMs). Before a mechanical prototype, incorporating an antagonistic setup of PAMs was developed. A feedback-based closed-loop angle and force controller was chosen to suit the desired system best with good tracking performance. Experiments on the orthosis demonstrated that the robot could assist the hand to move along a torque-sensitive trajectory with small errors and the differential forces were also kept stable.

10.1.3 Design and control of a soft ankle rehabilitation robot

A novel parallel robot has been proposed and developed for the treatment of musculoskeletal and neurological ankle injuries. While a range of robots have been developed and demonstrated to be effective for ankle rehabilitation [1], existing ankle devices suffer from a variety of limitations, including an incompatible robot structure that has misaligned rotation centre between the robot and the ankle joint, stiff actuation, a non-three-dimensional workspace and also the lack of real-time ankle assessment and adaptive interaction training schemes.

This research overcomes the above-mentioned limitations by developing a soft ankle rehabilitation robot (SARR). First, it has a compatible movement structure with aligned rotation centre with the human ankle. Secondly, four Festo fluidic muscles (FFMs) are adopted for soft actuation to make the robotic training safe and comfortable for patients. Thirdly, this robot has three rotational DOFs for comprehensive ankle training. These three DOFs are for ankle dorsiflexion/plantarflexion, inversion/eversion and adduction/abduction, respectively. Lastly, but importantly, real-time assessment function is integrated to facilitate the implementation of advanced interaction training strategies on the SARR. The assessment techniques used on the SARR was proposed based on a review [2]. Additionally, this robot has flexibility in adjusting the robotic range of motion (ROM) and placement for use on different patients. The developed SARR has some advantages, including soft actuation for safe human–robot interaction, aligned rotation centre between the robot and the ankle joint, three DOFs for three-dimensional rehabilitation exercises and the integration of real-time ankle assessment.

The position control is the basic requirement of rehabilitation robots to conduct training exercises. Satisfactory trajectory tracking performance cannot only guarantee safe and effective passive training; it also provides the basis for advanced interaction training. In Chapter 7, a cascade controller with position feedback in the outer loop and force feedback in the inner loop was developed and implemented on the SARR. This method can guarantee good tracking of the predefined trajectory, as well as allowing four FFMs to all be in tension during operations, which is safe for patients since robots may lose controllability with certain cables being slack. It must be noted that the implementation of the cascade controller involves the force distribution of each FFM for a given robotic torque. We adopted an analytic-iterative method that has less computation burden with respect to numerical algorithms and leads to less energy consumption with respect to analytic methods. Further, considering the cascade position controller in the low level, a high-level intelligent algorithm was proposed for adaptive interaction training. This intelligent strategy was implemented by defining an adaptive predefined trajectory based on the movement intention of the patient.

Experimental results demonstrated that the cascade position control can achieve good trajectory tacking performance, and guarantee FFMs in tension during the robotic operation. The intelligent algorithm aims to adapt the predefined trajectory based on the movement intention of the patient. If no movement intention is detected, the SARR operates in a passive mode along the predefined trajectory. If movement intention is detected, the SARR runs in an active interaction model based on the adapted trajectory, wherein the movement workspace, direction and velocity are adaptively adjusted. By the proposed virtual game-guided training together with the intelligent controller, the SARR can deliver virtual reality training based on the patient-robot interaction. The active training strategy is also expected to make the robotic training more interesting and effective and promote the outcomes. To summarise, the proposed the cascade position controller and the intelligent algorithm have the potential for clinical applications of ankle rehabilitation, especially when it is implemented on the SARR. With the consideration of the movement intention of the patient, this novel interaction training scheme can adaptively adjust the pre-defined trajectory to be in a safe range, and comfortable and effective for the patient. With the integration of a virtual-reality game the training can be more attractive and effective.

10.1.4 Design and control of a soft robotic GAit Rehabilitation EXoskeleton

A unilateral robotic GAit Rehabilitation EXoskeleton (GAREX) system has been designed and built. PAMs were adopted to actuate the sagittal plane rotations of exoskeleton's hip and knee joints. The two major design criteria of the exoskeleton are the capability of deliver task specific robotic gait rehabilitation and thoughtful hardware system to facilitate the control systems development towards safety and more effective gait training. Only a few PAM-driven gait rehabilitation robots have been reported and to the author's knowledge none of them have conducted detailed torque analysis to verify the system's ability to provide task-specific gait training. GAREX was designed with future clinical application in mind. The system is capable to provide sufficient torque for the knee and hip joint rotations in the sagittal planes to facilitate gait rehabilitation for a patient weighing up to 100 kg.

Four analogue valves were selected to allow detailed modelling of the entire controlled plant in the following research. Position, pressure and force sensors were installed for both control feedback and system monitoring. Safe training was achieved through the system monitoring as well as dedicated features such as mechanical stops and emergency stop buttons.

To ensure GAREX can provide training to a wide population range, the system was designed to be modular and telescopic. The knee and hip actuation modules' relative position can be adjusted to accommodate variable lengths of patients' lower limb segments. To fit subjects with different builds, the horizontal and vertical positions of the exoskeleton module to the trunk manipulation module was made adjustable, together with the vertical position of the trunk manipulation module relative to the supporting frame.

The task-specific criterion imposes joint torque, ROM and control bandwidth requirements to the exoskeleton design. These are trade-off between the ROM and torque a PAM-actuated joint can provide. Hence detailed design analysis was conducted to verify the exoskeleton design.

The PAM actuation system is highly nonlinear and subject to hysteresis behaviours. It is highly beneficial to model the entire system in order to better understand the system and help upcoming controller implementation. The system model consists of four sequential sub-models, which are the flow dynamics of the valve, the pressure dynamics of the PAMs, the force dynamics of the PAMs and the load dynamics of the mechanism. In previously developed PAM-driven rehabilitation robots, the first two sub-models had been ignored with the use of pressure-regulating valves, which could lead to unpredictable transient behaviour of the controlled PAM pressure.

During the process of exoskeleton development, it was also noticed that there were no dynamic force models for the FESTO PAM available for direct implementation. As a result, a new dynamic modelling approach of PAM actuators has been developed based on the original model developed in [3]. The linear dynamic model was developed for McKibben PAM. To better represent the behaviours of the FESTO PAM, the model in [3] was modified to a piece-wise linear form, which is still in a simple form for further usage in controller development. Moreover, experimental procedures and data processing have been fully automated, so the model can be quickly obtained for PAMs with different sizes.

One major contribution of Chapters 8 and 9 is the novel application of the multiple inputs multiple outputs (MIMO) sliding mode (SM) control system for both trajectory tracking and average pressure control of a rotational joints actuated by antagonistic PMs. The MIMO SM controller was developed based on the model of the complete system of the exoskeleton. It was hypothesised that lower average PM pressure leads to less compliant joint. The MIMO SM controller was initially implemented to the knee joint mechanism and extensive experiments were conducted either without subject or with healthy subject to investigate its performance. Apart from investigating the ability of simultaneous angular trajectory and average pressure tracking, novel experiments were performed by five healthy subjects to demonstrate that the MIMO SM controller was able to adjust the joint compliance by controlling the average PM pressure.

10.2 Future work

10.2.1 Modelling and fabrication process of the Peano muscle

In Chapter 3 the model of the Peano muscle's static force generation was presented and validated. It models four physical effects not found in previous physics-based Peano muscle models, increasing its accuracy for control and design over these existing modelling approaches. However, its accuracy was limited by the goodness of fit of its material property parameters and its inability to model Peano muscle hysteresis. In the future, we plan to address these issues through more rigorous muscle characterisation experiments and the addition of a suitable hysteresis model.

Chapter 4 presents a method for sensing the physical state of the reactive Peano muscle, without compromising its form or behaviour. This method is useful for controlling the motion and force of the actuator in a rehabilitation device as well as enabling that device with the ability to monitor the rehabilitation progress and detect the movement intention of its wearer. On characterising the reactive Peano muscle and its embedded sensors, it was found that the muscle had a relatively low maximum inflation pressure. We also found the muscles' sensors were limited by their significant hysteresis and sensitivity to quantities other than the desired measurement quantity. These problems could be fixed by refining the fabrication process of the muscle: degassing its silicone, selection of low hysteresis sensor materials, more seamless integration of the sensors in the muscle structure and providing the sensors' wires with suitable stress relief. Hence, future work on the reactive Peano muscle will focus on an improved fabrication process.

10.2.2 Two-degrees of freedom for the wrist rehabilitation robot

While the developed wrist rehabilitation robot has shown potentials for the functionalities of assessment and rehabilitation, there are some we can do in future for comfortable and comprehensive wrist training. The most promising update to the present device is the incorporation of additional DOF by adding another pair of soft actuators. To reduce the joint friction of the prototype, the motion accuracy would also be improved. Different control strategies should also be brought in for different training modes on a subject-specific basis. Clinical evaluation of the proposed robotic system by recruiting a large sample of patients can be then conducted with more stable structure and multifunctional training schemes.

10.2.3 Optimisation and improvement of the soft ankle rehabilitation robot

While the developed SARR of this book is flexible in generating varying ROMs, driven torque and the overall placement of the robot, it suffers from a few limitations in terms of mechanical design. Three of these limitations are discussed further and potential improvements during future work are proposed. The distance between the upper platform and the robotic end effector is too long; this distance is not conveniently and easily adjusted. Pure robotic training for ankle adduction/abduction is impracticable based on the current layout of the FFMs. Finally, the installation of the FFMs is not robust. Therefore, future work can focus on the optimisation and improvement of the current SARR in relation to the following aspects.

Mechanically, (1) designing more flexibility to allow for the adjustment of the height and inclination angle of the rehabilitation robot, to allow the robot to be set to any posture according to the requirements of different patients; (2) replacing the cables used for connecting FFMs by ball joints or universal joints to make the actuation system more stable and accurate and (3) decreasing the distance between the upper platform and the robotic end effector to allow the patient to easily interface with the robot (may be achieved by using shorter actuators, removing single-axis load cells or other methods such as structure optimisation).

Functionally, the achieved robotic ROM and the driven torque can be improved by optimising the connection point of the FFMs. In brief, in the process of the commercialisation of the SARR, mechanical design optimisation and improvements must still occur. A friendly robot appearance will also help with obtaining buy-in from patients during commercialisation.

While proposed control schemes are both capable of conducting passive and active training, further research should be conducted to compare the effectiveness of these training schemes. Future work will further optimise the proposed control methods through clinical trials involving a large sample of participants with injured ankles when evaluating its therapeutic effects.

10.2.4 Control and validation of the GAREX

The authors recommend two tracks for the further work. One track is to develop more sophisticated control strategies for more effective gait rehabilitation. Being soft and intrinsically compliant, the GAREX system is a good platform for implementing and testing various control strategies especially those to realise the assistance-as-needed (AAN) concept.

Integrating ground reaction force (GRF) sensing capability into the GAREX could open new possibilities for control strategy development. The stance and swing phase of a gait cycle can be easily identified with GRF sensing. A straightforward possible development is to have different joint compliances for the stance and swing phase. The knee and hip joints' torque requirements are much higher during the stance phase than the swing phase due to the need to support bodyweight. Therefore, the exoskeleton could be controlled to be stiff during the stance phase and compliant during the swing phase. Bio-signals, such as electromyography (EMG), could be integrated into the control system for detecting the patient's intention or patient ability assessment. A patient-specific EMG-driven neuromuscular model by Ma *et al.* [4] could potentially be integrated with the GAREX system. During robotic gait training, a patient's joint torque can be calculated by the model in real-time, which would help the system better estimate the patient's ability or participating level in order to benefit AAN control development.

Another track is the further system development towards clinical trials. The exoskeleton design will need more attention than current prototype. When designing the current exoskeleton, it was aimed to build a robust working system in a short period of time. As a result, the current exoskeleton is not optimal in terms of weight, durability and user-friendliness. One of the advantages of the PAM actuators is being lightweight and reducing the inertia of the exoskeleton will increase the bandwidth of the control system. The current exoskeleton was designed with flat aluminium parts and machined steel parts for robustness and quick fabrication, but it also led to a heavy exoskeleton. Hence, the weight of the current design could be significantly trimmed by careful material selection and design analysis.

In clinical setting, the preparation time for the experiment need to be as short as possible. Currently, the exoskeleton has a modular design and can be adjusted to fit anthropometric data of most of the population. However, the adjustments require time-consuming procedures including bolting and unbolting. Hence, mechanisms that allow quick adjustment are also worthy to consider. It is also necessary to have a body weight support (BWS) system for clinical trials. The BWS system not only ensures the safety and stability of patient during gait rehabilitation training, but also can be used as means of adjusting assistant [5]. It is also valuable to investigate the cooperation between the GAREX and BWS systems.

Finally, the current exoskeleton is of a unilateral design. Once the redesign of the hardware system is completed, GAREX could be extended to a bi-lateral system. A bilateral system can facilitate gait training on a larger variety of patients than a unilateral system.

10.3 Summary

This chapter summarises the major outcomes and contributions achieved in this book, and points out some work that can be further explored in future. The major contributions achieved in this book are identified as: (1) the modelling and development of a soft actuator (the Peano muscle); (2) design and control of a soft wrist rehabilitation robot; (3) design and control of the SARR for ankle therapy and (4) design and control of the GAREX for gait exercises. These prototypes have been developed to advance robot-assisted rehabilitation techniques, and an obvious advantage is the use of soft actuators for safe human–robot interaction. Future work will mainly focus on the validation of the proposed techniques, as well as their clinical effectiveness for healthcare applications. By using the developed techniques in this book, robot-assisted healthcare techniques are expected to be safer, more comprehensive and efficient.

References

[1] Zhang M, Davies TC, Xie S. Effectiveness of robot-assisted therapy on ankle rehabilitation–a systematic review. J Neuroeng Rehabil. 2013;10:30. doi: 10.1186/1743-0003-10-30.

[2] Zhang M, Davies TC, Zhang Y, Xie S. Reviewing effectiveness of ankle assessment techniques for use in robot-assisted therapy. J Rehabil Res Dev. 2014;51(4):517–34.

[3] Reynolds D, Repperger D, Phillips C, Bandry G. Modeling the dynamic characteristics of pneumatic muscle. Ann Biomed Eng. 2003;31(3):310–17.

[4] Ma Y, Xie S, Zhang Y. A patient-specific EMG-driven neuromuscular model for the potential use of human-inspired gait rehabilitation robots. Comput Biol Med. 2016;70:88–98.

[5] Frey M, Colombo G, Vaglio M, Bucher R, Jorg M, Riener R. A novel mechatronic body weight support system. IEEE Trans Neural Syst Rehabil Eng. Sept. 2006;14(3):311–21.

Index

www.ingramcontent.com/pod-product-compliance
Lightning Source LLC
LaVergne TN
LVHW011800200926
848484LV00003B/740

www.ingramcontent.com/pod-product-compliance
Lightning Source LLC
LaVergne TN
LVHW011749200926
848484LV00003B/655